BIOCHEMICAL EFFECTS OF ENVIRONMENTAL POLLUTANTS

BIOCHEMICAL EFFECTS OF ENVIRONMENTAL POLLUTANTS

edited by

S. D. LEE

Health Effects Research Laboratory
Environmental Research Center
U.S. Environmental Protection Agency
Cincinnati, Ohio

with the assistance of

Bruce Peirano

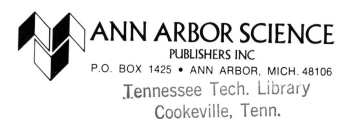

ANN ARBOR SCIENCE
PUBLISHERS INC
P.O. BOX 1425 • ANN ARBOR, MICH. 48106

PREFACE

This volume derived from a symposium organized to emphasize the value of understanding the biochemical effects of environmental pollutants. Detection of early biochemical lesions that are related to subsequent changes in structure and physiology would be useful as early signs of environmental hazards that produce disease in humans. Too often in the past such hazards have been defined only after outbreaks of human cases have occurred. Epidemiologic studies identifying cadmium, methyl mercury, asbestos and kepone are only recent and publicized examples of the after-the-fact approach to environmental protection.

Perhaps even more important in the long term, basic understanding of the mechanisms by which environmental chemicals produce their effects appears as the only rational basis for predicting the hazards associated with the mixtures of chemicals encountered in the real world. Empirical testing of all possible pollutant combinations is decidedly unachievable because of the sheer volume and expense of such an enterprise. Consequently, prediction based on detailed knowledge of the biochemical and pharmacodynamic properties of individual chemicals appears to be the only viable alternative for making regulatory decisions.

Trace metal and oxidant pollutant toxicology were chosen as the general areas of discussion because they have been researched sufficiently to begin their assessment in light of the general aims stated above. Incorporation of these separate fields results in a certain degree of discontinuity. However, all the presentations made have directly or indirectly assessed these major questions—some have emphasized the interaction of nutritional factors in modifying the effects of toxic substances, and others deal with the multiplicity of mechanisms often possible which interfere with particular systems of even single enzymes. Finally, specific interactions between environmental chemicals have been demonstrated. A comprehensive classification of chemical effects of predictive value remains illusive. The main reason is that most research emphasizes purely

v

empirical goals with little regard for the general knowledge which should arise out of any toxicologic study. These goals are not at all contradictory. They simply involve formation of specific and testable hypotheses which go beyond the overly simplistic question of "effect" and "no effect" concentrations of chemicals. Such an approach would serve to channel research in productive directions, avoiding the expensive comprehensive approach more aptly called the "shotgun rationale" which seems to guide a major share of efforts in environmental health.

Responsibility for the scientific content of each contribution lies with the authors, although the authors cooperated in a considerable effort toward editorial clarification.

Sincere gratitude is extended to Dr. R. John Garner, Director, Health Effects Research Laboratory, EPA, Cincinnati, for his support. We are indebted for the time and efforts of Drs. Donald Tierney, Harold Petering, Milos Chvapil, Vincent Finelli, and R. S. Bhatnagar for the organization of the symposium and to the individual contributors who made the entire effort a success. A special acknowledgment is necessary for the tireless assistance provided by Mr. Bruce Peirano and Mrs. Carol Haynes.

Si Duk Lee
Cincinnati, Ohio

CONTENTS

Dedicated to better health
and a brighter future.

CHAPTER 1

BIOCHEMICAL EFFECTS OF ENVIRONMENTAL POLLUTANTS

KEYNOTE ADDRESS

D. S. Barth

Deputy Assistant Administrator for Health
Health and Ecological Effects
U.S. Environmental Protection Agency
Washington, D.C. 20460

INTRODUCTION

In order to put the subject of this Symposium into perspective, I deem it necessary to spend some time discussing the objective of EPA, how this objective is being attained, and how outputs from health effects research contribute to the attainment of this objective. I will then discuss the importance of biochemical effects research in relation to health effects research in general.

EPA'S OBJECTIVES

The subjects dealt with by EPA include air pollution, water pollution, pesticides, solid waste management, radiation, noise and toxic substances. In brief, the objective of EPA is to abate or control environmental pollution to socially acceptable levels. The role of research and development then is to provide a body of research information sufficient to enable an informed judgment to be made with regard to acceptable levels for various environmental pollutants.

The laws that EPA must implement are many and varied. However, the intent of Congress in each law is aimed at the protection and enhancement of the environment. This implies that required controls are generally designed to abate adverse effects on health or welfare to

1

acceptable levels or to prevent the occurrence of new adverse effects. In all instances health effects are deemed to be of primary importance, with welfare effects being secondary but still of major concern.

EPA'S OFFICE OF RESEARCH AND DEVELOPMENT PROGRAMS TO MEET OBJECTIVES

The research and development program of EPA is generally concerned with the following subject areas:

> effects
> environmental exposure levels
> predictive models linking source emissions to exposure levels
> control technology

Effects research includes development of exposure-effect relationships for selected environmental pollutants, acting singly or in combination, on selected populations of receptors for both health and welfare effects.

The documentation of environmental exposure levels is essentially a monitoring task. Such exposure monitoring data are necessary to determine where and to what extent environmental exposure levels exceed acceptable values and to measure the efficacy of control programs as they are implemented. Validated predictive models linking source emissions to exposure levels are required to design the most cost-effective control plans for source emissions to reduce exposure levels to acceptable values. Control technology must be available to control major emission sources adequately. In many cases this requires extensive research and development and demonstration programs.

Let us now consider in somewhat more detail the outputs required from our health effects research programs and the research methods and approaches used to obtain those outputs. As already mentioned, we seek exposure-effect relationships for selected pollutants, acting singly or in combination, on selected populations at risk.

Principal factors to be considered in the selection of pollutants for study include:

> our present state of knowledge for both regulated and unregulated pollutants
> known or suspected seriousness of adverse effects from over-exposure
> availability of adequate measurement methods
> size of the populations at risk and estimates of exposure levels
> occupational health experience with pollutants under consideration

Principal factors to be considered in the selection of populations for study include:

> most sensitive populations at risk
> higher exposure levels for most sensitive populations

likelihood of the presence of contributing factors not related to environmental pollutant(s).

Approaches used to perform health effects research in EPA include epidemiological, toxicological and clinical studies. Whenever possible, all three approaches are used in a coordinated fashion. Biochemical studies may be included in any or all of the three approaches.

Our recently implemented program to assess the contribution of environmental carcinogens to cancer incidence in the general population is an example of the meshing of these areas in a comprehensive study. The initial thrust of this program will include media transport assessment, inter- and intramedia transformation, measurement methodology, exposure monitoring, dose assessment, and retrospective estimation of exposure, all conducted under a rigorous quality assurance program in areas of high and low cancer incidence. After this initial phase, the coordinated data base will generate a requirement for targeted epidemiological and toxicological studies. Finally, the information will provide values for the construction and validation of a predictive model.

ROLE OF BIOCHEMICAL EFFECTS
RESEARCH IN ORD PROGRAM

A distinction can be made in biochemical effects research between "effects monitoring" and "health effects." The former is a requirement for the final stages of environmental exposure monitoring, such as exposure/dose assessment. The latter involves establishing a meaningful relationship between a biochemical change and the health or well-being of the exposed population.

Toxicological lethality studies have long been used to evaluate the hazards of various chemicals; however, such methods are relatively gross because of the comparatively large doses required to produce observable effects within the short life spans of the experimental animals. It is here that the study of biochemical effects may offer an advantage. Such effects undoubtedly precede such end points as the LD_{50} and, if thoroughly understood, not only may explain the mechanism of the hazard but also may indicate methods of control or reversal. These considerations suggest that possible hazards may be identified and their effects estimated long before the results of chronic toxicity or epidemiological studies are available. This would be particularly true for carcinogenic chemicals that produce their end effects only after a long latent period and for those, such as lead, that may accumulate slowly to an end-effect level with continued exposure.

Some results along this line are already appearing; for example, the relationship among blood-lead levels, ALA-D, and urinary homovanillic acid concentration and the somewhat tenuous relationship between mutagenesis and carcinogenesis that is the basis for the proposed use of the bacterial mutagenesis test for detection of carcinogens. To expand on these somewhat, if the indication of nerve damage suggested by the biochemical detection of increased homovanillic acid excretion can be confirmed, then an early indication of harmful effects may be possible so that control can be established before permanent harm ensues. Erythrocyte ALA-D, on the other hand serves as a convenient "effect" for relating environmental exposure to dose assessment. The subject of mutagenesis was addressed in the December 1975 Nobel lecture by Dulbecco, who advocated widespread use of bacterial mutagenicity tests before releasing any new compound to the public. The feasibility of such a program is strengthened by the finding that most of the commonly available substances are not promutagens.

The foregoing are examples of biochemical effects used in different applications. The sensitivity, and even specificity, of such tests hold great promise for the future. If developed to full potential, biochemical changes related to the assessment of human health and welfare effects would significantly aid the EPA in fulfilling its mandate to protect and enhance the environment.

FUTURE CHALLENGES

Some current and future problems of major concern to EPA's health effects research programs include:

> development of suitable animal models for extrapolation to humans
>
> development of adequate screening tests, *in vitro* or *in vivo,* to estimate toxic properties of environmental pollutants
>
> development of methods for determining effects in humans or experimental animals of long-term, low-level exposures
>
> development of methods for determining varying effects of different averaging times for different exposures
>
> development of methods for measuring and interpreting physiological or biochemical changes occurring as precursors to disease
>
> development of methods for biological monitoring to quantitate exposure levels
>
> development of personal exposure meters to improve our ability to assess exposure to air pollutants
>
> development of biochemical exposure indicators to assess exposure by any route.

This symposium was convened to address some of the problems I have enumerated, and to assess current progress in the area of biochemical change as related to effects of environmental pollutants. We can expect much mutual education from the discussions.

CHAPTER 2

CELLULAR APPROACHES TO THE STUDY
OF ENVIRONMENTAL POLLUTANTS

N. A. Elson and R. G. Crystal

Pulmonary Branch
National Heart, Lung, and Blood Institute
Building 10, Room 6N260
Bethesda, Maryland 20014

INTRODUCTION

Epidemiologic and animal studies strongly suggest that airborne pollutants are commonly encountered in the urban environment in concentrations which are toxic to the lungs.[1-3] Detailed studies have resulted in
the identification of those pollutants which cause injury and the development of guidelines relating concentration, form and time of exposure
to the relative toxicity for each pollutant.[2] With this kind of animal
data available as a groundwork, workers in the respiratory pollutant
field are turning their attention toward validating animal toxicity studies
by evaluating humans exposed to airborne pollutants; identifying the
mechanisms by which airborne pollutants cause lung injury; and determining how pollutant-related pulmonary injury can be circumvented or
treated.[4]

There are formidable obstacles to the solution of these problems.
Direct biopsy evaluation of human lung under controlled conditions is
impossible, and so to validate animal toxicity studies, only safe, and
hence indirect, methodologies can be used. Even in animal studies, the
task of identifying the pathogenic mechanisms is complex, since the lungs
of animals exposed to pollutants show the results of multiple injuries.
This yields a montage of the secondary effects of inflammation, clearance

mechanisms and repair processes, occurring simultaneously or in overlapping sequence to the primary toxic effect of the pollutant. Thus, to expand our understanding of the effects of airborne pollutants, it is necessary to develop new methodologies on two fronts: (1) safe, noninvasive methods to evaluate the effect of pollutants on man; and (2) approaches which will simplify the evaluation of the mechanisms of pollutant-related lung injury.

To accomplish these goals, most attention is being focused on the cells of the lung. While it is conceivable that environmental pollutants directly affect the pulmonary extracellular matrix, most available evidence suggests the earliest injury is at the cellular level.[1] By developing methodologies to evaluate the cells of the lung, we can gain insight into how the lung responds to inhaled pollutants, and thus determine safe limits of exposure and pathogenic mechanisms of pollutant-related lung injury. The solutions to these problems will eventually form the basis of a rational approach to prevention, diagnosis and treatment of pollutant-related respiratory disease.

INDIRECT STUDIES OF LUNG CELLS

While population studies implicate the toxicity of airborne pollutants on the human lung, it is only through carefully controlled exposure chamber studies that specific information can be developed. As discussed at this conference, short exposure to low concentrations of ozone can result in functional abnormalities manifested by mild obstruction to airflow.[5-6] Since this phenomenon is presumably secondary to the primary effects of ozone on the constituent cells of the lung*, evaluation of lung cells in these individuals would provide several important pieces of information: (1) which cells are involved; (2) how the pollutant affects each cell; and (3) the mildest exposures which cause cellular dysfunction. The last is of particular importance, since it is probable that cellular dysfunction precedes physiologic dysfunction. Although our laboratory has not specifically studied the effects of airborne pollutants in humans, we have utilized several methods which yield information on the status of lung cells in man, particularly those cells concerned with inflammatory and immune mechanisms.

---

*"Lung cells" will be used to refer to any cell comprising the parenchyma, airways or blood vessels of lung, plus blood-derived cells that may reside in lung.[7-9] In the normal individual, the latter refers to monocytes (or their daughter macrophages) and lymphocytes. In diseased lungs, neutrophils, eosinophils and/or basophils may also be present.

Bronchoalveolar Lavage

The fiberoptic bronchoscope has greatly expanded acess to the lung.[10] Besides its use in diagnosing tumors and infection, this instrument can be used to sample the cells and fluids which bathe the bronchoalveolar epithelial surface. This procedure, termed bronchoalveolar lavage, is simple, safe and rapid and has been performed on many normal volunteers without complications (Figure 2.1).[11,12] The bronchoscope is positioned in a subsegmental airway of the lingula and 100 ml of saline

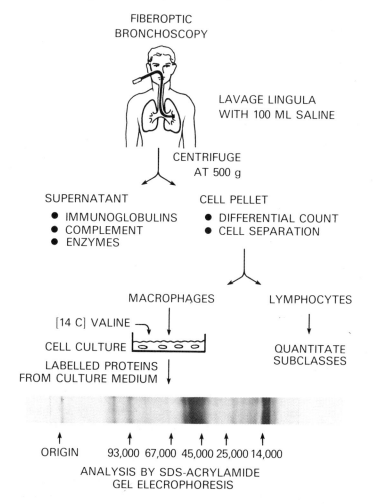

FIBEROPTIC
BRONCHOSCOPY

LAVAGE LINGULA
WITH 100 ML SALINE

CENTRIFUGE
AT 500 g

SUPERNATANT

- IMMUNOGLOBULINS
- COMPLEMENT
- ENZYMES

CELL PELLET

- DIFFERENTIAL COUNT
- CELL SEPARATION

MACROPHAGES

[14 C] VALINE

CELL CULTURE

LABELLED PROTEINS
FROM CULTURE MEDIUM

LYMPHOCYTES

QUANTITATE
SUBCLASSES

ORIGIN   93,000 67,000 45,000 25,000 14,000

ANALYSIS BY SDS-ACRYLAMIDE
GEL ELECROPHORESIS

Figure 2.1. Schematic of the procedure of bronchoalveolar lavage and subsequent analysis of lavage cells and proteins.

is used to "wash out" the bronchoalveolar surface. The material obtained can be analyzed in many different ways; our interest has been toward its cellular and protein constituents, with particular emphasis on those aspects which evaluate inflammatory and immunologic aspects of lung injury.[13]

Analysis of the cellular constituents of lavage fluid demonstrates that from the normal, nonsmoking human, 100 ml of lavage fluid yields approximately 10^7 cells.[11-13] On the average, these cells are alveolar macrophages (80%) and lymphocytes (20%) with rare (<1%) neutrophils; eosinophils and basophils are almost never found. Smoking subjects have more alveolar macrophages (85%), fewer lymphocytes (12%) and a few neutrophils (3%).[11-13]

When these methods are applied to patients with idiopathic pulmonary fibrosis (IPF)*, a different cell population is found.[13] On the average, patients with IPF have a significantly greater number of neutrophils (32%), a small but consistent presence of eosinophils (3%) and a smaller proportion of both macrophages and lymphocytes than normal (50% and 12% respectively). Importantly, the relative number of neutrophils found in the lavage fluid of these patients correlates with the degree of inflammation found on open-lung biopsy specimens of the same patients. Thus, bronchoalveolar lavage can be used to gauge the extent of active inflammation ("alveolitis") in the pulmonary parenchyma. Of interest is the fact that with corticosteroid treatment, the relative percentage of neutrophils in IPF lavage fluid returns toward normal, suggesting such therapy is efficacious in diminishing alveolitis.

Pulmonary fibrosis is a final pathway of lung injury which may result from many different causes. Some causes involve local responses to injury very different from that found in IPF. For example, chronic hypersensitivity pneumonitis (CHP) is a disorder that results from repeated exposures to aerosolized organic antigens, resulting in alveolitis, granulomas and fibrosis in the pulmonary parenchyma.[15] In these individuals, the parenchymal inflammation manifests itself in bronchoalveolar lavage fluid with a striking number of lymphocytes (62%) together with neutrophils (8%) and eosinophils (1%).[13] The macrophages are much reduced from normal (30%) and their morphology takes on a "foamy" appearance. In addition, not only are the lymphocytes in great abundance, but their subclasses are markedly different

---

* IPF is a fatal pulmonary disorder beginning with alveolitis which leads to diffuse pulmonary fibrosis. The patient develops restrictive lung disease and resting hypoxemia which worsens with exercise. The average patient survival is 4 years from the onset of symptoms.[14]

from normal. Using conventional surface marker methods, both T and B lymphocytes can be identified in normal bronchoalveolar lavage fluid in the same ratio as that found in peripheral blood (2.5-3.0 to 1).[16] In chronic hypersensitivity pneumonitis, however, there is a marked increase in the bronchoalveolar lavage T/B ratio (15 to 1) while the peripheral blood lymphocytes remain in the ratio of 2.5-3.0 to 1.[13] Thus, analysis of bronchoalveolar lavage cells in these patients suggests that the lung can operate as a relatively independent immune organ and that "inflammation" in the lung is manifested differently in diverse disorders such as IPF and CHP.

One of the primary manifestations of airborne pollutant toxicity may be the direct effects of the pollutant on the cells comprising the broncho-alveolar epithelium and the cells in the bronchoalveolar fluid. Long before these cells are destroyed by the pollutant, they may be qualitatively altered such that they are unable to carry out their differentiated functions properly. One sensitive monitor of the differentiated state of cells is the type of proteins the cell will synthesize and secrete.[17-19] For example, the human alveolar macrophage secretes a variety of proteins ranging in molecular weight from 14,000 to 150,000 (Figure 2.1). This molecular weight "map" of the proteins produced by this cell may well be altered even with mild injury. This type of analysis is adaptable to *in vitro* studies, *e.g.,* cultured alveolar macrophages obtained by lavage of normal volunteers can be exposed to low concentrations of specific pollutants *in vitro*.[20-22] Alternatively, the effect of *in vivo* exposure of a normal volunteer to a specific pollutant may be gauged by comparing the proteins secreted by alveolar macrophages harvested from serial lavages obtained before and after exposure.[23-25]

In addition to cellular analysis, bronchoalveolar lavage fluid can be examined for specific protein components. Quantitative studies of lavage immunoglobulins have revealed that patients with IPF have elevated levels of IgG, while patients with CHP have elevated levels of IgG and IgM.[13] The proteins of lavage fluid can also be analyzed for enzymatic activity. For example, enzymes such as β-glucuronidase, lysozyme and collagenase can be found in lavage fluid. Presumably, such analyses are a reflection of the status of the cells of the lung within the alveolus or lining the bronchoalveolar surface. If airborne pollutants disturb the function of these cells, it is possible that the proteins of lavage fluid are significantly altered by these agents.

Gallium Scanning

An alternative method for evaluating the extent of alveolitis is to utilize a radioactive tracer which accumulates in regions of active pulmonary parenchymal inflammation. [67]Gallium-citrate is particularly suited for this approach, since it is a short-lived isotope which is taken up by neutrophils and emits γ-rays easily detected by available clinical nuclear scanning devices. Forty-eight hours following intravenous administration of [67]gallium-citrate, the isotope is found in areas of pulmonary inflammation as well as in bone and liver (Figure 2.2). The relative quantity of ^{67}Ga accumulation in the lung fields can be ranked by accounting for the percentage of lung involved, the density and texture of the scan. Evaluation of a number of patients with IPF compared with controls have shown that 60-70% of patients with IPF accumulate ^{67}Ga in the lung compared to 5% of controls.[26] The quantitative ranking of ^{67}Ga in these patients correlates with the degree of alveolitis found in open lung biopsy as well as the percentage of neutrophils found on bronchoalveolar lavage of the same individuals. These data suggest that scanning with [67]gallium-citrate may be a useful, safe, non-invasive method to follow pulmonary inflammation and its response to therapeutic intervention. If, in fact, airborne pollutants cause parenchymal inflammation, this methodology may prove useful for evaluating controlled exposures in humans.

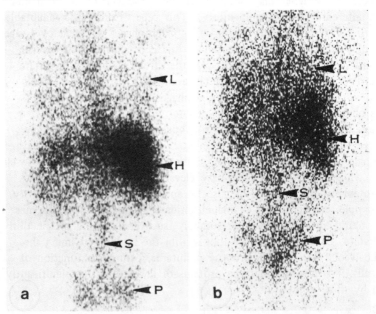

Figure 2.2. [67]Gallium scintiscans of: A. a normal individual; and B. a patient with idiopathic pulmonary fibrosis. The lung fields (L), hepatic image (H), spine (S), and pelvis (P) are viewed from the posterior aspect. Increased pulmonary uptake of [67]gallium is apparent in the fibrotic patient.

DIRECT STUDIES OF LUNG CELLS

While bronchoalveolar lavage and [67]gallium-citrate scanning could be used to evaluate the effects of airborne pollutants on humans, these methods focus on the cells free in the fluid bathing the bronchoalveolar epithelial surface or blood-borne cells brought to the lung as part of the inflammatory state. They do not get at the critical question of the action of pollutants on the normal cells of the parenchyma, airways and blood vessels. As discussed previously, because of the complexity of the response of lung cells to pollutants, we must significantly reduce the number of variables in each experimental situation before we can begin to identify pathogenic mechanisms. One approach is to utilize methodologies which evaluate lung cells *in vitro*. These model systems, mostly capitalizing on techniques of tissue culture, enable the investigator to focus on lung cells in a controlled milieu so that the earliest effects of the pollutants could be identified. Using current technology, basically two methods could be exploited: lung explant culture and lung cell culture.

Lung Explant Culture

Explants are fragments (0.5-1.0 mm) of parenchyma, tracheobronchial tree or blood vessels which are incubated in culture medium without serum for periods ranging from 1 to 48 hr. During this period labeled metabolic precursors of proteins, carbohydrates or lipids can be added, and the synthesis or degradation of specific products assayed.[27] Studies of this kind have three major advantages: (1) the explants are easy to prepare, even from a human lung biopsy; (2) the results can be assumed to have relevance to the *in vivo* lung, since the complex structure of differentiated lung tissue is still relatively intact; and (3) the environment of the explant can be controlled, thus significantly reducing the number of mostly unknown variables present in the intact experimental subject. On the other hand, use of the explant has disadvantages: (1) it is difficult to identify which cell types are responsible for the biologic process under study; and (2) the presence of multiple tissue compartments may affect the uniform delivery of oxygen, airborne pollutants and/or metabolic precursors to all cells in the explant and may impede the recovery of products produced by the cells.

Our major use of the lung explant has been to use it to evaluate the synthesis of connective tissue, the predominant material of the extracellular space.[28-33] The components of connective tissue (collagen, elastic fibers and proteoglycans) give the lung a structural framework and significantly contribute to lung mechanical properties. In addition, the pulmonary connective tissue plays a critical role in the pathogenesis and functional abnormalities of common pulmonary disorders such as emphysema and fibrosis. Since the production of connective tissue is so vital to the maintenance of normal lung structure and function, it is quite possible that a major effect of atmospheric pollutants on pulmonary cellular dysfunction is the altered production or destruction of these macromolecules.

The explant system can be easily adapted to evaluate the effect of an *in vivo* manipulation on the synthesis of lung components such as collagen. For example, unilateral pneumonectomy in the two-month-old rabbit induces rapid lung growth in the remaining lung, manifested by an increased number of alveoli[34] with a proportional increase in the number of lung cells, total protein and collagen (Figure 2.3A).[35] This growth is reflected in explants of lungs of these animals, which demonstrate that pneumonectomy induces the cells of the remaining lung to rapidly increase their average rate of collagen synthesis.[35] Insight into the mechanisms involved in this induction of lung growth comes from the observation that intrathoracic replacement of the volume of the excised lung with

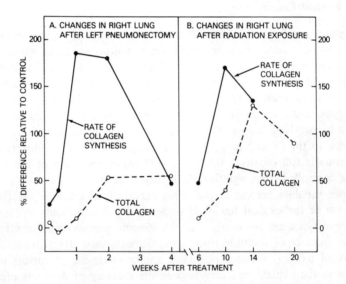

Figure 2.3 A. Effects of unilateral pneumonectomy in the 10-week-old rabbit on the rate of collagen synthesis (●——●) and total collagen content (○---○) of the remaining lung. B. Changes in the rate of collagen synthesis (●——●) and total collagen content (○----○) in the right lung of a 10-week-old rabbit after exposure to 3000 rads of X-radiation. The methods used in 2.3A and 2.3B were identical, and the data is expressed as percentage increase over age-matched controls where percent increase = [experimental-control] x 100/control.

wax completely eliminates the compensatory growth of the remaining lung. This suggests that the control of lung growth may be modulated by mechanical factors such as the dimensions of the chest wall.[35]

Another example of the use of the explant system to evaluate *in vivo* events is the induction of pulmonary fibrosis by external X-radiation.[36] Unilateral exposure of the ten-week-old rabbit lung to 3000 rads of radiation results in gradual development of pulmonary fibrosis. The gradual increase in collagen concentration found in these lungs is, in part, due to the radiation-induced increases in the average rate of collagen synthesis (per cell) as measured in explant cultures of exposed animals (Figure 2.3B).

In both examples discussed, increases in lung collagen concentration followed increases in the average rate of synthesis of collagen by lung cells, suggesting a causal relationship between the two. However, in other situations, the level of collagen in rabbit lung parenchyma is obviously not controlled by synthesis alone. For example, in normal neonatal lung growth, rabbit lung collagen concentration increases steadily while the rate of collagen synthesis decreases (Figure 2.4A).[28] In addition, once maturity is reached, collagen synthesis continues at a low, but steady rate, but the concentration of collagen does not increase (it remains constant). In both situations it is apparent that collagen concentration is not controlled solely by synthesis, but that the quantity of collagen present must be the result of a blanace between synthetic and degradative mechanisms.

A similar conclusion is reached after comparing the concentration of lung parenchymal glysocaminoglycans* to the average rate of synthesis of these macromolecules (Figure 2.4B).[33, 37] Here, too, an increase in a parenchymal connective tissue component (*i.e.*, glycosaminoglycan concentration from 45 to 180 days after birth) cannot be controlled by synthetic mechanisms alone, since the average rate of glycosaminoglycan synthesis actually decreases during this period. Thus, the rate of degradation of macromolecules must also be considered whenever evaluating the metabolism of these components.

Since it has been suggested that atmospheric pollutants may cause connective tissue destruction and/or proliferation,[38-39] these types of explant studies may be useful in defining the effects of exposure of

---

* Glycosaminoglycans are the large carbohydrate side chains of proteoglycans; in the pulmonary parenchyma, the glycosaminoglycans include hyaluronic acid, chondroitin 4 and 6 sulfate, dermatan sulfate, heparan sulfate and heparin. In the studies under discussion, the term "glycosaminoglycans" refers to all of these components.[33]

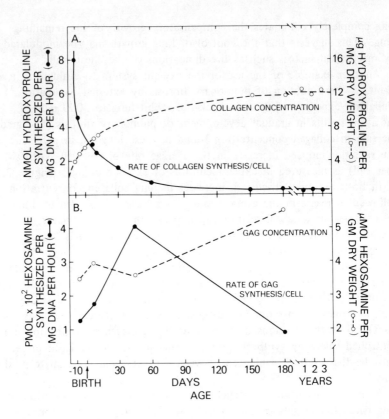

Figure 2.4 Rate of synthesis and concentration of collagen and glycosaminoglycans (GAG) in explants of lung parenchyma from rabbits of various ages. A. The average rate of collagen synthesis per cell was quantitated as the incorporation of [^{14}C] proline into [^{14}C] hydroxyproline by the cells of the explant (●——●). The collagen concentration is proportional to the amount of hydroxyproline per unit dry weight of parenchyma (○---○).[29-32] B. The average rate of GAG synthesis per cell quantitated as the incorporation of [1-^{14}C] glucosamine into parenchymal explants (●——●). GAG concentration is proportional to hexosamine per unit dry weight (○---○).[31,33,37]

animals on the maintenance of lung connective tissue by lung cells. In addition, these methods may be adapted to evaluating other functions of lung cells including energy production,[40] glucose metabolism,[41] lipid metabolism,[42] and the synthesis of other structural proteins or enzymes.[19]

Lung Cell Culture

Although studies of lung explants provide an important groundwork for an understanding of the function of lung cells, they cannot specify the role of individual cells in the synthesis, maintenance and degradation of lung structure. There are approximately forty different cell types comprising the lung[7]; therefore, lung explants contain many types of differentiated cells. For example, an explant of lung parenchyma would contain the major cells of the alveoli including alveolar type I, alveolar type II, endothelial and mesenchymal cells, while an explant of the pulmonary artery would include endothelial, smooth muscle and mesenchymal cells. Thus, in order to simplify the evaluation of lung cells in lung injury, it is necessary to turn to cell culture methods.

The major advantages of working with cells in culture are[19]: (1) single-cell types can be cultured and thus the cell type responsible for the observed effects are known; (2) uniform access to the cell by the culture environment is assured; (3) cell-cell interactions can be controlled; and (4) secreted products of the cells can be separated from intracellular products of the cells (something that is very difficult with explant systems). There are, however, disadvantages to cell culture methods. Isolation of the relevant cell types in adequate yield, viability and purity can be a formidable problem. In addition, the results obtained from cell culture must always be interpreted with caution, since removal of cells from the lung and their subsequent culture may result in substantial changes in their *in vivo* differentiated state.

The most easily isolated lung cell is the alveolar macrophage. It can be obtained in high yield and purity by bronchoalveolar lavage of animals or humans.[13,43] Since macrophages adhere to surfaces, plating the lavage fluid cells in plastic culture dishes overnight, followed by rinsing, results in a pure culture of alveolar macrophages (Figure 2.5). Alveolar macrophages isolated in this way will live for several weeks in culture, but do not divide under usual conditions.

Another readily available cell is the lung mesenchymal cell, usually referred to as a fibroblast (Figure 2.5). It adapts well to tissue culture conditions, and this property can be used as an isolation and purification step. This is accomplished by dispersing fragments of lung into a uniform cell suspension by a combination of mechanical and enzymatic disruption, followed by culture through several passages.[19,44] The fibroblast will usually dominate the culture to the exclusion of other cell types, although some preparations will appear to be heterogeneous through several subcultivations. Further purification can be achieved, if necessary, by cloning cells from the heterogeneous mixture to obtain a fibroblast line descended from a single cell.

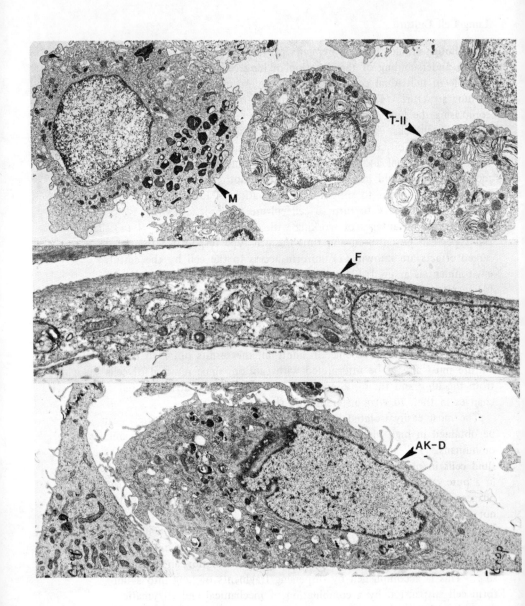

Figure 2.5   Electron micrographs of lung cells in culture. Top: freshly isolated adult
rabbit lung alveolar macrophages (M) and alveolar type II cells (T-II) (x3675).[18]
Middle: newborn rabbit lung fibroblast (F) at subcultivation 15 (x7350).[19,44]
Bottom: cloned cat lung epithelial cell (AK-D) (x4900).[17]

Since dispersions of lung tissue obviously contain cells other than fibro-blasts, cloning methods can be used to obtain nonfibroblast cell lines. Success in obtaining such lines is sometimes limited by their poor growth under tissue culture conditions, but several laboratories have succeeded in growing cells with epithelial rather than fibroblast morphology.[17,45] For example, an epithelial cell (termed AK-D) derived from the fetal-cat lung obtained late in gestation is easily maintained in culture.[17] This cell has very different morphologic characteristics than the fibroblast (Figure 2.5) and may be the culture representative of an alveolar type I cell or perhaps a type II cell in transition to a type I cell. Using methods developed for other organs, it may soon be possible to culture other specific lung-cell types including endothelial cells[46] and smooth-muscle cells.[47]

The technical impediments and uncertainties of cloning have led several laboratories to attempt to isolate pure populations of specific lung cells directly from the lung. Varying degrees of success have been reported using enzymatic digestion, heavy particle phagocytosis, and gradient sedi-mentation. For example, it is now possible to isolate relatively pure populations of alveolar type II cells from the lung of animals (Figure 2.5).[18,48,49] Studies with these cells have shown they synthe-size and secrete dipalmitoyl phosphotidylcholine (the major lipid of surfactant)[50,51] as well as a number of proteins characteristic of this cell.[18] However, current isolation methods do not give consistent results both as to purity and viability and thus type II cells are available only with a great deal of laboratory effort.

Once a cell type is isolated in sufficient yield, purity and viability, metabolic studies can be carried out at a more sophisticated level than is possible in the explant. Each cell synthesizes a large number of biologi-cally important macromolecules; some are common to every cell, while others are related to the differentiated functions of a given cell type. In particular, the products which the cell secretes into the extracellular space are a specific reflection of the differentiated function of the cell. Thus, when cells are damaged or their differentiated state is altered, the products which the cell secretes are likely to be altered as well. Changes in the differentiated state secondary to maturation, exposure to mediators, infection or toxic environmental exposure could, therefore, be characterized at the cellular level by observing changes in the pattern of macromolecular secretion.

Among the many different kinds of cellular secretory products, we have been particularly interested in proteins and glycosaminoglycans. In the case of proteins, a number of different approaches can be used. As shown above in the example of the human alveolar macrophage, the overall distribution of secreted proteins can be examined by electrophoresis on sodium dodecyl sulfate acrylamide gels, which separates proteins according to their molecular weight. Such analysis yields molecular-weight maps of secreted proteins, akin to a "biochemical fingerprint" of the differentiated state of the cell (Figure 2.1).[17-19] This can be used to identify cells in culture and determine changes in the differentiated state, for example in the presence of environmental pollutants.

Although the overall pattern of secreted proteins is a sensitive monitor of cellular changes, more specific information on cell function can be gained by evaluating the synthesis of individual proteins. For example, our interest in the synthesis and degradation of lung connective tissue has led us to examine the metabolism of collagen in tissue culture in some detail. Results indicate that approximately 5% of the total protein synthesized by rabbit lung fibroblasts in confluent culture is collagen. Further analysis reveals this collagen consists of two types, termed Type I and Type III.[44] Type I collagen is the common fibrillar collagen seen on electron micrographs; Type III collagen forms loosely associated fibrils, referred to in the older literature as reticulin.[31] The significance of the synthesis of both types of collagen by the lung fibroblast is underlined by recent data which suggests that there is a shift in the proportion of Type I and Type III collagens in pulmonary fibrosis.[52] If loss of lung function is in part due to this relative change in collagen types in the alveolar interstitium, then an understanding of the cellular basis behind it will be a major step forward in understanding this disease. Possible ways for this change to occur via collagen synthetic mechanisms include changes in the differentiated state of a given population of lung cells or replacement of one population of lung cells by another.

The protein products of cell secretion include not only connective tissue proteins, but also specific enzymes which act in the extracellular space. For example, collagenase is produced by several cells in culture: the fibroblast,[53,54] alveolar macrophage,[55] monocyte[54] and neutrophil.[56] Of particular interest is the recent observation that these collagenases have different substrate specificities. The fibroblast and macrophage enzymes attack both Type I and Type III collagens, while the neutrophil enzyme is relatively specific for Type I.[57] This observation is relevant to the possibilities of shifts of collagen types in pulmonary inflammation. It raises the possibility that the composition of the lung connective tissue can be altered not only by control over collagen synthesis, but also by control of selective enzymatic degradation.

Glycosaminoglycans secreted by cells in culture can be evaluated by methods similar to those used in the explant. As in the explant, they can be labeled with relatively specific precursors and individually quantitated. Preliminary results indicate that lung fibroblasts in culture synthesize heparan sulfate, dermatan sulfate, chondroitin sulfate and hyaluronic acid.[58] In addition, the quantitative patterns of synthesis and secretion of the glycosaminoglycans may differ between different cell types. For example, about 20–25% of the glycosaminoglycans secreted by normal cat lung fibroblasts is dermatan sulfate. On the other hand, cat lung epithelial cell (AK-D), makes very little dermatan sulfate, and secretes it in barely detectable amounts (<1%).[58]

The synthesis of connective tissue proteins and enzymes which degrade them all represent complex differentiated functions performed by the cells of the lung. These cells do not act in a vacuum, but as part of the appropriate coherent response of the organ to growth, injury and repair. It is likely that at least some of these responses are orchestrated through soluble mediators produced by one cell type to modulate the function of another. The use of appropriate populations of isolated lung cells can help determine how these mediators act, and what their role is in lung disease.

CONCLUSIONS

From the above discussion it should be apparent how these methodologies might apply to the study of the effect of environmental pollutants on lung cellular function. The lung is a complex organ which can be damaged by many different processes, including environmental pollutant exposure. Frequently, such damage evolves into a non-specific picture of lung injury which leaves a few clues as to the original cause. Present methods for evaluation of lung damage, such as histopathology and physiologic testing, have frequently not been helpful in pinpointing the pathogenesis of these disorders. We have described newer methods which may help to characterize the metabolic and biochemical processes of the lung at the cellular level, both in the normal state and in response to disease. With a detailed knowledge of these processes, it should be possible to begin to understand how the multiple environmental assaults on the lung produce their damage, and how to avoid or reverse these effects.

REFERENCES

1. Stern, A.C., ed., *Air Pollution.* (New York: Academic Press, 1976).
2. "Health Hazards of the Human Environment." World Health Organization, Geneva (1972).
3. Fennelly, P.F. "The Origin and Influence of Airborne Particulates," *Amer. Scient.* 64:46-56 (1976).

4. Aharonson, E. F., A. Ben-David and M. A. Klingberg, Eds. *Air Pollution and the Lung* (New York: John Wiley and Sons, 1976).

5. Kerr, H. D., T. J. Kulle, M. L. McIlhany and P. Swidersky. "Effects of Ozone on Pulmonary Function in Normal Subjects," *Amer. Rev. Resp. Dis.* 111:763-773 (1975).

6. Buckley, R. D., J. D. Hackney, C. Posin and K. Clark. "Effects of Gaseous Pollutants," Chapter 11, this volume (1977).

7. Kuhn, C. "The Cells of the Lung and their Organelles," in *The Biochemical Basis of Pulmonary Function*, R. G. Crystal, Ed. (New York: Marcel Dekker, 1976), pp. 3-48.

8. Fulmer, J. D. and R. G. Crystal. "The Biochemical Basis of Pulmonary Function," in *The Biochemical Basis of Pulmonary Function*, R. G. Crystal, Ed. (New York: Marcel Dekker, 1976), pp. 419-466.

9. Crystal, R. G. "Biochemical Processes in the Normal Lung," in *Lung Cells in Disease*, A. Bouhuys, Ed. (Amsterdam: North Holland, 1976), pp. 17-38.

10. Ikeda, S. *Atlas of Flexible Bronchofiberoscopy.* (Baltimore: University Park Press, 1974).

11. Reynolds, H. Y. and H. H. Newball. "Analysis of Proteins and Respiratory Cells Obtained from Human Lungs by Bronchial Lavage," *J. Lab. Clin. Med.* 84:559-573 (1974).

12. Reynolds, H. Y. and H. H. Newball. "Fluid and Cellular Milieu of the Human Respiratory Tract," in *Immunologic and Infectious Reactions in the Lung.* C. H. Kirkpatrick and H. Y. Reynolds, Eds. (New York: Marcel Dekker, 1976), pp. 3-27.

13. Reynolds, H. Y., J. D. Fulmer, J. A. Kazmierowski, W. C. Frank and R. G. Crystal. "Analysis of Bronchoalveolar Lavage Fluid from Patients with Idiopathic Pulmonary Fibrosis and Chronic Hypersensitivity Pneumonitis," *J. Clin. Invest.* 59:165-175 (1977).

14. Crystal, R. G., J. D. Fulmer, W. C. Roberts, M. L. Moss, B. R. Line and H. Y. Reynolds. "Idiopathic Pulmonary Fibrosis: Clinical, Histological, Radiographic, Physiologic, Nuclear, Cytologic and Biochemical Aspects," *Ann. Int. Med.,* in press (1976).

15. Fink, J. N. "Hypersensitivity Pneumonitis," in *Immunologic and Infectious Reactions in the Lung.* C. H. Kirkpatrick and H. Y. Reynolds, Eds. (New York: Marcel Dekker, 1976), pp. 229-241.

16. Daniele, R. P., M. D. Altose and D. T. Rowlands, Jr. "Immunocompetent Cells from the Lower Respiratory Tract of Normal Human Lungs," *J. Clin. Invest.* 56:986-995 (1975).

17. Elson, N., K. Bradley, A. Hance, A. Kniazeff, S. Breul, A. Horwitz and R. Crystal. "Synthesis of Collagen in Cultured Lung Cells," *Clin. Res.* 23:346A (1975).

18. Elson, N. A., J. B. Karlinsky, J. A. Kelman, R. A. Rhoades and R. G. Crystal. "Differentiated Properties of the Type 2 Alveolar Cell: Partial Characterization of Protein Content, Synthesis and Secretion," *Clin. Res.* 24:464A (1976).

19. Collins, J. F. and R. G. Crystal. "Protein Synthesis," in *The Biochemical Basis of Pulmonary Function*, R. G. Crystal, Ed. (New York: Marcel Dekker, 1976), pp. 171-212.

20. Weissbecker, L., R.D. Carpenter, P.C. Luchsinger and T.S. Osdene. *"In Vitro* Alveolar Macrophage Viability: Effect of Gases," *Arch. Environ. Health.* 18:756-759 (1969).

21. Hurst, D.J. and D.L. Coffin. "Ozone Effect on Lysosomal Hydrolases of Alveolar Macrophages *In Vitro," Arch. Int. Med.* 127:1059-1063 (1971).

22. Huisingh, J.L., J.A. Cambell and M.D. Waters. "Evaluation of Trace Element Interactions Using Cultured Alveolar Macrophages," *Hanford Biology Symposium.* 16:35 (1976).

23. Alpert, S.M., D.E. Gardner, D.J. Hurst, T.R. Lewis and D.L. Coffin. "Effects of Exposure to Ozone on Defensive Mechanisms of the Lung," *J. Appl. Physiol.* 31:247-252 (1971).

24. Plopper, C.G., D.L. Dungworth and W.S. Tyler. "Ultrastructure of Pulmonary Alveolar Macrophages *In Situ* in Lungs from Rabbits Exposed to Ozone," *Amer. Rev. Resp. Dis.* 108:632-638 (1973).

25. Katz, G.V. and S. Laskin. "Effect of Irritant Atmospheres on Macrophage Behavior," *Hanford Biology Symposium.* 16:36A (1976).

26. Line, B.R., J.D. Fulmer, A.E. Jones, H.Y. Reynolds, W.C. Roberts and R.G. Crystal. "[67]Gallium Scanning in Idiopathic Pulmonary Fibrosis: Correlation with Histopathology and Broncho-Alveolar Lavage," *Amer. Rev. Resp. Dis.* 113(4, part 2):244 (1976).

27. Cowan, M.J., J.F. Collins and R.G. Crystal. "Collagen and Lung Growth: A prototype of Connective Tissue Differentiation," in *Eukaryotes at the Subcellular Level.* (New York: Marcel Dekker, 1976), pp. 257-313.

28. Bradley, K.H., S.D. McConnell and R.G. Crystal. "Lung Collagen Composition and Synthesis: Characterization and Changes with Age," *J. Biol. Chem.* 249:2674-2683 (1974).

29. Bradley, K., S. McConnell-Breul and R.G. Crystal. "Lung Collagen Heterogeneity," *Proc. Nat. Acad. Sci.* 71:2828-2832 (1974).

30. Bradley, K., S. McConnell-Breul and R.G. Crystal. "Collagen in the Human Lung," *J. Clin. Invest.* 55:543-550 (1975).

31. Hance, A.J. and R.G. Crystal. "The Connective Tissue of Lung," *Amer. Rev. Resp. Dis.* 112:657-711 (1975).

32. Hance, A.J., and R.G. Crystal. "Collagen," in *The Biochemical Basis of Pulmonary Function,* R.G. Crystal, Ed. (New York: Marcel Dekker, 1976), pp. 215-271.

33. Horwitz, A.L., N.A. Elson and R.G. Crystal. "Proteoglycans and Elastic Fibers," in *The Biochemical Basis of Pulmonary Function,* R.G. Crystal, Ed. (New York: Marcel Dekker, 1976), pp. 273-311.

34. Langston, C., P. Sachdeva, M.J. Cowan, J. Haines, R.G. Crystal and W.M. Thurlbeck. "Alveolar Multiplication in the Contralateral Lung Following Unilateral Pneumonectomy in the Rabbit," *Amer. Rev. Resp. Dis.* 115:7-13 (1977).

35. Cowan, M.J. and R.G. Crystal. "Lung Growth After Unilateral Pneumonectomy: Quantification of Collagen Synthesis and Content," *Amer. Rev. Resp. Dis.* 111:267-277 (1975).

36. Wagner, W.M. "The Effects of X-Ray Energy and Absorbed Dose on the Production of Pulmonary Fibrosis in Rabbits," Thesis, The Johns Hopkins School of Hygiene and Public Health, Baltimore (1976).

37. Horwitz, A. L. and R. G. Crystal. "Content and Synthesis of Glycosaminoglycans in the Developing Lung," *J. Clin. Invest.* 56: 1312-1318 (1975).
38. Hussain, M. Z., M. G. Mustafa, C. K. Chow and C. E. Cross. "Ozone-Induced Increase of Lung Proline Hydroxylase Activity and Hydroxyproline Content," *Chest.* 69 (suppl.):273-275 (1976).
39. Bhatnagar, R. S. "Role of Superoxide in Oxidant Induced Pulmonary Fibrosis," Chapter 5, this volume (1977).
40. Fisher, A. B. "Oxygen Utilization and Energy Production," in *The Biochemical Basis of Pulmonary Function,* R. G. Crystal, Ed. (New York: Marcel Dekker, 1976), pp. 75-104.
41. Tierney, D. F. and S. E. Levy. "Glucose Metabolism," in *The Biochemical Basis of Pulmonary Function,* R. G. Crystal, Ed. (New York: Marcel Dekker, 1976), pp. 105-125.
42. Mason, R. J. "Lipid Metabolism," in *The Biochemical Basis of Pulmonary Function,* R. G. Crystal, Ed. (New York: Marcel Dekker, 1976), pp. 127-169.
43. Myrvik, Q. N., E. S. Leake and B. Fariss. "Studies on Pulmonary Alveolar Macrophages from the Normal Rabbit: A Technique to Procure Them in a High State of Purity," *J. Immunol.* 86:128-132 (1961).
44. Hance, A. J., K. Bradley and R. G. Crystal. "Lung Collagen Heterogeneity. Synthesis of Type I and Type III Collagen by Rabbit and Human Lung Cells in Culture," *J. Clin. Invest.* 57:102-111 (1976).
45. Douglas, W. H. J. and M. E. Kaighn. "Clonal Isolation of Differentiated Rat Lung Cells," *In Vitro* 10:230-237 (1974).
46. Jaffee, E. A., R. L. Nachman, C. G. Becker and C. R. Minick. "Culture of Human Endothelial Cells Derived from Umbilical Veins. Identification by Morphologic and Immunologic Criteria," *J. Clin. Invest.* 52:2745-2756 (1973).
47. Ross, R. "The Smooth Muscle Cell. II. Growth of Smooth Muscle in Culture and Formation of Elastic Fibers," *J. Cell. Biol.* 50:172-186 (1971).
48. Kikkawa, Y. and K. Yoneda. "The Type II Epithelial Cell of the Lung," *Lab. Invest.* 30:76-84 (1974).
49. Mason, R. J., M. C. Williams and J. A. Clements. "Isolation and Identification of Type 2 Alveolar Epithelial Cells," *Chest.* 67 (Suppl.):36S-37S (1975).
50. Kikkawa, Y., K. Yoneda, F. Smith, B. Packard and K. Suzuki. "The Type II Epithelial Cells of the Lung. II. Chemical Composition and Phospholipid Synthesis," *Lab. Invest.* 32:295-302 (1975).
51. Mason, R. J. "Secretion of Disaturated Phosphatidyl Choline by Primary Cultures of Type II Alveolar Cells," *Hanford Biology Symp.* 16:30A (1976).
52. Hutcheson, E. T. and A. H. Kang. "Collagen Polymorphism in Idiopathic Chronic Pulmonary Fibrosis," *J. Clin. Invest.* 57:1498-1508 (1976).
53. Werb, Z. and M. C. Burleigh. "A Specific Collagenase from Rabbit Fibrobasts in Monolayer Culture," *Biochem. J.* 137:373-385 (1974).

54. Horwitz, A. L., J. A. Kelman, S. C. Brin and R. G. Crystal. "Collagenase Production by Cells in Culture," *Fed. Proc.* 35:1740 (1976).

55. Horwitz, A. L. and R. G. Crystal. "Collagenase from Rabbit Pulmonary Alveolar Macrophages," *Biochem. Biophys. Res. Comm.* 69:296-303 (1976).

56. Lazarus, G. S., R. S. Brown, J. R. Daniels and H. Fullmer. "Human Granulocytic Collagenase," *Science* 159:1483-1485 (1968).

57. Horwitz, A. L., A. J. Hance and R. G. Crystal. "Granulocyte Collagenase: Selective Digestion of Type I and Type III Collagen," *Proc. Nat. Acad. Sci.* 74:897-901 (1977).

58. Karlinsky, J. B., N. A. Elson, A. L. Horwitz and R. G. Crystal. "Lung Cells in Culture: Glycosaminoglycan Synthesis and Secretion by a Fetal Cat Fibroblast and Epithelial Cell," In preparation.

CHAPTER 3

INJURY AND CELL RENEWAL IN
RAT LUNGS EXPOSED TO OZONE

M. J. Evans and G. Freeman

Stanford Research Institute
333 Ravenswood Avenue
Menlo Park, California 94025

INTRODUCTION

In a previous study by Evans et al.,[1] pulmonary cell renewal was studied in rats exposed to low levels of ozone (O_3). Epithelial cells were the principal cells affected by the gas. In the alveoli, the initial tissue damage occurred to Type 1 cells. This was followed by proliferation of Type 2 cells. A peak of Type 2 cell proliferation occurred after 2 days of exposure, which then declined to near control levels by the fourth day. Since Type 1 cells exhibited no further damage despite continuous exposure to O_3, they appeared to have become tolerant to that concentration of O_3. A similar result was observed previously in animals exposed to NO_2.[2]

To test how well the tissue had adapted to the O_3, another series of experiments was performed in which rats tolerant to one concentration of O_3 were reexposed to a higher concentration of O_3. The results showed partial protection against injury on reexposure to elevated concentrations of O_3. The degree to which the rats were protected was related to the initial concentration of O_3 to which they were exposed and the concentration of O_3 on reexposure. That is, higher initial concentrations of O_3 afforded more protection against reinjury than lower initial concentrations when the rats were reexposed to twice the initial concentration.

The basis for the increased resistance to O_3 is not known. Because the principal cell damaged by O_3 is the Type 1 cell, changes associated with the increased resistance should ultimately relate to these cells.

The purpose of the present study was to determine if renewed Type 1 cells were resistant to O_3 injury on reexposure. To accomplish this, we utilized tritiated thymidine (^{3}H-TdR) labeling of dividing cells and autoradiography to identify the cells. Because Type 2 cells take up ^{3}H-TdR before division and can transform into Type 1 cells following division, new Type 1 cells formed in this manner will also be labeled. In the following experiments, animals were exposed to O_3 for 2 days and labeled with ^{3}H-TdR. The Type 2 cells were then allowed to transform into Type 1 cells (2 to 3 days after labeling). These animals were reexposed to higher concentrations of O_3, and the labeled new Type 1 cells remaining after reexposure were studied.

MATERIALS AND METHODS

A group of 30-day-old male Sprague-Dawley rats (Hilltop Lab Animals, Inc.), each weighing approximately 100 g, was exposed to 0.5 ± 0.05 ppm O_3 in air for 2 days. Following exposure, the rats were each injected with 500 μCi of ^{3}H-TdR (specific activity, 6.7 Ci/mMole, New England Nuclear) and were allowed to recover in clean air. After 3 days of recovery, one-half of the animals were reexposed to 1.0 ± 0.05 ppm O_3 for 1 day. Five of the reexposed group and 5 of the control animals were then sacrificed. The lungs of animals from both groups were then prepared for light and electron microscopic autoradiography by previously described methods.[2,3] For light microscopy, the alveoli were scanned and all labeled epithelial cells were counted. Labeled cells present in the epithelium were Type 1, Type 2, and intermediate cells (Figures 3.1, 3.2 and 3.3, respectively). Each cell type was then expressed as a proportion of the total labeled epithelial cell population.[3] For electron microscopy, only Types 1 and 2 cells were studied.

RESULTS AND DISCUSSION

In rats not reexposed to O_3 (controls), labeled cells were distributed throughout the tissue, more of them appearing in alveoli near the openings of the terminal bronchioles. There was no evidence of tissue damage. In rats reexposed to O_3 (experimentals), the distribution of labeled cells was similar; however, in alveoli near the openings of terminal bronchioles, the epithelium exhibited damage. Labeling indexes (LIs) from both control and experimental animals are presented in Table 3.1.

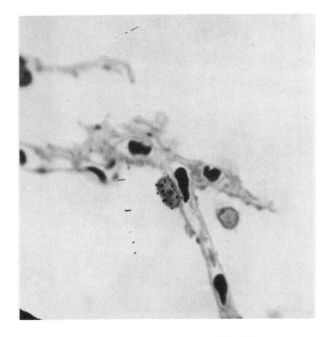

Figure 3.1   Labeled Type 1 cell (X 1,250).

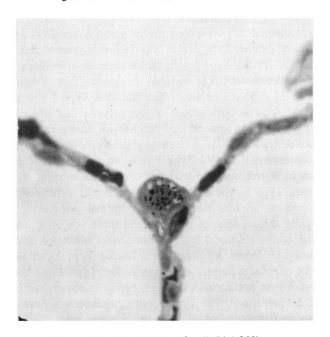

Figure 3.2   Labeled Type 2 cell (X 1,250).

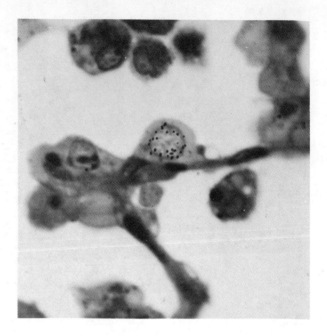

Figure 3.3   Labeled intermediate cell (X 1,250).

In experimental rats reexposed to 1.0 ppm O_3 for 24 hr, the average proportion of labeled Type 1 cells was 16.8. In control rats, the average proportion of labeled Type 1 cells in the alveolar epithelium was 18.9. Previous studies showed that maximal damage to Type 1 cells occurred after 24 hr of exposure to O_3.[4] The fact that Type 1 cell LIs are essentially the same in both groups of rats suggests that labeled Type 1 cells were not injured and did not desquamate during reexposure to the higher concentration of O_3. Electron microscopic autoradiography was used to determine if labeled Type 1 cells were damaged. Preliminary observations in alveoli near the openings of terminal bronchioles revealed that labeled Type 1 cells and labeled Type 2 cells were intact. Labeled Type 1 cells at this time had a relatively normal cytoplasm. The cells were slightly thicker than in controls, and there was some evidence of interstitial edema (Figure 3.4). However, some unlabeled Type 1 cells were damaged. Figure 3.5 illustrates a labeled Type 2 cell adjacent to a portion of exposed basement membrane. The Type 1 cell that presumably had covered that portion of membrane before exposure had been damaged and had desquamated. The Type 2 cell cytoplasm was normal and appeared to be flattening out to cover the exposed area.

Table 3.1   Proportion of Labeled Epithelial Cell Types[a]

Schedule	Sacrifice	N	% of Type 1	Mean	% of Type 2	Mean	% of Intermediate	Mean
Control group	Day 5	161	19.9		72.0		3.1	
		126	14.3		80.4		2.1	
		193	30.0	18.9	65.6	77.2	4.4	2.1
		266	13.8		85.0		0.9	
		252	16.7		83.2		0.1	
	Day 6	142	18.2		79.0		2.8	
		143	17.5		74.2		8.3	
		162	16.1	14.0	83.9	83.2	0	2.8
		47	4.3		95.7		0	
Experimental group, reexposure for 24 hr to 1.0 ppm O$_3$	Day 5 (1 hr of recovery)	88	19.3		71.6		1.6	
		143	19.6	16.8	78.4	74.3	2.0	6.1
		131	13.8		78.0		8.2	
		77	14.3		68.2		17.5	
	Day 6 (24 hr of recovery)	241	8.7		40.9		51.5	
		175	4.8		29.2		65.0	
		198	4.0	6.8	63.2	54.3	33.0	38.6
		119	5.7		68.0		26.3	
		167	13.0		70.0		17.0	

[a]All rats were exposed to 0.5 ppm O$_3$ for 2 days, labeled with ^{3}H-TdR, and allowed to recover for 3 days before reexposure to 1.0 ppm.

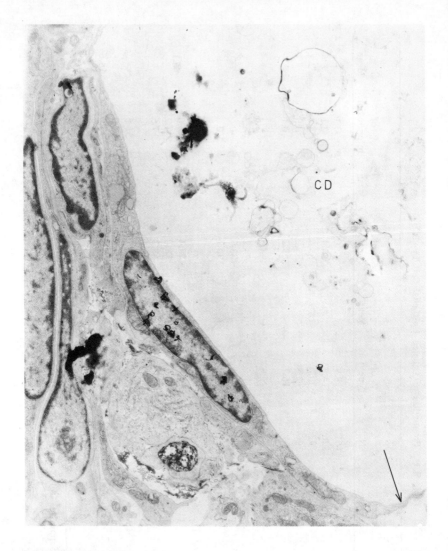

Figure 3.4 Labeled Type 1 cell 1 hr following reexposure for 24 hr to 1.0 ppm O_3 (X 9,500). Note the cellular debris (CD) in the alveoli and a portion of the Type 1 cell lifting off the basement membrane (arrow).

After 1 day of recovery, the group reexposed to O_3 for 24 hr had an average Type 1 cell LI of 6.8. The control group had an average Type 1 cell LI of 14.0. These data would suggest at first that labeled Type 1 cells in the experimental rats were being lost from the tissue. However, it was previously demonstrated that Type 2 cells would have

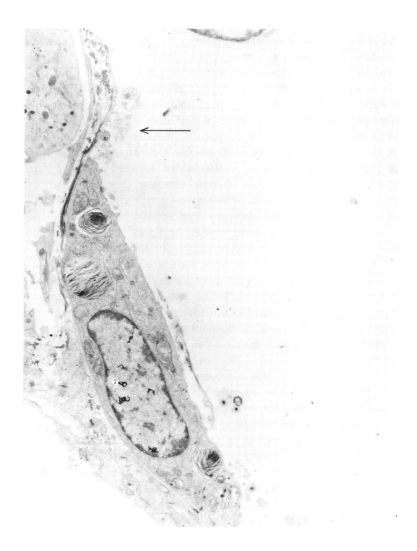

Figure 3.5 Labeled Type 2 cell 1 hr following reexposure for 24 hr to 1.0 ppm O_3 (X 9,000). Note the exposed basement membrane (arrow) where a Type 1 cell had been damaged and sloughed off.

begun to divide again at this time, resulting in a large increase in labeled intermediate cell types in the epithelium. Since Type 1 cells do not divide, the increased number of labeled cells would result in a reduction in the proportion of labeled Type 1 cells in the tissue. Thus, the decreased Type 1 cell LI probably does not represent injury and sloughing of labeled Type 1 cells but rather an increased rate of division of Type 2 cells. This viewpoint is supported by the large increase in labeled intermediate cells at this time. Electron microscopic autoradiography of these labeled Type 1 cells is currently in progress to determine if they are morphologically different from the cells of the previous group sacrificed immediately after exposure.

This study has shown that new Type 1 alveolar cells, as indicated by ^{3}H-TdR labeling, were not morphologically altered or decreased in number immediately following reexposure to a higher concentration of O_3. Since Type 1 cells are the main cell type affected by O_3, and the labeled Type 1 cells in this study resulted from the initial exposure, their persistence during reexposure suggests they were resistant to the O_3. The basis for their resistance to O_3 is not known. Other investigators have reported increased activities of various enzymes in the lung during oxidant exposure, which coincide with the appearance of an epithelium tolerant to the oxidant.[5,6]   Thus, increases in enzyme activity could be associated with tolerance in the new Type 1 cells. The increased enzyme activity could have occurred through the formation of new, altered cells or simply as a characteristic of newly formed cells.[7]   Since there was considerable cell division following the initial injury, most of the cells in the affected area are relatively young with respect to their life span, so either situation is possible.

In a previous study, it was concluded that tolerance was associated with a degree of change in the affected cells.[1]   Such a change is compatible with the concept of increasing protective enzyme activities and with the evidence presented here that some cells were injured on reexposure to higher concentrations of O_3 while others in the same area were not. However, another possible explanation of the data is that an increase occurred in the total number of epithelial cells. How this increase may relate to the tissue's ability to tolerate O_3 on reexposure is obscure, although such an increase is a common occurrence in animals exposed to oxidants. We are currently studying changes in the volume of epithelial cells during oxidant exposure in an attempt to further understand this problem.

ACKNOWLEDGMENT

This research was supported by PHS Grants ES 00842 and HL 16330 from the U.S. Department of Health, Education and Welfare.

REFERENCES

1. Evans, M. J., L. V. Johnson, R. J. Stephens and G. Freeman. "Cell Renewal in the Lungs of Rats Exposed to Low Levels of Ozone," *Exp. Mol. Pathol.* 24:70 (1976).
2. Evans, M. J., R. J. Stephens, L. J. Cabral and G. Freeman. "Cell Renewal in the Lungs of Rats Exposed to Low Levels of NO_2," *Arch. Environ. Health* 24:180 (1972).
3. Evans, M. J., L. J. Cabral, R. J. Stephens and G. Freeman. "Transformation of Alveolar Type 2 Cells to Type 1 Cells Following Exposure to NO_2," *Exp. Mol. Pathol.* 22:142 (1975).
4. Stephens, R. J., M. F. Sloan, M. J. Evans and G. Freeman. "Early Response of Lungs to Low Levels of Ozone," *Amer. J. Pathol.* 74:31 (1974).
5. Chow, C. K. and A. L. Tappel. "Activities of Pentose Shunt and Glycolytic Enzymes in Lungs of Ozone-Exposed Rats," *Arch. Environ. Health* 26:205 (1973).
6. Tierney, D., L. Ayers, S. Herzog and J. Yang. "Pentose Pathway and Production of Reduced Nicotinamide Adenine Dinucleotide Phosphate," *Amer. Rev. Respir. Dis.* 108:1348 (1973).
7. De Lucia, A. J., M. C. Mustafa, C. G. Plopper, C. E. Cross, D. L. Dungworth and W. S. Tyler. "Biochemical and Morphological Alterations in the Lung Following Ozone Exposure," *Amer. Inst. Chem. Eng. Air*—Part I (1973).

CHAPTER 4

NUCLEIC ACID METABOLISM
IN NORMAL AND DAMAGED LUNG

H. P. Witschi

Départment de Pharmacologie
Faculté de Médecine
Université de Montréal
Montréal, P.Q., Canada

INTRODUCTION

During the past decade, a substantial amount of information has become available on the early biochemical changes related to the development of certain human diseases. Disturbances in nucleic acid metabolism have been linked to the development of several well-defined pathologic conditions. It is safe to assume that interference with synthesis, structure and degradation of cellular DNA and RNA often plays a key role in the causing of disease. Much of the available evidence has recently been summarized.[1] A full and thorough understanding of the "pathology of transcription and translation" may ultimately help to predict the hazards of environmental agents.

Normal and pathologic nucleic acid metabolism of eucaryotic cells has been studied predominantly in homogeneous cell populations maintained in culture. In the whole animal, most experiments have been done with a few selected organs, most often the liver. For lung, comparatively little information is available. The cellular heterogeneity of lung does not make it an attractive organ for a detailed analysis of RNA and DNA metabolism. Nevertheless, some information exists and should be taken into account if one considers the interaction of environmental agents with the lung.

RNA METABOLISM

Toxic agents quite often alter the rate of *in vivo* RNA synthesis. It is possible to evaluate this by measuring the incorporation of a suitable radioactive precursor into RNA. When the kinetics of incorporation of orotic acid into total cellular RNA were examined in rat lung and compared to rat liver, it was found that hepatic RNA was labeled about 20 times more than lung RNA.[2]   On the other hand, injection of uridine preferentially labeled lung RNA. An estimation of the specific activity and of the pool size of uridine nucleotides, the immediate precursors of RNA, revealed that the rate of RNA synthesis was about the same in both liver and lung, despite the large differences in the specific activity of the final product. In hamster, the rate of pulmonary RNA synthesis appeared to be about half the rate of hepatic RNA synthesis.[3]

A determination of the kinetic constants of some enzymes involved in pyrimidine metabolism showed that the apparent K_m (10^{-3} M) were very similar: for uridine kinase 0.19 in liver and 0.15 in lung; for OMP decarboxylase 0.002 in liver and 0.001 in lung. A calculation of the apparent V_{max} per tissue unit showed that the average lung cell could handle as much uridine as the average liver cell, but would be about 15 times less effective in handling orotic acid.[3]   These findings, although unconfirmed, might point out a true biochemical difference between liver and lung cells: liver seems better equipped to synthesize pyrimidines *de novo*, whereas the capability to utilize preformed pyrimidines via the salvage pathway appears to be equal in both organs.

RNA synthesis in lung is inhibited by actinomycin D within less than an hour. The degree of inhibition depends on the dose.[2,3]   Other agents may interfere with hepatic RNA synthesis, but do not do so in lung. Examples are diethylnitrosamine[4] and nickel carbonyl.[2]   The observation made with diethylnitrosamine (DEN) is probably not too surprising: DEN causes extensive liver necrosis and this might account for the decreased RNA synthesis. No profound acute effect of DEN on lung parenchyma has been described. For nickel carbonyl, there is at least some indirect evidence that the compound interferes with transcription in lung.[5,6]   This is accompanied by an inhibition of hepatic RNA synthesis.[7]   The failure to verify the same phenomenon in lung most likely reflects the inadequacy of *in vivo* incorporation studies when it comes to detect changes in a small population of pulmonary cells or when biochemical signs of cell damage may be superceded by events associated with tissue repair, as occurs soon in lung after injection of nickel carbonyl.[8]

Virtually no information is available on the effects of pollutants and gases on RNA metabolism. Ozone has been found to decrease the incorporation of radioactive precursors into total pulmonary RNA.[9] Oxygen does not inhibit the incorporation of uridine into pulmonary monoribosomes in newborn guinea pigs[10] and does not interfere with the incorporation of orotic acid into RNA in adult rat lung (Table 4.1).

Table 4.1   RNA Synthesis in the Lung of Rats Exposed to 100% Oxygen

Duration of Exposure to O_2 (hr)	dpm/mg RNA[a]		
6	Controls:	507 ± 44	(4)
	O_2-exposed:	531 ± 42	(4)
24	Controls:	413 ± 77	(6)
	O_2-exposed:	458 ± 64	(8)

[a] 5 μCi orotic acid - ^{14}C i.v., animals killed 15 min later.   Mean $\pm$ S.E.M., number of animals in parenthesis.

Occasionally, toxic agents will produce an increase in pulmonary RNA. Exposure to ozone[11] or to cadmium aerosol[12] is followed by a net increase in pulmonary RNA. Similar observations have been made in lungs after partial pneumonectomy.[13,14]   A determination of the RNA/DNA ratio allows one to decide whether the increase in lung RNA is due to cellular hypertrophy or to hyperplasia; hypertrophy of lung cells is accompanied by an increase in the RNA/DNA ratio, whereas the ratio remains unchanged in hyperplasia.

Estimation of whether cellular hypertrophy in the lung is preceded or accompanied by increased rates of RNA synthesis is difficult. In mouse lung, the antioxidant butylated hydroxytoluene (BHT) produces, within a few days, a proliferation of pulmonary alveolar cells.[15]   Biochemically, the events are characterized by a net increase in pulmonary RNA and pulmonary DNA; however, RNA accumulates faster and to a larger extent than does DNA and, from 4 days after BHT on, the RNA/DNA ratios are twice as high as those found in control lungs (Table 4.2).

In vivo incorporation studies show that the specific activity of RNA, after a 15-minute incorporation time, is substantially lower in the lungs of BHT-treated animals than in controls (Table 4.3).

However, this most probably does not indicate a decreased rate of synthesis, but reflects changes in the amount of RNA present in lung as well as alterations in specific activity and pool size of RNA precursors. It has not yet been possible to measure, with accuracy, precursor pool size in mouse lung. To what extent the increased amount of RNA after

Table 4.2   RNA/DNA in Mouse Lung After BHT

Days After BHT 400 mg/kg	mg RNA/mg DNA	
	BHT	Controls
1	0.42 ± 0.01(6)	0.42 ± 0.03(5)
2	0.69 ± 0.04(4)[b]	0.52 ± 0.02(3)
3	0.74 ± 0.03(6)[b]	0.49 ± 0.05(6)
4	0.80 ± 0.02(5)[b]	0.41 ± 0.01(5)
5	0.92 ± 0.03(5)[b]	0.50 ± 0.02(5)
6	0.93 ± 0.03(6)[b]	0.47 ± 0.03(6)
7	0.86 ± 0.05(5)[b]	0.52 ± 0.04(3)

[a]Means ± S.E.; number of animals in parenthesis.
[b]$p < 0.05$ vs. controls.

Table 4.3   Specific Activity of Mouse Lung RNA After BHT[a]

Days After BHT[b]	dpm/mg RNA 10^{-3}	
	BHT	Controls
1	13.2 ± 2.1(6)	12.2 ± 0.8(5)
2	8.5 ± 1.6(4)[c]	13.7 ± 1.6(3)
3	6.7 ± 0.7(6)[c]	10.1 ± 0.9(6)
4	5.9 ± 0.5(5)[c]	10.8 ± 0.7(5)
5	5.5 ± 0.3(5)	8.5 ± 1.7(5)
6	7.0 ± 0.7(6)[c]	11.5 ± 1.0(6)
7	8.0 ± 1.0(5)[c]	12.2 ± 1.2(3)

[a]10 μCi orotic acid - [14]   i.p., animals killed 15 min. later.
[b]Means ± .E., number of animals in parenthesis.
[c]$p < 0.05$ vs. controls.

BHT is due to enhanced synthesis, impaired breakdown or a combination of the two remains to be established.

The few studies done on the influence of environmental agents on RNA metabolism in lung have not yet given too many tangible results. However, it should not be overlooked that quantitative and qualitative changes in RNA metabolism probably underlie pulmonary carcinogenesis. Urethane alters the activity of RNA polymerase in rat lung nuclei.[16] Nuclear RNA isolated from human lung cancer differs slightly from normal pulmonary RNA.[17,18] In vitamin A-deficient animals, qualitative changes in tracheal RNA synthesis can be correlated with morphologic alterations.[19,20]

Human bronchial epithelium, if maintained in organ culture, remains viable over several weeks while actively synthesizing RNA, among other macromolecules.[21]

To discuss all the implications of these studies goes beyond the scope of the present article. However, they show that an in-depth analysis of the interaction of environmental agents with RNA metabolism is clearly warranted and of great interest.

DNA METABOLISM

Changes in pulmonary DNA metabolism have received somewhat more attention than RNA metabolism. It was mentioned earlier that quantitative and qualitative alterations in lung RNA might underlie the development of malignant tumors, caused by environmental agents. It is thought that modification, damage and repair of DNA might play an equal, if not more important, role. The interaction of lung-specific carcinogens with DNA is a field of considerable research activity[22-25] and no attempt will be made to review further this particular topic.

Interactions of environmental agents with the lung can be detected by monitoring DNA synthesis. Usually, DNA synthesis occurs only in cells that are preparing to divide. It is detected by measuring the incorporation of radioactive thymidine into DNA. Occasionally, thymidine is incorporated into preexisting DNA as a repair process following DNA damage; this has been called "unscheduled DNA synthesis." However, most of the time increased incorporation of thymidine into pulmonary DNA indicates that pulmonary cells prepare to divide and will multiply.

Radioautographic techniques have been shown to be a most powerful experimental tool to monitor DNA synthesis in lung. Our present information on Type 2 cell proliferation as a repair mechanism following Type 1 cell damage is based on such studies.[26-29] Autoradiography has two very attractive features: the cell types that proliferate may be precisely identified and, by counting the number of cells synthesizing DNA, quantitative information concerning the extent of cell proliferation can be obtained.

Compared to autoradiography, biochemical analysis is at a disadvantage: it does not allow the identification of which pulmonary cell types proliferate. On the other hand, biochemical procedures are technically simple and allow the processing of large numbers of samples in a comparatively short time. We have taken advantage of this approach in some studies with the antioxidant BHT.

The initial lesion produced by BHT in mouse lung is a degeneration of Type 1 alveolar cells. This is followed by an intensive repair phase. On days 2 and 3 after BHT, it is predominantly Type 2 alveolar cells that proliferate. On days 4 to 6, interstitial cells and capillary endothelial cells divide. Seven days after BHT and later, the initial lesions are fully repaired, although the newly formed Type 1 cells, derived from dividing Tyep 2 cells, retain remnants of lamellar and multivesicular bodies as well as some peroxisomes.[30,31]

These events can be followed and quantitated by determining the increase of pulmonary DNA content and by measuring DNA synthesis.[32] The activity of several pulmonary enzymes also increases following BHT. Determination of pulmonary thymidine kinase allows the establishment of good relationships between the amount of BHT administered and the extent and duration of the repair phase. On the other hand, DNA polymerase is detected in lung with difficulty, even at a time when a substantial number of cells are proliferating.[33]

BHT appears to be a convenient tool to produce substantial cell growth in mouse lung. This provides an opportunity to examine whether environmental agents may affect tissue repair in lung. It has recently been suggested that oxygen could interfere with compensatory lung growth following partial pneumonectomy.[34] We undertook several experiments in which we examined the effects of 100% oxygen on the lungs of mice treated with BHT.

Animals were injected i.p. with 400 mg/kg of BHT and DNA synthesis was measured 3 days later. From 90 min to 24 hr prior to death, some animals were kept in 100% O_2, and controls in a similar chamber ventilated with air. An exposure of 16 or 24 hr to oxygen significantly depressed DNA synthesis, and some inhibitory effect was observed already after 4 and 10 hr (Table 4.4).

Table 4.4   Inhibition of DNA Synthesis in Mouse Lung by Oxygen[a]

Duration of Exposure to O_2 (hr)	In Vivo DNA Synthesis (% of controls)
1.5	88 ± 11 (7)
4	71 ± 5 (5)
10	68 ± 12 (9)
16	51 ± 7 (22)[b]
24	37 ± 8 (8)[b]

[a]All animals injected with 400 mg/kg of BHT; DNA synthesis measured 3 days later

[b]$p < 0.05$ vs. corresponding controls

The data confirm earlier observations made with autoradiographic methods.[35-37] In the next series of experiments we examined the effects of oxygen 2 days after BHT, at a time when most proliferating cells are Type 2 alveolar cells, and after 4 days when the cells in division consist of approximately an equal number of Type 2 alveolar and interstitial cells. It was found that 2 days after BHT, DNA synthesis was inhibited as early as 10 hr after O_2; at 24 hr, it was 26% of controls. Four days after BHT, a significant inhibition was seen only after 24 hr exposure to O_2 and it was 63% of control values (Table 4.5).

Table 4.5   Inhibition of DNA Synthesis by Oxygen 2 and 4 Days After BHT[a]

Days After BHT	Duration of O_2 Exposure (hr)	In Vivo DNA Synthesis (% of controls)
2	10	71 ± 9 (10)[b]
	24	26 ± 2 (10)[b]
4	10	81 ± 16 (6)
	24	63 ± 4 (10)[b]

[a]All animals injected with BHT, 400 mg/kg on day O.
[b]$p < 0.05$ vs. corresponding controls

The data invite an interesting speculation: proliferating Type 2 alveolar cells might be more susceptible to 100% oxygen than proliferating interstitial cells. If this is so, then other oxidant gases might have similar effects. This could mean that oxidant pollutants not only induce cell damage in lung, but might also interfere with the subsequent tissue repair. This could be of some importance if primary damage to the alveolar zone is caused by drugs and agents that reach the lung via the bloodstream. The primary damage might not cause symptoms and thus go unnoticed, since lung has so many functional units arranged in parallel. However, the repair phase following injury might be compromised by inhalants such as oxygen, ozone, nitrogen dioxide or tobacco smoke. Repetition of this sequence of events could lead to the development of chronic lung damage. There are at least two examples of acute drug-induced lung damage aggravated by oxygen.[38,39] Future experiments will have to show whether this speculation can be substantiated.

CONCLUSIONS

Analysis of nucleic acid metabolism in lung could have two main purposes: to understand mechanisms of disease and to recognize that a potentially damaging event has occurred. The fundamental aspects of RNA metabolism in lung are an unexplored field. With the possible exception of studies concerned with tracheobronchial carcinogenesis, not much more than simple *in vivo* incorporation experiments have been done. The available data are not much help when it comes to recognizing pathologic events, let alone understanding them.

DNA metabolism is better explored. Substantial contributions have been made in clarifying the cellular events underlying tissue damage and repair in lung. More recently, biochemical techniques have contributed to examining the dose-effect and time-effect relationships between environmental agents and the lung.

ACKNOWLEDGMENT

This work was supported by the Medical Research Council, MRC Group in Drug Toxicology.

REFERENCES

1. Farber, E. *The Pathology of Transcription and Translation.* (New York: Marcel Dekker Inc., 1972).
2. Witschi, H. P. "A Comparative Study of *In Vivo* RNA and Protein Synthesis in Rat Liver and Lung," *Cancer Res.* 32:1686 (1972).
3. Witschi, H. P. "Qualitative and Quantitative Aspects of the Biosynthesis of Ribonucleic Acid and of Protein in the Liver and the Lung of the Syrian Golden Hamster," *Biochem. J.* 136:781 (1973).
4. Witschi, H. P. "The Effects of Diethylnitrosamine on Ribonucleic Acid and Protein Synthesis in the Liver and Lung of the Syrian Golden Hamster," *Biochem. J.* 136:789 (1973).
5. Sunderman, F. W., Jr. "Inhibition of Induction of Benzpyrene Hydroxylase by Nickel Carbonyl," *Cancer Res.* 27:950 (1967).
6. Sunderman, F. W., Jr. and C. K. Leibman. "Nickel Carbonyl Inhibition of Induction of Aminopyrine Demethylase Activity in Liver and Lung," *Cancer Res.* 30:1645 (1970).
7. Beach, D. J. and F. W. Sunderman, Jr. "Nickel Carbonyl Inhibition of ^{14}C-Orotic Acid Incorporation into Rat Liver RNA," *Proc. Soc. Exp. Biol. Med.* 131:321 (1969).
8. Hackett, R. L. and F. W. Sunderman, Jr. "Pulmonary Alveolar Reaction to Nickel Carbonyl," *Arch. Environ. Health* 16:349 (1968).
9. Penha, P. D., L. Amaral and S. Werthamer. "Ultrastructural and Biochemical Alteration in Mouse Lung Exposed to Ozone," *Amer. J. Pathol.* 66:57a (1972).

10. Bieber, M. M., M. G. Cogan, T. C. Durbridge and R. C. Rosan. "Oxygen Toxicity in the Newborn Guinea Pig Lung," *Biol. Neonate* 17:35 (1971).

11. Scheel, L. D., O. J. Dobrogorski, J. T. Mountain, J. L. Svirbely and H. E. Stokinger. "Physiologic, Biochemical, Immunologic and Pathologic Changes Following Ozone Exposure," *J. Appl. Physiol.* 14:67 (1959).

12. Hayes, J. A., G. L. Snider and K. C. Palmer. "The Evolution of Biochemical Damage in the Rat Lung After Acute Cadmium Exposure," *Amer. Rev. Resp. Dis.* 113:121 (1976).

13. Romanova, L. K., E. M. Leikina and K. K. Antipova. "Nucleic Acid Synthesis and Mitotic Activity during Development of Compensatory Hypertrophy of the Lung of Rats," *Bull. Exp. Biol. Med.* 63:303 (1967).

14. Buhain, W. J. and J. S. Brody. "Compensatory Growth of Lung Following Pneumonectomy," *J. Appl. Physiol.* 35:898 (1973).

15. Marino, A. A. and J. T. Mitchell. "Lung Damage in Mice Following Intraperitoneal Injection of Butylated Hydroxytoluene," *Proc. Soc. Exp. Biol. Med.* 140:122 (1972).

16. Eker, P. "Effects of the Carcinogen Urethane on Nuclear RNA Polymerase Activities," *Europ. J. Cancer* 11:493 (1975).

17. Yazdi, E., F. Györkey, H. Busch and P. Györkey. "Biochemical Study of Nuclei Isolated from Normal Lung and from Lung Tumors. I. Isolation of Nuclei and Characterization of Nuclear RNA," *J. Natl. Cancer Inst.* 47:212 (1971).

18. Yazdi, E. and F. Györkey. "Biochemical Study of Nuclei Isolated from Normal Lung and from Lung Tumors. II. Nuclear RNAs of Low Molecular Weight," *J. Natl. Cancer Inst.* 47:765 (1971).

19. Kaufmann, D. G., M. S. Baker, J. S. Smith, W. R. Henderson, C. C. Harris, M. B. Sporn and U. Saffiotti. "RNA Metabolism in Tracheal Epithelium: Alteration in Hamsters Deficient in Vitamin A," *Science* 177:1105 (1972).

20. Kaufmann, D. G., M. S. Baker, C. C. Harris, J. M. Smith, H. Boren, M. B. Sporn, and U. Saffiotti. "Coordinated Biochemical and Morphologic Examination of Hamster Tracheal Epithelium," *J. Natl. Cancer Inst.* 49:783 (1972).

21. Barrett, L. A., E. M. McDowell, A. L. Frank, C. C. Harris and B. F. Trump. "Long-Term Organ Culture of Human Bronchial Epithelium," *Cancer Res.* 36:1003 (1976).

22. Harris, C. C., A. L. Frank, C. van Haaften, D. G. Kaufmann, R. Connor, F. Jackson, L. A. Barrett, E. M. McDowell and B. F. Trump. "Binding of (^{3}H) Benzo(a)pyrene to DNA in Cultured Human Bronchus," *Cancer Res.* 36:1011 (1976).

23. Cox, R. and C. C. Irving. "Damage and Repair of DNA in Various Tissues of the Rat Induced by 4-Nitroquinoline 1-oxide," *Cancer Res.* 35:1858 (1975)

24. Laishes, B. A., D. J. Koropatnick and H. F. Stich. "Organ-Specific DNA Damage Induced in Mice by the Organotropic Carcinogens 4-Nitroquinoline 1-oxide and Dimethylnitrosamine," *Proc. Soc. Exp. Biol. Med.* 149:978 (1975).

25. Ross, A. E., L. Keefer and W. Lijinsky. "Alkylation of Nucleic Acids of Rat Liver and Lung by Deuterated N-Nitrosodiethylamine," *J. Natl. Cancer Inst.* 47:789 (1971).

26. Evans, M. J., L. J. Cabral, R. J. Stephens and G. Freeman. "Transformation of Alveolar Type 2 Cells to Type 1 Cells Following Exposure to NO_2," *Exp. Mol. Pathol.* 22:142 (1975).

27. Stephens, R. J., M. F. Sloan, M. J. Evans and G. Freeman. "Early Response of Lung to Low Levels of Ozone," *Amer. J. Pathol.* 74: 31 (1973).

28. Adamson, I. Y. R. and D. H. Bowden. "The Type 2 Cell as Progenitor of Alveolar Epithelial Regeneration," *Lab. Invest.* 30:35 (1974).

29. Witschi, H. P. "Proliferation of Type II Alveolar Cells: A Review of Common Responses in Toxic Lung Injury," *Toxicology* 5:267 (1976).

30. Adamson, I. Y. R., O. H. Bowder, M. G. Coli and H. P. Witschi. "Lung Injury Induced by Butylated Hydroxytoluene Cytodynamic and Biochemical Studies in Mice," *Lab. Invest.* (in press).

31. Hirai, K. I., M. Yamauchi, H. P. Witschi and M. G. Coli. "Ultrastructural Evidence of Transformation of Alveolar Type II Cells to Type I Epithelial Cells in BHT Treated Mouse Lung," *J. Cell Biol.* 70:860 (1976).

32. Witschi, H. P. and W. Saheb. "Stimulation of DNA Synthesis in Mouse Lung Following Intraperitoneal Injection of Butylated Hydroxytoluene," *Proc. Soc. Exp. Biol. Med.* 147:690 (1974).

33. Witschi, H. P., S. Kacew, B. K. Tsang and D. Williamson. "Biochemical Parameters of BHT-Induced Cell Growth in Mouse Lung," *Chem.-Biol. Interactions* 12:29 (1976).

34. Brody, J. S. "Time Course of and Stimuli to Compensatory Growth of the Lung After Pneumonectomy," *J. Clin. Invest.* 56:897 (1975).

35. Evans, M. J., J. D. Hackney and R. F. Bils. "Effects of a High Concentration of Oxygen on Cell Renewal in the Pulmonary Alveoli," *Aerospace Med.* 40:1365 (1969).

36. Bowden, D. R. and I. Y. R. Adamson. "Reparative Changes Following Pulmonary Cell Injury: Ultrastructural, Cytodynamic and Surfactant Studies in Mice after Oxygen Exposure," *Arch. Pathol.* 92:279 (1971).

37. Northway, W. H., R. Petriceks and L. Strahinian. "Quantitative Aspects of Oxygen Toxicity in the Newborn: Inhibition of Lung DNA Synthesis in the Mouse," *Pediatrics* 50:67 (1972).

38. Fisher, H. K., J. A. Clements and R. R. Wright. "Enhancement of Oxygen Toxicity by the Herbicide Paraquat," *Amer. Rev. Resp. Dis.* 107:246 (1973).

39. Brodski, J. "Increased Susceptibility to Pulmonary Oxygen Toxicity After Cholesterol Biosynthesis Inhibition," *Aviat. Space Environ. Med.* 46:254 (1975).

CHAPTER 5

THE ROLE OF SUPEROXIDE IN OXIDANT-INDUCED PULMONARY FIBROSIS

Rajendra S. Bhatnagar

Laboratory of Connective Tissue Biochemistry
School of Dentistry
University of California
San Francisco, California 94143

INTRODUCTION

Oxidant gases such as oxides of nitrogen and ozone are becoming increasingly significant as a major health hazard in the environment. Photochemical reactions of nitrogen oxides and other components of automobile and certain industrial exhausts generate ozone[1,2] in concentrations that have been shown to be deleterious to organisms. Ozone comprises over 90% of measured oxidant in photochemical smog.[3] Although atmospheric oxidants may interact with other organ systems, their most obvious effects are in lungs because lungs present the largest exposed surface to the atmosphere. There is a considerable body of information linking pathophysiological alterations in the lungs to exposure to environmental oxidants. A very important sequel to ozone exposure is interstitial fibrous thickening, as seen by morphological[4,5] as well as biochemical[6,7] criteria. Such changes in the microarchitecture of lungs may arise as a result of biochemical injury and a subsequent reparative response leading to deposition of "scar tissue" and proliferation of connective tissue elements. Additionally such injury may involve a more direct, initial stimulation of collagen synthesis[6,7] and any structural changes accruing from this may provide a focal area with altered mechanical properties, thus contributing to tissue damage and subsequent reparative connective tissue proliferation.

47

The principal component of toxicity of oxygen and ozone is the superoxide free-radical.[8]   The enzyme superoxide dismutase is induced as a part of tissues' protective response to oxidant injury.[9]   Increased tolerance to oxygen is accompanied by increased concentrations of superoxide dismutase.[10,11]   Studies suggest that superoxide radicals may also play a role in the toxicity of ozone.   Previous studies in our laboratory have shown that superoxide is a reactant in the posttranslational processing steps during the synthesis of collagen.[12,13]   We have further investigated the role of superoxide radicals in the synthesis of collagen in cultures of WI-38 human embryonic lung fibroblasts.   Our studies suggest that superoxide may directly stimulate the synthesis of collagen in these cultures.

MATERIALS AND METHODS

WI-38 diploid fibroblasts, derived from fetal human lung, were obtained in the 20-22 passages from Grand Island Biological Co.   The cells were cultured in 60-mm petri dishes (Falcon plastics) in Eagles minimum essential medium with Earle's salts (Grand Island Biological Co.).   The medium contained 20% fetal calf serum and was supplemented with 2 mM glutamine.   The medium also contained 3.3 mM $NaHCO_3$.   All experiments were carried out between 27-30th passages.   At confluence the cells were transferred to a medium containing 2% fetal calf serum for all exposure and labeling procedures. $(3,4-^3H)$-L-proline (41 Ci/m mole) and $(U-^{14}C)$-L-proline (225 mC/m mole) were obtained from New England Nuclear Corp.   Highly purified, protease-free collagenase was a product of Advance Biofactures, Lynbrook, New York.   All chemicals and biochemicals used were obtained from commercial sources and were of the highest purity available.

Collagen synthesis was measured by following the synthesis of labeled hydroxyproline.   Hydroxyproline occurs in significant amounts only in collagen and is synthesized by the hydroxylation of proline already incorporated into the collagen sequence.   Thus, analysis for radioactive hydroxyproline synthesized from radioactive proline, gives a specific method for assaying collagen synthesis.   Radioactive hydroxyproline was measured in 6 N HCl hydrolysates of nondialyzable fractions from the cultures using a published procedure.[14]

Incorporation of radioactive proline into the collagen sequence was also assayed using a protease-free preparation of clostridial collagenase. This enzyme specifically cleaves collagen into dialyzable peptides.   Collagenase treatment was carried out as described previously[15] and the radioactivity dialyzed out after collagenase treatment was used as an index of collagen synthesis. Control experiments using proteins double-labeled with ^{14}C-proline and ^{3}H-tryptophan showed that there was no non-collagenolytic activity present in the collagenase preparation.

Levels of prolyl hydroxylase were assayed in the cells using a previously described procedure.[16] Medium was removed from the cultures and the cell layers were rinsed twice with 0.1 tris · HCl, pH 7.4. The cells were transferred to a tight-fitting glass-glass homogenizer, and were homogenized after swelling for 10 min in 1 ml of the above buffer containing 0.1% Triton X 100. The detergent was included to solubilize the membrane-associated enzyme. The homogenates were centrifuged briefly at 15,000 x G to remove cell debris and the supernatant was used for enzyme assay. The protein content of the enzyme preparation was determined using standard procedures.[17] The complete incubation mixture for prolyl hydroxylase assay contained approximately 1 mg culture supernatant protein, 0.5 mM ascorbate, 0.1 mM α-ketoglutarate, 0.1 mM ferrous ammonium sulfate and 10^5 dpm ^{3}H-proline labeled unhydroxylated collagen substrate, in a total volume of 2.0 ml. The reaction was carried out at 37° C for 10 min and was terminated by the addition of trichloracetic acid to a final concentration of 5%. Tritium is released in stoichiometric amounts during the hydroxylation reaction, and the hydroxylation was measured by assaying the radioactivity in tritiated water collected by vacuum distillation. The enzyme level data are expressed as dpm [3]HHO formed per mg protein.

Superoxide was generated in the culture medium either by the addition of ascorbate, or by the photochemical oxidation of riboflavin.[18] Appropriate amounts of riboflavin were added in the culture medium and the cultures illuminated with a 60 W tungsten lamp placed at 30 cm. Superoxide dismutase (Sigma Chemical Company) was used to eliminate superoxide from some cultures, to demonstrate the role of the free radical.[8]

RESULTS AND DISCUSSION

It has been known for a long time that cells in culture synthesize significant amounts of collagen only if ascorbate is included in the culture medium. However, the mechanism by which ascorbate stimulates collagen synthesis has remained unclear. Ascorbate is a cofactor required for the posttranslational hydroxylation steps in collagen synthesis and our previous studies showed that the hydroxylation reaction involves superoxide radicals, generated by the interaction between ascorbate, and the metal cofactor of the enzyme, Fe^{2+}.[13] Other studies in this laboratory showed that ascorbate may be replaced in the hydroxylation reaction by exogenous superoxide.[12] A test was made to see if the stimulatory effect of ascorbate on collagen synthesis in cell cultures involved superoxide. WI-38 cells were grown to confluence, in the absence of ascorbic acid. At confluence, test cultures were exposed to ascorbate and Fe^{2+} added as ferrous ammonium sulfate. As seen in Table 5.1, ascorbate + Fe^{2+} treated cultures synthesized nearly four times the amount of hydroxyproline synthesized by control cultures or by cultures exposed to Fe^{2+} alone. In order to examine if the increase in hydroxyproline synthesis was attributable to superoxide, superoxide dismutase (SOD) was added to ascorbate + Fe^{2+}-treated cultures. The removal of superoxide by SOD abolished the stimulatory effect seen in the presence of ascorbate, confirming the involvement of the free radical. SOD had no effect on hydroxyproline synthesis in control cultures.

Table 5.1   Role of Superoxide in Ascorbate Supported Collagen Synthesis in WI-38 Fibroblasts[a]

Additions	Percent of Incorporated Radioactivity in Hydroxyproline
None	2.42
Fe^{2+}, 0.15 mM	1.96
Fe^{2+}, 0.3 mM	2.10
Ascorbate 3.5 mM	8.27
Ascorbate 7.0 mM	8.30
Ascorbate, 3.5 mM + Fe^{2+}, 0.15 mM	8.20
Ascorbate, 3.5 mM + Fe^{2+}, 0.3 mM	8.18
Ascorbate, 7.0 mM + Fe^{2+}, 0.15 mM	10.51
Ascorbate, 3.5 mM + SOD, 0.1 unit/ml	3.20
Ascorbate, 7.0 mM + SOD, 0.1 unit/ml	3.40
Ascorbate, 7.0 mM + Fe^{2+}, 0.15 mM + SOD, 0.1 unit/ml	2.1
Ascorbate, 7.0 mM + Fe^{2+}, 0.30 mM + SOD, 0.1 unit/ml	2.3

[a]Cultures were grown to confluence as described in the Methods Section, exposed to the different additives and labeled with ^{3}H-proline, 1.0 μCi/ml. After 24 hr, the culture proteins were processed for ^{3}H-hydroxyproline determination.

As discussed above, earlier studies in our laboratory showed that superoxide is involved in the synthesis of hydroxyproline. It was of interest to see if the increased synthesis of hydroxyproline was caused by increased hydroxylation of collagen polypeptides, or if it resulted from increased synthesis of the polypeptides.   The data from this experiment are presented in Table 5.2. Confluent cultures treated with

Table 5.2   Effect of Superoxide Dismutase on the Incorporation of Proline
Into Collagen Sequence in the Presence of Ascorbate[a]

Additions	Percent of Total Incorporated Radioactivity in Collagen
None	5.8
Ascorbate, 3.5 mM	18.45
Ascorbate, 3.5 mM + Fe^{2+}, 0.15 mM	19.30
Ascorbate, 3.5 mM + Fe^{2+}, 0.3 mM	16.45
Ascorbate, 3.5 mM + SOD, 0.1 unit/ml	8.10
Ascorbate, 3.5 mM + Fe^{2+}, 0.15 mM + SOD, 0.1 unit/ml	10.1
Ascorbate, 3.5 mM + Fe^{2+}, 0.3 mM + SOD, 0.1 unit/ml	5.0

[a]Culture conditions and assay procedures were as described in the Methods Section. The cultures were labeled with ^{14}C-proline, 1 μCi/ml and the labeled proteins, and the incorporation of proline into the collagen sequence measured by the use of collagenase.

ascorbate and Fe^{2+} incorporated greater amounts of labeled proline into the collagen sequence than did control cultures. The increased incorporation corresponded with data presented in Table 5.1, and the stimulation of collagen polypeptide synthesis was comparable to the stimulation observed in the synthesis of hydroxyproline. The increase in collagen polypeptide synthesis was also completely abolished by SOD, confirming that superoxide free-radicals play a significant role in stimulating the synthesis of collagen.

Synthesis of collagen proceeds in several discrete steps in which the polypeptides initially synthesized are modified enzymatically. The first such posttranslational modification results in the hydroxylation of specific proline and lysine residues. The specific hydroxylating enzyme for proline, prolyl hydroxylase, has been shown to be modulated along with the ability to synthesize collagen. Prolyl hydroxylase levels are elevated in lungs exposed to ozone,[6] NO_2[19] and silica.[20] We examined levels of prolyl hydroxylase in WI-38 cells exposed to superoxide to determine if the observed increase in collagen synthesis was accompanied by a corresponding increase in the enzyme. In these experiments, superoxide was generated by the photochemical oxidation of riboflavin as described in the Methods section. This procedure was adopted because of conflicting suggestions concerning the role of ascorbate in increasing the levels of prolyl hydroxylase in cell cultures.[21,22] Photochemically generated superoxide increased the levels of prolyl hydroxylase in confluent cultures (Figure 5.1).

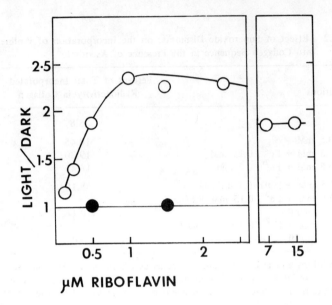

Figure 5.1   Superoxide-induced increase in prolyl hydroxylase in WI-38 cells. Riboflavin in the indicated concentration was added to confluent cultures, both in controls and superoxide-treated. The control cultures were kept in a light-tight incubator and the treated cultures were illuminated, as described in the Methods section. Some cultures also received superoxide dismutase (0.1 unit/ml). Prolyl hydroxylase levels were determined 24 hr after exposure. The data are expressed as ratios of enzyme level in the superoxide-treated (light) to the enzyme level in the corresponding control (dark). There were no significant differences between individual controls.

—O—O—   illuminated in the presence of riboflavin
—●—●—   illuminated in the presence of riboflavin and SOD.

Riboflavin is a normal component of the tissue culture medium (0.25 μM). Illumination of cultures without any further addition of riboflavin resulted in an increase in prolyl hydroxylase. Greater increases were observed, however, on supplementations of riboflavin in the medium. Increased levels of the enzyme were observed only in illuminated cultures, suggesting that photochemically generated superoxide rather than riboflavin itself was responsible for the increase. Cells illuminated in the presence of 0.5-2.5 μM riboflavin exhibited prolyl hydroxylase levels nearly 2.5-fold the corresponding nonilluminated controls. Concentrations of riboflavin, higher than 5 μM caused somewhat smaller increases in the enzyme. These levels were comparable to those observed at 1 μM and were approximately two times the levels in nonilluminated controls. The reason for the lowered response to the higher concentrations of riboflavin are not clear at present. Higher concentrations of superoxide generated in the presence of larger amounts of riboflavin may have contributed cytotoxic effects. Riboflavin in these concentrations itself was not toxic to the cells, and the levels of prolyl hydroxylase in the nonilluminated controls at these concentrations were comparable to those observed in nonilluminated controls containing lower concentrations of riboflavin.

Further confirmation of the role of superoxide in increasing prolyl hydroxylase levels was obtained by including SOD in some of the illuminated, riboflavin-containing cultures. As seen in Figure 5.1, SOD completely abolished the effect of illumination in the presence of riboflavin. Superoxide dismutase added in various control cultures did not have any effect on the enzyme levels, suggesting that the increased concentration of superoxide in the medium rather than intracellular factors were involved in increasing the prolyl hydroxylase content.

Studies on collagen synthesis indicated that superoxide stimulated its *de novo* synthesis. It was interesting to see if the increase in prolyl hydroxylase resulted from the stimulation of *de novo* synthesis or from activation of preexisting inactive enzyme. Confluent cultures of WI-38 cells were exposed to superoxide generated by the photochemical oxidation of riboflavin and the levels of the enzyme were determined as a function of length of exposure to superoxide. Increased levels of prolyl hydroxylase were not apparent until 18 hr after initial exposure. If the increase was caused by the activation of preexisting inactive enzyme, a much faster response would be expected. The time-lag in the appearance of the enzyme suggested that cellular events such as macromolecular synthesis were involved. Addition of cycloheximide, an inhibitor of protein synthesis, inhibited the increase in prolyl hydroxylase. These data suggest that a superoxide-induced increase in prolyl hydroxylase resulted from new protein synthesis rather than from activation of the enzyme.

In order to see if the increased synthesis of prolyl hydroxylase in the presence of superoxide involved transcriptional events, cultures were exposed to superoxide in the presence of Actinomycin D. As in the case of cycloheximide, no stimulatory effect on prolyl hydroxylase was observed in Actinomycin D-treated cultures, indicating that the enhanced synthesis of prolyl hydroxylase in cells exposed to superoxide was dependent on RNA synthesis (Figure 5.3).

Data in Figures 5.2 and 5.3 suggested that superoxide may induce *de novo* synthesis of collagen. As in other cases of enzyme induction, increased prolyl hydroxylase synthesis depended on transcriptional events occurring sometime during the lag period. We further investigated the kinetics of prolyl hydroxylase induction in experiments where transcription

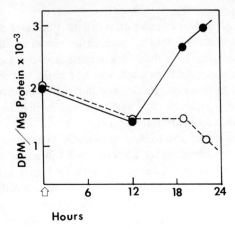

Figure 5.2 Time course of induction of prolyl hydroxylase by superoxide and its inhibition by cycloheximide. Confluent cultures were exposed to photochemically generated superoxide in the presence of 1.5 μM riboflavin. Cultures were terminated after the indicated exposures and prolyl hydroxylase levels determined. In order to determine if the increase in the enzyme was due to activation or *de novo* synthesis, one set of cultures was maintained in the presence of 1.0 μg/ml cycloheximide.

—●—●—   enzyme levels in superoxide exposed cultures.

—○—○—   enzyme levels in cultures exposed to superoxide in the presence of cycloheximide.

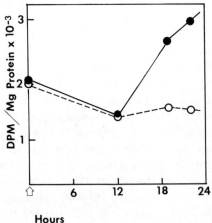

Figure 5.3 Induction of prolyl hydroxylase by superoxide and its inhibition by Actinomycin D. The experiment was carried out as described in the legend to Figure 5.2. In order to determine if the increase in prolyl hydroxylase involved in RNA synthesis, Actinomycin D, 1.0 μg/ml was included in one set of cultures.

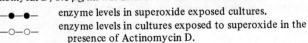

—●—●—   enzyme levels in superoxide exposed cultures.

—○—○—   enzyme levels in cultures exposed to superoxide in the presence of Actinomycin D.

was blocked 3 or 12 hr after the initial exposure to superoxide. As seen in Table 5.3, if Actinomycin D was administered 12 hr after initial exposure to superoxide, the cells continued to synthesize prolyl hydroxylase essentially on the same schedule as the cultures exposed to superoxide in the absence of the antibiotic (see data of Figure 5.3). However, if Actinomycin D was added to the culture medium 3 hr after exposure to the cultures to superoxide, the stimulatory response on prolyl hydroxylase synthesis was suppressed. These data suggest that the inductive effect of superoxide on prolyl hydroxylase involved early transcriptional events, resulting in the accumulation of specific messenger RNAs, which were translated with some delay.

Table 5.3   Effect of Actinomycin D on Superoxide-Induced Increase in Prolyl Hydroxylase[a]

	Hours After Exposure to Actinomycin D	Enzyme Activity dpm ^{3}H/mg Protein
Actinomycin D added 3 hr after exposure to riboflavin + light	6	2288
	12	5350
	18	3745
Actinomycin D added 12 hr after exposure to riboflavin + light	6	8037
	12	11741
	18	5220

[a]Confluent cultures were exposed to superoxide generated by illumination in the presence of riboflavin (0.5 μM). Actinomycin D 0.1 μg/ml was added 3 or 12 hr after exposure to superoxide. Prolyl hydroxylase levels were determined after indicated periods of exposure to Actinomycin D.

WI-38 cells served as an experimental model of aging.[23,24]   Experiments using "older" cultures in passages higher than the 35th showed that with increasing passage number, the cells became insensitive to the inducing effect of superoxide on collagen synthesis and prolyl hydroxylase synthesis.   Somewhat similar observations were reported by Paz and Gallop,[25] who found reduced ascorbate dependence of hydroxyproline synthesis in these cells in high passage.   In contrast to our observations, however, these workers found reduced synthesis of collagenous protein in "young" cells in the presence of ascorbate.

Our *in vitro* studies suggest that superoxide may play a direct role in enhancing collagen synthesis in addition to its participation in the post-translational processing of collagen.[12,13]   Several lines of evidence link superoxide to increased collagen deposition in lungs exposed to toxic levels of oxygen, ozone and other injury-causing agents. Increased oxygen consumption and superoxide generation accompanies tissue inflammation following injury.[26-28] Conditioning in sublethal concentrations of oxygen imparts some protection against oxygen toxicity, and this may be related directly to the induction of SOD.[11,19] SOD is induced as part of the protective action of aspirin and para amino benzoic acid against ozone-induced lipid peroxidation.[29] The deleterious effects of paraquat (methyl viologen) include interstitial fibrosis and appear to involve the generation of superoxide.[30,31] Superoxide also appears to be involved in other aspects of biochemical injury in the lungs, including the peroxidation of lipids and may be part of the mechanism of the toxicity of SO_2.[32]

At this time, the mechanism by which superoxide may exert its effects on cells, including the stimulation of collagen synthesis, is not known. The superoxide-free radical affects cell growth and differentiation.[33] Superoxide affects nucleoproteins, proteins and lipoproteins.[34] Such effects may involve the direct interaction between the free radical and informational macromolecules, leading to damage in genetic material.[35,36] Other possible modes of action of superoxide may include interaction with specific membrane receptors and alterations in membrane lipoproteins and other components[34] and may arise from the high reactivity of this radical.[8]

ACKNOWLEDGMENTS

Ms. Jamie McManus Long participated in many of these experiments. I thank Ms. Maximita Tolentino for expert technical assistance. Drs. M. Zamirul Hussain and S. D. Lee provided invaluable suggestions and much stimulating discussion during the course of this work. The assistance of Ms. Sandra Hodess is also acknowledged.

This research was supported in parts by EPA Contract 68-03-2005 and NIH Grants DE-03861 and HL-19668.

REFERENCES

1. Haagen-Smit, A. J. "Chemistry and Physiology of Los Angeles Smog," *Indus. Eng. Chem.* 44:1342 (1952).
2. Haagen-Smith, A. J., C. E. Bradley and M. M. Fox. "Ozone Formation in Photochemical Oxidation of Organic Substances," *Indus. Eng. Chem.* 45:2086 (1953).
3. Mueller, P. K. and M. Hitchcock. "Air Quality Criteria-Toxological Appraisal for Oxidants, Nitrogen Oxides and Hydrocarbons," *J. Air Pollut. Contr. Assoc.* 19:670 (1969).

4. Scheel, L. D., O. J. Dobrogorski, J. T. Mountain, J. L. Svirbely and H. E. Stokinger. "Physiologic, Biochemical, Immunologic and Pathologic Changes Following Ozone Exposure," *J. Appl. Physiol.* 14:67 (1959).

5. Witschi, H. "Exploitable Biochemical Approaches for the Evaluation of Toxic Lung Damage," *Essays Toxicol.* 6:125 (1975).

6. Hussain, M. Z., C. E. Cross, M. G. Mustafa and R. S. Bhatnagar. "Hydroxyproline Contents and Prolyl Hydroxylase Activity in Lungs of Rats Exposed to Low Levels of Ozone," *Life Sci.* 18:897 (1976).

7. Hussain, M. Z. and R. S. Bhatnagar. "Effect of Low Level Ozone Exposure on Lung Collagen Synthesis in Rats: Variation with Age," Submitted for publication.

8. Fridovich, I. "Superoxide Dismutases," *Advan. Enzymol.* 41:35 (1974).

9. Mustafa, M. G., S. M. Macres, B. K. Tarkington, C. K. Chow and M. Z. Hussain. "Lung Superoxide Dismutase: Stimulation by Low Level Ozone Exposure," *Clin. Res.* 23(2):138A (1975).

10. Crapo, J. D. and D. F. Tierney. "Superoxide Dismutase and Pulmonary Oxygen Toxicity," *Amer. J. Physiol.* 226:1401 (1974).

11. Crapo, J. D. "Superoxide Dismutase and Tolerance to Pulmonary Oxygen Toxicity," *Chest* 67:395 (1975).

12. Bhatnagar, R. S. and T. Z. Liu. "Mechanism of Hydroxylation of Proline," *Proc. IXth Intl. Congress Biochem.* 335 (1973).

13. Bhatnagar, R. S. and T. Z. Liu. "Evidence for Free-Radical Involvement in the Hydroxylation of Proline," *FEBS Letter* 26:32 (1972).

14. Juva, K. and D. J. Prockop. "A Modified Procedure for the Assay of [3]H- or ^{14}C-Labeled Hydroxyproline," *Anal. Biochem.* 15:77 (1966).

15. Rapaka, R. S., K. R. Sorensen, S. D. Lee and R. S. Bhatnagar. "Inhibition of Hydroxyproline Synthesis by Palladium Ions," *Biochim. Biophys. Acta* 429:63 (1976).

16. Bhatnagar, R. S., R. S. Rapaka, T. Z. Liu and S. M. Wolf. "Hydralazine-Induced Disturbances in Collagen Biosynthesis," *Biochim. Biophys. Acta* 271:125 (1972).

17. Lowry, O. H., N. J. Rosebrough, A. L. Farr and R. J. Randall. "Protein Measurement with the Folin Phenol Reagent," *J. Biol. Chem.* 193:265 (1951).

18. Paine, A. J. and A. E. M. McLean. "Role of Adenochrome in Aryl Hydrocarbon Hydroxylase Induction by Epinephrine in Rat Liver Cell Culture," *Biochem. Pharmacol.* 23:1910 (1974).

19. Hacker, A. D. "Effects of Nitrogen Dioxide on Collagen Metabolism," Ph.D. Thesis, University of California, Los Angeles (1975).

20. Halme, J., J. Uitto, K. Kahanpaa, P. Karhunen and S. Lindy. "Protocollagen Proline Hydroxylase Activity in Experimental Pulmonary Fibrosis of Rats," *J. Lab. Clin. Med.* 75:535 (1970).

21. Stassen, F. L. H., G. J. Cardinale and S. Udenfriend. "Activation of Prolyl Hydroxylase in L-929 Fibroblasts by Ascorbic Acid," *Proc. Natl. Acad. Sci.* 70:1090 (1973).

22. Levine, C. I. and C. J. Bates. "Ascorbic Acid and Collagen Synthesis in Cultured Fibroblasts," *Ann. N.Y. Acad. Sci.* 258:288 (1975).

23. Holliday, R. and G. M. Tarrant. "Altered Enzymes in Aging Human Fibroblasts," *Nature* 238:26 (1972).

24. Hayflick, L. "Aging Under Glass," *Exp. Gerontol.* 5:291 (1970).

25. Paz, M. A. and P. M. Gallop. "Collagen Synthesized and Modified by Aging Fibroblasts in Culture," *In Vitro* 5:302 (1975).

26. Babior, B. M., R. S. Kipnes and J. T. Curnutte. "Biological Defense Mechanisms. The Production by Leukocytes of Superoxide, a Potential Bacterial Agent," *J. Clin. Invest.* 52:74 (1973).

27. Johnston, R. B., Jr. B. B. Keele, Jr., H. P. Misra, L. S. Webb, J. E. Lehmeyes and K. V. Rajagopalan. "Superoxide Anion Generation and Phagocytic Bacterial Activity," In *The Phagocytic Cell in Host Resistance,* J. H. Bellanti and D. H. Dayton, Eds. (New York: Raven Press, 1975), p. 61.

28. McCord, J. M. and M. L. Salin. "Free-Radicals and Inflammation: Studies on Superoxide-Mediated NBT Reduction by Leukocytes," In *Erythrocyte Structure and Function,* G. J. Brown, Ed. (New York: Alan Liss, Inc., 1975), p. 731.

29. Khandwala, A. S. and J. B. L. Gee. "Superoxide Dismutase Induction by Enzyme-Inducing Agents," *Fed. Proc.* 34:427 (1975).

30. Bus, J. S., S. D. Aust and J. E. Gibson. "Superoxide and Singlet Oxygen-Catalyzed Lipid Peroxidation as a Possible Mechanism for Paraquat (Methyl Viologen)Toxicity ," *Biochem. Biophys. Res. Comm.* 58:749 (1974).

31. Autor, A. P. "Reduction of Paraquat Toxicity by Superoxide Dismutase," *Life Sciences* 14:1309 (1974).

32. Kaplan, D., C. McJillan and D. Luchtel. "Bisulfate-Induced Lipid Oxidation," *Arch. Environ. Health* 30:507 (1975).

33. Michelson, A. M. and M. E. Buckingham. "Effects of Superoxide Radicals on Myoblast Growth and Differentiation," *Biochem. Biophys. Res. Comm.* 58:1079 (1974).

34. Lavelle, F., A. M. Michelson and L. Dimitrijevic. "Biological Protection by Superoxide Dismutase," *Biochem. Biophys. Res. Comm.* 55:350 (1973).

35. Van Hemmen, J. J. and W. J. A. Menling. "Inactivation of Biologically Active DNA by γ-Ray Induced Superoxide Radicals and Their Dismutation Products—Singlet Molecular Oxygen and Hydrogen Peroxide," *Biochim. Biophys. Acta* 402:133 (1975).

36. Ishida, R. and T. Takehashi. "Increased DNA Chain Breakage by Combined Action of Bleomycin and Superoxide Radical," *Biochem. Biophys. Res. Comm.* 66:1432 (1975).

CHAPTER 6

BIOCHEMICAL EFFECTS OF ENVIRONMENTAL OXIDANT POLLUTANTS IN ANIMAL LUNGS

Mohammad G. Mustafa, Allen D. Hacker and Jean J. Ospital

The Center for the Health Sciences
University of California
Los Angeles, California 90024

M. Zamirul Hussain

The Laboratory of Connective Tissue Biochemistry
University of California
San Francisco, California 94143

Si Duk Lee

The Health Effects Research Laboratory
U.S. Environmental Protection Agency
Cincinnati, Ohio 54268

INTRODUCTION

The pulmonary effects of inhaled oxidants have received wide attention ever since it became known that ozone and nitrogen oxides were present in the atmosphere of large urban areas. Early studies performed with experimental animals have dealt with rather large concentrations of oxidants that were capable of causing severe lung injury and death.[1-3] In recent years, however, attention has been focused on the effects of ambient or near-ambient levels of oxidants, and evidence is accumulating that significant biochemical and morphological changes in the lung result from various low-level exposures of less than 1 ppm O_3 or 5 ppm NO_2. Morphologically, the characteristic changes appear to be damage of squamous epithelial cells in the bronchiolar and adjacent alveolar regions,

59

and replacement of damaged cells by an increased number of thick cuboidal cells.[4,5] Biochemical parameters measured following low-level exposures to O_3 or NO_2 seem to show an augmentation, reflecting metabolic alterations in lung tissue.[6-14]

The objective of this study was to determine the quantitative biochemical changes in the lung after exposure of animals to environmental oxidants. An attempt was made to examine the metabolic profile of lung tissue after acute, high-level exposure of rats to O_3 and chronic, low-level exposure to O_3 or NO_2. Acute exposures, which caused an extensive injury to lung tissue, were conducted to gain a better understanding of the possible mechanisms of oxidant damage. Low-level exposures, on the other hand, were designed to approach the oxidant concentrations that occur in moderate to severe episodes of photochemical smog. The overall goal was to provide the following lines of information: the nature of biochemical lesions from oxidant exposure, including the possible mechanisms involved; the degree of biochemical lesions as a function of oxidant dosage and exposure time; and the development of possible metabolic adaptation and its physiological significance.

EXPERIMENTAL PROCEDURE

Animal Exposures

In this study male Sprague-Dawley rats, 60-70 days old and weighing 300-350 g, were used. To minimize the influence of preexisting respiratory disease on lung biochemical parameters, the rats were obtained from a colony free of chronic respiratory disease (Hilltop Animal Labs).

The exposure protocols are presented in Table 6.1. For routine studies rats were exposed to 0.8 ppm O_3 for periods between 1 and 30 days. In selected experiments rats were exposed to a relatively high concentration of O_3 (2 or 3 ppm) for a short time in order to cause an acute injury to the lung. Likewise, rats were exposed to 0.5 or 0.2 ppm O_3 for a week in order to assess the low-level oxidant effects. The low concentrations of O_3 (0.2, 0.5 or 0.8 ppm) approximately represented oxidant levels in moderate to severe episodes of smog in urban environments. Details of exposure chambers, generation of O_3 and flow rates, and conditions for exposure of control and experimental animals have been reported previously.[8,10] The concentrations of NO_2 chosen were 15 ppm, an arbitrary level expected to cause extensive lung injury, and 5 ppm, representing the Threshold Limit Value (TLV). The exposure conditions for NO_2 were the same as those for O_3, except that NO_2 was obtained from a compressed gas tank (5% NO_2 in nitrogen, Liquid Carbonic) and

Table 6.1   Protocols for Oxidant Exposure

Oxidant Concentration (ppm)	Length of Exposure
Ozone	
3	Continuous for 4 or 8 hr
2	Continuous for 8 hr
0.8	Continuous for 1 to 30 days or intermittent[a] for 7 days
0.5	Continuous or intermittent[a] for 7 days
0.2	Continuous for 7 days
Nitrogen dioxide	
5	Continuous for 8 hr to 4 days
15	Continuous for 1 to 7 days

[a]Intermittent refers to 2-, 4-, 6- or 8-hr daily exposure

diluted with filtered room air to achieve the desired concentration in the chamber.

Tissue Preparation

At the end of each exposure an appropriate number of control and exposed animals were anesthetized with sodium pentobarbital, a thoractomy was performed and the lungs removed. To prepare lung slices, the lobes were separated, rinsed in cold saline, blotted on a filter paper and weighed. The lobes were then sliced with a McIlwain tissue slicer at 1-mm thickness, and a weighed portion of the slices was transferred to individual flasks for assay.

Lung homogenate, mitochondria, microsomes and cytosol were prepared as follows. Immediately after exposure, rats from control and exposed groups were killed. Each lung, while still in the chest cavity, was perfused and (as appropriate) lavaged with cold saline. Vascular perfusion, carried out by introducing 15-20 ml of saline via the pulmonary artery, resulted in removal of blood, giving essentially a white lung. Alveolar lavage, carried out by introducing 30 ml of saline (in 10 ml aliquots) through the trachea, resulted in removal of 1-2 millions of alveolar free cells. These cells from the lavage fluid were later collected by centrifuging at 200 xg for 10 min. The lung was then removed, trimmed of cartilage and connective tissue, and rinsed with an ice-cold medium containing 0.15 M sucrose, 0.15 M mannitol, 1 mM Tris-chloride and 1 mM Tris-EDTA at pH 7.5 (hereafter referred to as sucrose-mannitol medium).

The lung was then minced, washed once, and homogenized in a glass-Teflon®* homogenizer (0.15-mm clearance) using the sucrose-mannitol medium and allowing two strokes of the pestle. The homogenate (approximately 8% w/v) prepared separately from each lung was filtered through a two-layer cheesecloth, and made to a final volume of 10 ml. The overall operation starting from animal killing to this stage required about 4 min.

To isolate mitochondria, an 8-ml aliquot of filtered lung homogenate was centrifuged first at 700 xg for 10 min to remove the nuclei and broken cell debris, and then at 9000 xg for 10 min to sediment the mitochondrial fraction. The mitochondrial fraction** thus obtained was washed once by resuspending it in sucrose-mannitol medium and again centrifuging it at the speeds outlined above. The final pellet was resuspended in a 2-ml volume.

The mitochondria-free supernatant was then diluted 1:1 with cold distilled water, and centrifuged at 40,000 xg for 30 min. The residue obtained was referred to as the microsomal fraction and the supernatant as cytosol. The microsomal residue was resuspended in a 2-ml volume.

Assays

For measurement of oxygen consumption, lung tissue slices (200 mg) were transferred to Gilson respirometer flasks containing 4 ml of Krebs-Ringer phosphate buffer (pH 7.4), including 0.2% glucose. A series of flasks also contained 0.1 mM 2,4-dinitrophenol. The flasks were attached to a Gilson differential respirometer and shaken at a frequency of 120 cycles/min in a bath maintained at 37°C. The flasks were gassed with 100% O_2 for 7 min at a rate of 1 liter/min/flask, and then allowed to equilibrate for 20 min. Readings of oxygen uptake at constant barometric pressure were then taken every 10 min for 1 hr, and a least squares program was used to calculate the slope (μl O_2/hr). Oxygen consumption

---

* Registered trademark of E. I. duPont de Nemours & Company, Inc., Wilmington, Delaware.

** As reported in a previous study,[15] lung mitochondrial preparations thus obtained were characterized for purity. From marker enzyme activities—acid phosphatase for lysosomes and NADPH-cytochrome c reductase for microsomes—the mitochondrial preparations were contaminated approximately 10% by lysosomes and 15% by microsomes. The degree of contamination was the same for mitochondrial preparations from control and exposed rat lungs. The purity of preparations employed in this study, as judged from the rate of substrate oxidation per mg of mitochondrial protein, was comparable to that reported earlier.[16,17] The yield of mitochondria, based on total respiratory activity per lung in homogenate and isolated mitochondria, was approximately 50% from each lung.

in tissue slices was also determined polarographically at $37°C$ using an oxygraph (Gilson, Model KI-C) and a Clark electrode. The values obtained by these two means of determination agreed well.

Measurement of oxygen consumption in lung homogenate and mitochondria was made polarographically at $30°C$. The reactions were carried out in medium (1.5 ml, pH 7.5) containing 100 mM sucrose, 100 mM mannitol, 25 mM Tris-chloride, 2 mM phosphate and 1-2 mg protein equivalent of tissue preparations per ml (10 mM glucose, 1 mM ATP and 20 μg hexokinase per ml were also added to achieve maximal respiration rates); concentrations of substrates were 15 mM each except Wurster's blue, which was 0.1 mM.

Monoamine oxidase activity was determined in lung homogenate, mitochondria and microsomes polarographically at $30°C$. The reaction mixture (1.5 ml, pH 7.5) contained 50 mM phosphate, approximately 3 mg protein equivalent of tissue preparations and a substrate, *e.g., n*-amylamine (12 μmol), benzylamine (12 μmol), tyramine (12 μmol), or 3-hydroxytyramine (9 μmol).

Determination of glucose consumption and production of pyruvate and lactate were carried out by incubating lung slices (200 mg/flask) in 4.5 ml of Krebs-Ringer bicarbonate buffer (pH 7.4) containing 0.2% glucose at $37°C$ for 90 min with the gas phase consisting of 5% CO_2 in oxygen. The amount of glucose consumed was determined in filtered medium at the end of incubation using the Worthington glucostat reagent set (Worthington Biochemicals). Likewise, the pyruvate and lactate produced were determined according to Bucher *et al.*[18] and Hohorst,[19] respectively.

Cytochrome *c* reductase activities pertaining to succinate, NADH and NADPH were determined spectrophotometrically at $23°C$ by following the reduction of ferricytochrome *c* at 550 nm (Beckman DBG-T recording spectrophotometer). The assay medium (1 ml, pH 7.5) contained 50 mM phosphate, 50 μM ferricytochrome *c*, 1 mM cyanide, and 0.2-0.3 mg protein equivalent of tissue preparation; concentrations of substrates were 20 mM succinate, 0.25 mM NADH or 0.15 mM NADPH.

Glucose-6-phosphate dehydrogenase (G6PD), 6-phosphogluconate dehydrogenase (6PGD) and isocitrate dehydrogenase (ICDH) activities were determined spectrophotometrically at $23°C$ by following the reduction of $NADP^+$ at 340 nm. The assay medium for G6PD (1 ml, pH 8.3) contained 50 mM triethanolamine-HCl, 5 mM $MgCl_2$, 1.25 mM glucose-6-phosphate, 0.125 mM $NADP^+$ and 0.2-0.3 mg protein equivalent of cytosol; the medium for 6PGD (1 ml, pH 8.3) contained 50 mM triethanolamine-HCl, 5 mM $MgCl_2$, 0.125 mM $NADP^+$, 1.25 mM 6-phosphogluconate and 0.2-0.3 mg protein equivalent of cytosol; and the medium for ICDH (1 ml, pH 7.8) contained 100 mM Tris-chloride, 1 mM

$MnCl_2$, 0.25 mM D-isocitrate, 0.3 mM $NADP^+$ and 0.2-0.3 mg protein equivalent of cytosol.

Glutathione reductase activity was determined spectrophotometrically at 23°C by following the oxidation of NADPH at 340 nm. The assay medium (1 ml, pH 6.6) contained 66 mM phosphate, 0.4 mM oxidized glutathione, 0.3 mM NADPH, and 0.2-0.3 mg protein equivalent of cytosol.

Disulfide reductase activity was determined essentially as described by Tietze.[20] The assay medium (1 ml, pH 7.5) contained 100 mM phosphate, 5 mM EDTA, 2 mM DTNB (5, 5'-dithionitrobenzoic acid), 0.3 mM NADPH, and 0.4-0.5 mg protein equivalent of cytosol. The reduction of DTNB (a disulfide) in the reaction cuvette was followed spectrophotometrically (23°C) at 412 nm against the reference cuvette containing all the reagents but NADPH.

Glutathione-disulfide transhydrogenase activity was determined according to the procedure of Tietze.[20] The assay medium (1 ml, pH 7.5) contained 100 mM phosphate, 5 mM EDTA, 1 mM cystamine, 1 mM glutathione, 0.3 mM NADPH, 0.6 units of glutathione reductase, and 0.4-0.5 mg protein equivalent of cytosol. The reaction was initiated by adding cystamine, and the oxidation of NADPH was measured spectrophotometrically (23°C) at 340 nm.

Superoxide dismutase (SOD) activity was determined spectrophotometrically (23°C) by following the percentage of inhibition in the reduction of ferricytochrome c at 550 nm. The assay medium (1 ml, pH 7.8) contained 50 mM phosphate, 0.1 mM Tris-EDTA, 10 μM ferricytochrome c, 0.15 mM xanthine, 15 μl xanthine oxidase preparation (an amount that would yield cytochrome c reduction at an observed rate of 0.1 absorbance unit per minute) and 15-25 μg protein equivalent of tissue preparations. A 50% inhibition in the reduction of cytochrome c was taken as 1 unit of SOD activity.

Glutathione peroxidase activity was determined spectrophotometrically (23°C) by coupling peroxide reduction to NADPH oxidation through the glutathione reductase reaction.[21] The assay medium (1 ml, pH 7.6) contained 100 mM phosphate, 0.25 mM glutathione, 0.15 mM NADPH, 0.2 mM cumene peroxide, 0.6 units of glutathione reductase, and 0.1-0.2 mg protein equivalent of cytosol.

Protein synthesis in lung tissue was assessed by determining the rate and extent of incorporation of labeled amino acids into lung proteins. For *in vitro* incorporation, a 1-ml aliquot of lung homogenate from each control and exposed animal was centrifuged at 15,000 xg for 30 min, and the resultant supernatant was employed for the amino acid incorporation reaction according to the method described by Massaro *et al.*[22] with minor modifications. The assay medium (0.5 ml) contained 50 mM

Tris-chloride (pH 7.4), 100 mM KCl, 10 mM $MgCl_2$, 1 mM GSH, 1 mM ATP, 0.5 mM GTP, 4 mM creatine phosphate, 0.15 mg creatine phosphokinase, 0.05 mM uniformly labeled L-leucine-^{14}C or L-phenylalanine-[14]C (60 mC/mmole), a standard mixture of leucine- or phenylalanine-free amino acids to give a 0.025 mM concentration for each amino acid, and 0.4-0.5 mg protein equivalent of tissue preparation. The reaction mixture was incubated for 30 min at $37°C$ after which the reaction was stopped by addition of cold 10% trichloroacetic acid, and the product was assayed according to Massaro et al.[22]

For in vivo protein synthesis, 0.1 mC of L-leucine-4,6-^{3}H with a specific activity of 5 C/mmol in 0.2 ml of saline was injected into anesthetized rats via the femoral vein of the hind left leg. After exactly 20 min, the rats were sacrificed and the lungs, after vascular perfusion and endobronchial lavage, were removed and homogenized as described in the Tissue Preparation section. A 0.2-ml aliquot of each lung homogenate from control and exposed rats was treated with 2 ml of cold 10% trichloroacetic acid. The precipitate was collected, washed and counted for radioactivity as described by Massaro et al.[22] A 0.2-ml aliquot of whole blood collected from each rat was also treated with trichloroacetic acid and the resultant precipitate counted for radioactivity as above.

Nonprotein sulfhydryls were determined by the method of Sedlak and Lindsay[23] as adapted to our laboratory.[24] Glutathione was determined enzymatically by the method of Klotsch and Bergmeyer[25] as modified previously.[26] Determination of protein was made in lung homogenate, mitochondria, microsomes and cytosol according to the modified Lowry microanalysis.[27]

Results are expressed as units per mg protein of homogenate, mitochondria, microsomes or cytosol as well as units per lung, and the values given are means ± standard deviations.

Chemicals

Chemicals used were the reagent grades commercially available. Wurster's blue was made from N,N,N',N'-tetramethyl-p-phenylenediamine and crystallized essentially by the method of Michaelis and Granick.[28]

RESULTS AND DISCUSSION

Various aspects of lung metabolism have been studied after an exposure of animals to a given concentration of O_3 or NO_2. In order to keep the presentation relatively simple the results have been described, for the most part, under the subheadings of various metabolic parameters.

Effect on Oxidative and Energy Metabolism

Alterations of physiologic functions in the lung caused by O_3 or NO_2 exposure have been amply documented. We intended to determine whether oxidants would interact with lung cells and intracellular organelles by affecting their biochemical functions.

In this regard, lung mitochondrial oxidative and energy metabolism and microsomal electron transport activities were examined. There were several other considerations for this study. Since mitochondria isolated from tissues under various physiologic conditions have been found to differ with respect to biochemical properties,[29-31] it was thought possible that O_3 or NO_2 inhalation would affect lung mitochondrial functions. Mitochondrial functions are critical to cellular terminal oxidative processes and energy production. Oxidant inhalation causing lung mitochondrial injury would, therefore, have detrimental consequences on the metabolism of lung cells. Activities of numerous enzymes in mitochondria have functional sulfhydryl groups, and mitochondrial membranes are rich in unsaturated lipids. Both sulfhydryl groups and unsaturated lipids are susceptible to attack by oxidants. It is possible that mitochondria in lung cells would be targets for oxidant reactions, as was shown with the chloroplasts and mitochondria of plant cells.[32-35] Functions of lung mitochondria, therefore, offer sensitive parameters for detection and assessment of oxidant effects on lung cells.

Our previous studies[8,17,36] have shown that short-term exposure of rats to O_3 (2 ppm for 8 hr or 4 ppm for 4 hr) caused a 20-25% depression of lung mitochondrial oxygen consumption, using 2-oxoglutarate, succinate and glycerol-l-phosphate as substrates. Under these exposure conditions, both coupled phosphorylation and respiratory control of lung mitochondria were affected. Exposure of rats to 4 ppm O_3 for 4 hr resulted in a 25-35% decrease in ADP:0 ratios (the numerical expression of the degree of coupling between phosphorylation of ADP to ATP and mitochondrial oxygen consumption) and a 30% loss of respiratory control. Permeability of isolated lung mitochondria was examined by their ability to oxidize added NADH. Lung mitochondria from control animals were relatively impermeable to added NADH, but those from O_3-exposed animals showed an increased permeability as judged from NADH oxidation at a rate three-fold higher than the control. Concomitant with the loss of mitochondrial functions there was an oxidative loss (20%) of mitochondrial sulfhydryl groups after O_3 exposure (4 ppm for 4 hr). In addition, lung mitochondria and microsomes from exposed animals exhibited a 30-40% loss of activities for several marker enzymes, namely, cytochrome c reductases pertaining to succinate, NADH and NADPH.

These results have led to the conclusion that acute O_3 exposure adversely affects lung mitochondrial and microsomal functions and that the functional alterations may be attributed to one or all of the following: oxidative loss of SH groups that are functional constituents of many enzymes; lipid peroxidation-mediated damage of membranes and membrane-dependent enzymes; and loss of intramitochondrial components (*e.g.,* NAD) due to structural damage. Interference of O_3 with mitochondrial oxidative and energy metabolism may significantly contribute to the overall lung damage that results from acute exposure of animals to this oxidant.

In contrast to the inhibitory effects of high-level, short-term O_3 exposures, low-level, long-term exposures resulted in an augmentation of lung cellular oxidative metabolism. Figure 6.1 shows that lung tissue slices from rats exposed to 0.8 ppm O_3 for 7 days exhibited a 48% ($p < 0.05$) increase in oxygen consumption relative to control. In the presence of 2,4-dinitrophenol, which permitted the maximal rate of respiration in lung tissue slices, the relative difference in the rates between control and exposed animals remained significant (24%, $p < 0.05$). This suggested that lung tissue from exposed rats indeed had a relatively greater capacity to utilize oxygen.

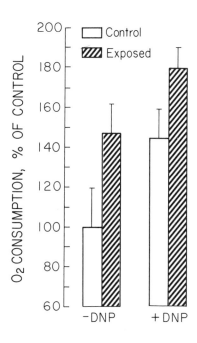

Figure 6.1   Effect of 0.8 ppm ozone exposure on oxygen consumption in lung tissue slices. Control values ($\mu l\ O_2/hr \cdot$ lung) were: 1138 ± 241 in absence of DNP and 1650 ± 231 in presence of DNP.

The changes in the relative rates of oxygen consumption are further illustrated in Figure 6.2. Oxidation of several mitochondrial substrates—2-oxoglutarate, succinate, glycerol-1-phosphate and ascorbate-Wurster's blue—was examined in lung homogenate after exposure of rats to 0.8 ppm for up to 30 days. As judged from oxygen consumption, the rates were slightly depressed (5-10%, nonsignificant) after exposure for 1 day. After 2 days of exposure a significant increase occurred, which attained a maximum (35-50% increase over control, $p < 0.001$) between 3 and 4 days and remained at an elevated level for as long as 30 days of continuous exposure. It may be noted that of all four substrates, oxidation of succinate seemed to show consistently the greatest augmentation.

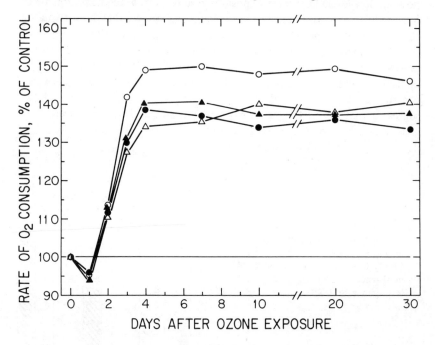

Figure 6.2 Effect of 0.8 ppm ozone exposure on oxygen consumption in lung homogenate. Control values (nmol O_2/min · lung) were: 605 ± 68 for succinate oxidase (O - O), 465 ± 52 for 2-oxoglutarate oxidase (● - ●), 422 ± 50 for glycerol-1-phosphate oxidase (△ - △) and 680 ± 73 for ascorbate-Wurster's blue oxidase (▲ ▲).

Oxygen consumption was also examined in isolated lung mitochondria from both control and exposed rats. On the basis of per mg of mitochondrial protein there was a small (15%, nonsignificant) increase in the rates of substrate oxidation in lung mitochondria from exposed rats relative to control. However, there was a significant increase (20-25%, $p < 0.05$) in the yield of isolated lung mitochondria from exposed rats relative to control as determined by the total protein content of the mitochondrial preparation. The increased rates of oxygen consumption in lung homogenate from exposed rats, therefore, would be attributable primarily to an increase in the population of lung mitochondria.

The increase of lung mitochondrial population was substantiated morphologically. Sections of lung tissue were examined by transmission electron microscopy. From the electron micrographs it did not appear that there was any general increase in the number of mitochondria per cell in the lungs of exposed animals. However, the lung sections from exposed animals (0.8 ppm, 7-10 days) showed approximately a three-fold greater abundance of alveolar Type 2 cells compared to control animals.[8] Since Type 2 cells contain numerous mitochondria and are thought to represent approximately 10% of normal lung cellular population, their proliferation in alveolar epithelium may significantly increase the overall population of mitochondria in the lung. In this regard, an important contribution may also result from bronchiolar (cuboidal) epithelial cells, which proliferate after O_3 or NO_2 exposure.[4,5]

Under conditions of low-level (0.8 ppm) O_3 exposure, no significant change was observed in coupled phosphorylation or respiratory control indexes. An ADP:0 ratio of 1.8 and respiratory control index of 3.0 were observed for oxidation of succinate in isolated lung mitochondria from both control and exposed rats (0.8 ppm for 7 days).

In addition, activities of several marker enzymes in lung mitochondria and microsomes were examined. As shown in Figure 6.3, cytochrome c reductase activities pertaining to succinate, NADH and NADPH (partial reactions of mitochondrial and microsomal electron transport chains) were augmented 40-50% ($p < 0.001$) after exposure of rats to 0.8 ppm O_3. As judged from protein content, the yield of lung microsomal fraction from exposed rats was 20-25% ($p < 0.05$) greater than that from control rats, thus accounting for the increased enzyme activities in exposed rat lung.

Oxygen consumption in lung homogenate was also determined after exposure of animals to 15 ppm NO_2 for up to 7 days. The rate of oxygen consumption for succinate oxidation showed an increase as a function of exposure time and reached a peak (approximately 80% over control, $p < 0.05$) after 3 days.

Augmentation of mitochondrial enzyme activities has been shown to occur in lung tissue under pathological conditions, namely succinate dehydrogenase and succinate oxidase activities in mouse lungs infected with tubercle bacilli;[37] oxidase and dehydrogenase activities pertaining to

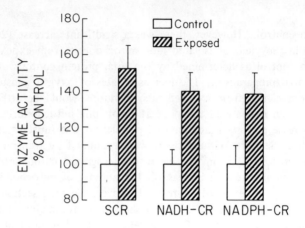

Figure 6.3 Effect of 0.8 ppm ozone exposure on cytochrome *c* reductase activities
in lung mitochondria and microsomes. Control values (nmoles cytochrome *c*
reduced/min · lung) were: 1250 ± 130 for succinate-cytochrome *c* reductase (SCR)
in mitochondria; and 16250 ± 840 for NADH-cytochrome *c* reductase (NADH-CR)
and 800 ± 78 for NADPH-cytochrome *c* reductase (NADPH-CR) in microsomes.

succinate, malate, 2-oxoglutarate and isocitrate in guinea-pig lungs after
exposure to silica dust;[38],[39] and oxygen consumption in human lung
tissue with a proliferative disease.[40],[41] Increased oxidative metabolism
of lung mitochondria after low-level oxidant exposures seems to offer
another example of proliferative conditions in lung tissue.

Mitochondrial functions are critical to the sustenance of cells. It is
known that mitochondria undergo division and are also synthesized *de
novo* in synchrony with cell division and growth.[42],[43] In regenerating,
repairing or proliferating tissue, they may undergo hyperplasia, and their
enzymatic activities may be augmented in response to work demand.
Morphologic studies suggest that cell renewal and hyperplasia are important
processes in the repair of injured lung.[4],[5],[44]-[47] Increase of mitochondrial
population, *vis-a-vis* an increase of oxidative and energy metabolism which
may be a consequence of cell renewal and hyperplasia, may have important functional implications for repair of injured lung tissue.

Effect on Glucose Metabolism

Although the lung functions in a relatively more aerobic environment
than other organs, lung tissue consumes large quantities of glucose via the
glycolytic pathway. In an aerobic tissue, glycolysis results in the formation
of pyruvate, which is then available for utilization via the mitochondrial
tricarboxylic acid cycle pathway. In the lung, however, a substantial
amount of glucose breakdown results in the production of lactate, which

may be influenced by oxidant stress. In this study glucose consumption and production of pyruvate and lactate in lung tissue slices were examined after exposure of rats to O_3 or NO_2. In addition, distribution of ^{14}C from labeled glucose was determined in the lipid and protein fractions of lung tissue in order to assess the biosynthetic pattern that might be affected by oxidant exposure.

Ozone effects on glucose consumption in lung tissue were determined after exposure of rats to 0.8 ppm O_3 for up to 4 days. As shown in Figure 6.4, the rate of glucose consumption in tissue slices increased 59% ($p < 0.02$) over control after 4 days of exposure. Under these conditions, both the rates of pyruvate and lactate production increased 43% ($p < 0.02$). However, in terms of absolute values, the amount of lactate produced (22.2 μmol/hr · lung), far exceeded the amount of pyruvate produced (3.7 μmol/hr · lung) by lung slices from exposed animals.

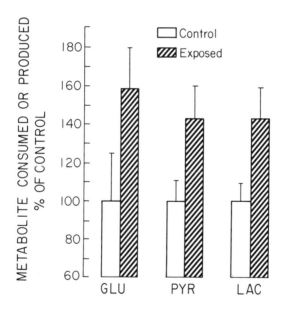

Figure 6.4 Effect of 0.8 ppm ozone exposure on glucose consumption and production of pyruvate and lactate in lung tissue slices. Control values (μmol/hr · lung) were: 30.6 ± 20.3 for glucose (GLU), 2.6 ± 0.2 for pyruvate (PYR) and 15.5 ± 5.6 for lactate (LAC).

To study the effects of NO_2 on glucose metabolism rats were exposed to 5 ppm NO_2 for up to 4 days. As measured in lung tissue slices, an 8-hr exposure resulted in a 32% ($p < 0.05$) increase in the mean consumption of glucose, and 6% (nonsignificant) and 43% ($p < 0.05\%$) increases in the mean production of pyruvate and lactate, respectively. The increase in glucose metabolism for this short-term exposure did not appear to be associated with any increase in the activity of either the hexose mono-phosphate shunt, as measured by the production of $^{14}CO_2$ by lung slices incubated with glucose-1-^{14}C, or the activity of the tricarboxylic acid cycle, as measured by the production of $^{14}CO_2$ from glucose-6-^{14}C. The incorporation of radioactive carbon from glucose-6-^{14}C was deter-mined in the total lipid and protein fractions of lung tissue, which showed, respectively, 26% and 13% increases relative to corresponding controls. With exposure for 1-4 days, the mean glucose consumption remained elevated at 50-60% ($p < 0.05$) above control values; the mean pyruvate production was not appreciably altered (up to 9% increase, nonsignificant) but the mean lactate production was elevated 20-25% ($p < 0.05$).

The results suggest that low-level oxidant exposure causes an alteration of glucose metabolism in the lung. Of note is the increased consumption of glucose with a concomitant rise in the production of lactate. These results are in agreement with the general observation that glucose consump-tion and lactate production in the lung are augmented due to pulmonary infection, hyperoxia and exposure to various agents.[48-53]

Effect on Monoamine Oxidase Activity

Monoamine oxidase (MAO) catalyzes the oxidative deamination of amines, and is of major importance in the regulation of metabolic degrada-tion of biological amines. The MAO activity in the lung is another index of this organ's diverse metabolic functions. The enzyme is membrane-bound, and located predominantly in the mitochondrial fraction, but the microsomal fraction also contains appreciable activity. The enzyme is capable of acting upon a number of aliphatic and aromatic amine sub-strates. In this study n-amylamine, benzylamine, tyramine and 3-hydroxy-tyramine were used as substrates.

Rats were exposed to O_3 either acutely (2 ppm for 8 hr) or chronically (0.8 ppm for 7 days). MAO activity was determined in lung homogenate, mitochondria and microsomes. Figure 6.5 shows that acute exposure re-sulted in a 30-40% ($p < 0.05$) depression of MAO activity in all three tissue preparations. Chronic exposure (Figure 6.6), on the other hand, resulted in a 20-35% ($p < 0.05$) increase of MAO activity. Activities of two marker enzymes—mitochondrial succinate-cytochrome c reductase and microsomal NADH-cytochrome c reductase—were determined in conjunc-tion with MAO activity. These enzyme activities were also depressed approximately 30% ($p < 0.05$) after acute exposure, and elevated 25-30%

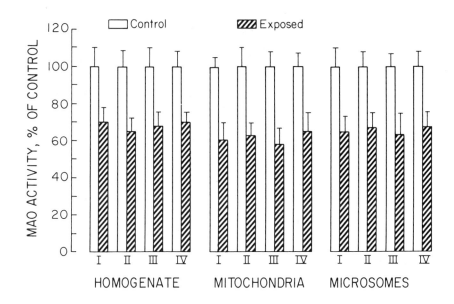

Figure 6.5 Effect of 2 ppm ozone exposure on monoamine oxidase (MAO) activity in lung tissue. Control values (nmol O_2/min·lung) were: 75 ± 8 for n-amylamine (I), 60 ± 8 for benzylamine (II), 52 ± 7 for tyramine (III) and 58 ± 8 for 3-hydroxytyramine (IV) in homogenate; 42 ± 5 for I, 33 ± 3 for II, 28 ± 4 for III and 32 ± 4 for IV in mitochondria; and 20 ± 3 for I, 16 ± 2 for II, 15 ± 2 for III and 15 ± 2 for IV in microsomes.

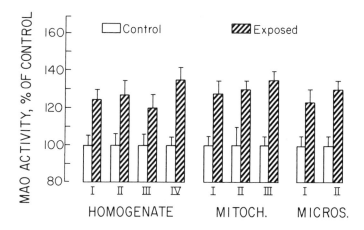

Figure 6.6 Effect of 0.8 ppm ozone exposure on monoamine oxidase (MAO) activity in lung tissue. Control values were as in legend to Figure 6.5

($p < 0.05$) after chronic exposure. The results suggest that O_3 exposure influences MAO activity, and that the acute effect can be explained on the basis of adverse reactions of oxidant with mitochondrial and microsomal membranes. The effect of chronic exposure can be explained on the basis of a general increase in the number of cells containing abundant mitochondria and endoplasmic reticula.

Effect on Enzymatic Activities Generating
Reducing Equivalents (NADPH)

Activities of a number of enzymes that furnish the reducing equivalents in the form of NADPH were studied. Of these enzymes the activities of glucose-6-phosphate dehydrogenase (G6PD) and 6-phosphogluconate dehydrogenase (6PGD) represent two important steps of the hexose monophosphate (HMP) shunt for glucose metabolism, and provide NADPH from $NADP^+$. In addition, the activity of cytosolic (NADP-specific) isocitrate dehydrogenase (ICDH) is an important source for NADPH. In many tissues NADP-specific malate dehydrogenase is also an important source for NADPH; however, no significant activity of this enzyme is found in lung cytosol.

As shown in Figure 6.7, G6PD activity was slightly depressed (7%, nonsignificant) after 1 day of exposure to 0.8 ppm O_3. After 2 days of exposure a significant increase occurred, which peaked between

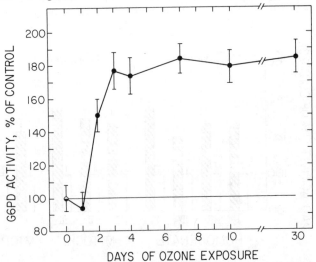

Figure 6.7   Effect of 0.8 ppm ozone exposure on glucose-6-phosphate dehydrogenase (G6PD) activity in lung cytosol. Control value was 2198 ± 190 nmol $NADP^+$ reduced/min · lung.

3 and 4 days, attaining a 60-80% (p < 0.001) augmentation over control, and remained essentially at a plateau thereafter for as long as 30 days of continuous exposure. Activities of other enzymes–6PGD and ICDH (Figure 6.8)–show 25-55% (p < 0.02) increases after a 7-day exposure to 0.8 ppm O_3.

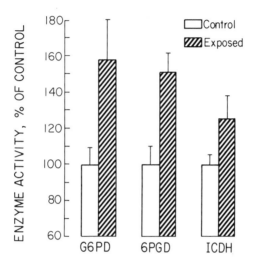

Figure 6.8   Effect of 0.8 ppm ozone exposure on marker enzyme activities in lung cytosol. Control values (nmol NADPH formed/min · lung) were: 2930 ± 280 for glucose-6-phosphate dehydrogenase (G6PD), 1760 ± 170 for 6-phosphogluconate dehydrogenase (6PGD) and 3590 ± 190 for isocitrate dehydrogenase (ICDH).

The augmentation of G6PD and 6PGD activities, *i.e.*, increased formation of NADPH from $NADP^+$ via the HMP shunt, has been observed in a variety of tissue injury, inflammation and repair processes,[54-56] including lung tissue injury and repair.[6,7,9,10,12,14,49,57,58] Although $NADP^+$ reduction may occur via the activity of other enzymes as well (*e.g.*, ICDH), the reactions catalyzed by G6PD and 6PGD have frequently been used as a marker for the occurrence of reparative processes in injured lung tissue. The significance of augmented G6PD and 6PGD activities probably relates to an increased operation of the HMP shunt required for reparative processes in the lung, *e.g.*, increased production of NADPH for biosynthetic processes including lipids and proteins, and increased production of pentoses for nucleic acid synthesis. However, the overall production of NADPH via the HMP shunt or the activity of ICDH may also have an important implication for development of tolerance to oxidant lung injury. For example, in previous studies the ability of lung tissue to augment G6PD activity in hyperoxia was found to correlate with the ability of animals to withstand O_2 toxicity,[49] and $NADP^+$ reduction in lung tissue via this enzyme activity increased with the length of O_2 or O_3 exposure.[6,7,9,10,14,49,57]

Effect of Enzyme Activities Related to Antioxidant Protection

Oxidant toxicity is thought to involve superoxide (O_2^-), and the enzyme superoxide dismutase (SOD) catalyzes its dismutation, thereby decreasing its harmful effects.[59] Since O_3 is a powerful oxidant, a study was undertaken to examine if O_3 exposure would alter superoxide dismutase activity in lung tissue, as had been observed for O_2 exposure.[60]

Superoxide dismutase activity is predominantly located in the cytosol and mitochondria. As shown in Figure 6.9, exposure of rats to 0.8 ppm O_3 for a week resulted in 38% and 46% ($p < 0.05$) increases, respectively, in the lung cytosol and mitochondrial fractions. In another exposure

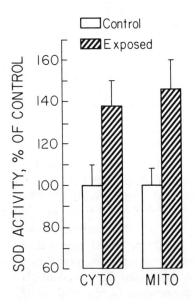

Figure 6.9   Effect of superoxide dismutase (SOD) activity in lung tissue. Control values (units/lung) were: 388 ± 36 in cytosol (CYTO) and 130 ± 16 in mitochondria (MITO).

protocol, in which O_3 levels were increased stepwise from 0.8 ppm for 72 hr to 1.5 ppm for 24 hr and finally to 3 ppm for 8 hr, the increases in SOD activity were, respectively, 15%, 25% and 50% in cytosol, and 50%, 67% and 118% in mitochondrial fraction relative to corresponding controls (Figure 6.10). The results demonstrate that SOD activity is

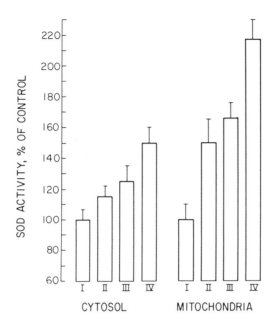

Figure 6.10 Effect of varying concentrations of ozone on superoxide dismutase (SOD) activity. Conditions for ozone exposure were: I - 0 ppm; II - 0.8 ppm for 3 days; III - 0.8 ppm for 3 days and then 1.5 ppm for 1 day; IV - 0.8 ppm for 3 days, 1.5 ppm for 1 day and then 3 ppm for 8 hr.

augmented in O_3-exposed rat lungs and that its response is proportional to dosage of O_3.

Free radical-mediated lipid peroxidation is considered to be an important mechanism of oxidant damage in the lung, and the activity of glutathione peroxidase is thought to lessen the lipid peroxidation in tissue.[7,9,21] Since O_3 possesses radiomimetic properties and is known to induce lipid peroxidation, a study was undertaken to examine if O_3 exposure would alter the activity of glutathione peroxidase in lung tissue. As shown in Figure 6.11, we observed an increase in glutathione peroxidase activity in the lung, 35% in cytosol and 47% in mitochondria ($p < 0.05$), after a week-long exposure of rats to 0.8 ppm O_3.

The augmentation of superoxide dismutase and glutathione peroxidase activities are in conformity with that of other enzyme activities in the lung seen after oxidant exposure. The significance of this augmentation might relate to adaptive changes leading to a diminution of oxidant toxicity.

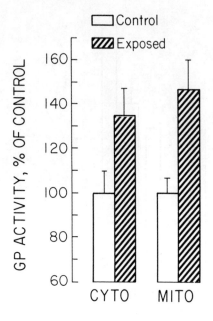

Figure 6.11 Effect of 0.8 ppm ozone exposure on glutathione peroxidase (GP) activity in lung tissue. Control values (nmol NADPH oxidized/min · lung) were: 1870 ± 290 in cytosol (CYTO) and 980 ± 88 in mitochondria (MITO).

Effect on Sulfhydryl Metabolism

Soluble or nonprotein sulfhydryl (NPSH) compounds, especially reduced glutathione (GSH), constitute a major pool of cellular reducing equivalents and may be important in determining the cellular redox state. GSH is thought to play specific roles in mitotic cells, and may therefore be essential for regenerating, repairing or proliferating systems. GSH is also considered to play a protective role against free radical-mediated or peroxidative damage.[2,6,7,9,10,21] In addition to GSH or NPSH, SH groups of enzymes and proteins (PSH) have important functional roles, and in order to maintain the functional integrity of SH-dependent enzymes and proteins these groups must remain in the reduced form, even under an oxidant stress. The levels of PSH and NPSH in lung tissue may therefore be crucial in oxidant injury.

Oxidation of SH groups may be an important mechanism by which oxidants cause cell injury.[2,61-66] Several authors have demonstrated that acute O_3 exposure results in an oxidation of GSH or NPSH in lung tissue and an inhibition of enzymes that are dependent on SH groups for their activities.[6,67,68] It is therefore conceivable that O_3 or NO_2 may interfere with lung cellular metabolism by oxidizing SH groups either directly or via free radical reactions.

A normal rat lung (weighing approximately 1 g) contains an average of 1.6 μmol of NPSH, of which up to 90% may be GSH. Our previous studies have shown that acute O_3 exposure resulted in a diminution of lung tissue SH levels.[6,10,24] Rats exposed to 2 ppm O_3 for 8 hr exhibited a decrease of approximately 40% in NPSH and 20% in PSH. For rats exposed to 4 ppm O_3 the NPSH level in lung tissue decreased as a function of exposure time, reaching a level as low as 50% of control after a 6-hr exposure. The level of GSH decreased 40% under these conditions but without a concomitant rise in the level of oxidized glutathione (GSSG).

Further studies revealed that NPSH or GSH oxidation during O_3 exposure resulted in the formation of mixed disulfides (PSSG) with other SH groups of lung tissue. It was also observed that PSSG formation was a transient phenomenon, $i.e.$, the levels of GSH or NPSH and PSH in lung tissue returned to control values after the animals were removed from the O_3 chambers and allowed to recover in air for a few days. Thus, mixed disulfide formation in lung tissue under oxidative stresses may represent a protective mechanism rather than a harmful event. For example, mixed disulfide formation prevents the oxidation of GSH to GSSG, which may then diffuse out from lung cells. Likewise, by forming mixed disulfides with PSH, GSH as well as PSH may be protected from oxidation beyond the $-SS-$ state. Although the binding of GSH with PSH may interfere with cellular enzymatic activities requiring SH groups, enzymatic or nonenzymatic mechanisms for disulfide reduction apparently exist in the lung and may lead to regeneration of the respective SH groups as conditions become favorable.

In contrast to acute O_3 exposure, which decreased the level of SH groups in lung tissue, low-level exposure to O_3 or NO_2 resulted in an elevation of GSH or NPSH in lung tissue. As shown in Figure 6.12, continuous exposure of rats to 0.8 ppm O_3 for 1 day resulted in a small (5%) decrease of NPSH level. After 2-7 days of exposure a significant rise (40%, $p < 0.001$) in the NPSH level was evident. The level of GSH, which followed a similar pattern, increased approximately 30% ($p < 0.001$). The level of GSSG, which represents 1-2% of the total glutathione in lung tissue, remained unchanged throughout the exposure period. As a function of O_3 concentrations (Figure 6.13), the increases in NPSH level for a 7-day exposure were 15%, 30% and 40%, respectively, for 0.2, 0.5 and 0.8 ppm O_3. The level of NPSH was also examined after NO_2 exposure. Exposure of rats to 15 ppm NO_2 for 7 days resulted in a 140% increase of NPSH in lung tissue.

In view of the elevation of GSH and NPSH levels, activities of several enzymes related to SH metabolism were examined. Figure 6.14 shows

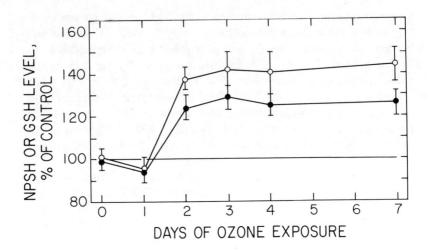

Figure 6.12   Effect of 0.8 ppm ozone exposure on nonprotein sulfhydryl (NPSH) or glutathione (GSH) level in lung tissue.   Control values (nmol/lung) were: 1550 ± 320 for NPSH (○ - ○) and 1290 ± 180 for GSH (● - ●).

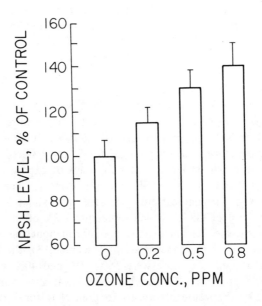

Figure 6.13   Effect of varying concentrations of ozone exposure on nonprotein sulfhydryl (NPSH) level in lung tissue.   Control value was 1550 ± 320 nmol/lung.

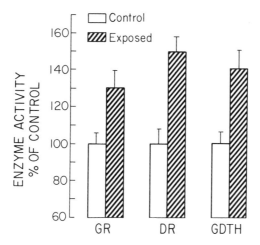

Figure 6.14   Effect of 0.8 ppm ozone exposure on the activities of
sulfhydryl metabolizing enzymes in lung cytosol. Control values
(nmol NADPH oxidized/min · lung) were: 1820 ± 230 for
glutathione reductase (GR), 1680 ± 180 for disulfide reductase
(DR) and 950 ± 110 for glutathione-disulfide transhydrogenase (GDTH).

these enzymes: (1) glutathione reductase (GR), which specifically catalyzes
the reduction of GSSG to GSH and is not inhibited by arsenite; (2) disulfide reductase (DR), which catalyzes the reduction of a broad spectrum
of disulfides (mixed disulfides); and (3) glutathione disulfide transhydrogenase (GDTH), which catalyzes the reduction of a disulfide via transfer
of a hydrogen from GSH. After exposure of rats to 0.8 ppm O_3 for up
to 7 days, a 30-50% (p < 0.02) rise in activity was observed for all three
enzymes.

The results demonstrate that low-level oxidant exposures result in an
elevation of GSH or NPSH. The concomitant increase in enzymatic activities related to SH metabolism might serve to enhance the replenishment
of SH groups in lung cells. An increased supply of GSH or similar reducing substances might serve to lessen the sensitivity of lung cells to oxidant
damage.

Effect on Protein Synthesis

Enhancement of enzymatic activities in lung tissue of rats exposed to
oxidant as described in earlier sections may be due to increased synthesis
of enzymes and/or activation of enzymes. While the study of activation
mechanisms requires isolation and purification of enzymes, the increase

in enzyme (protein) synthesis may be conveniently assessed from the incorporation of labeled amino acids into proteins.

In this study we have examined the extent of amino acid incorporation, *i.e.*, protein synthesis, in lung tissue of rats after exposure, to a low level of O_3. As shown in Figure 6.15, exposure of rats to 0.8 ppm O_3 for 1 day resulted in no differential incorporation of labeled amino acid *in vitro* for exposed and control lung tissues. After 2 and 3 days of

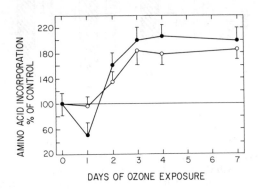

Figure 6.15   Effect of 0.8 ppm ozone exposure on amino acid incorporation into lung tissue proteins under *in vitro* (○ - ○) and *in vivo* (● - ●) conditions.

exposure, respectively, 35% and 84% increases in incorporation occurred relative to control. Continuation of the exposure for 4-7 days resulted in the same degree of incorporation as observed for 3 days. Under *in vivo* conditions (Figure 6.15), the incorporation after 1 day of exposure was 50% lower than the control, but increased 60% and 100%, respectively, after 2 and 3 days of exposure. The incorporation remained augmented at approximately 100% above the control level when the exposure was continued for 4-7 days. Thus, under both *in vitro* and *in vivo* conditions the highest incorporation was observed after 3 days of O_3 exposure, and this peak level was maintained during continued exposure for up to 7 days.

In order to determine whether the labeled amino acid was incorporated into proteins, the incorporation was studied in the presence of puromycin, an inhibitor of protein synthesis. As shown in Table 6.2, the increase in leucine incorporation observed in exposed lungs was abolished when the animals were treated with puromycin. Under *in vitro* conditions also, puromycin completely blocked the incorporation into acid-precipitable product in both exposed and control lung samples.

It is known that under these conditions of O_3 exposure collagen is synthesized in increased amounts. However, only up to 2% of the total

Table 6.2   Effect of Puromycin on Leucine Incorporation into Proteins

Puromycin Treatment	Leucine Incorporation CPM/Lung
Untreated control	7,000
Treated control	2,880
Untreated exposed	11,500
Treated exposed	2,570

After a 7-day exposure to 0.8 ppm O_3, rats from both control and exposed groups received 25 mg of neutralized puromycin (in saline) intraperitoneally. After 2 hr they received 100 μC of L-leucine-4,6-^{3}H intravenously. The rats were then sacrificed in exactly 20 min and the radioactivity in the acid-insoluble fraction of lung tissue was determined. Data represent averages of results from 5 rats in each group.

incorporation into proteins could be accounted for by collagen synthesis.[69,70]   Therefore, most of the amino acid incorporation seen in these experiments represented noncollagenous proteins, presumably including enzymes.

It should be pointed out that under *in vivo* conditions no radioactive incorporation was obtained in the acid-insoluble precipitate from blood or from pulmonary alveolar macrophages (as obtained by endobronchial lavage), suggesting that labeled proteins were synthesized within lung tissue, and were neither transported from the blood nor contributed by the macrophages. Our data are in confirmation with the observations of Massaro *et al.*[22]

Biochemical Changes due to Oxidant Concentration and Continuous Versus Intermittent Exposure

Having observed that considerable biochemical changes occur in the lung after 0.8 ppm O_3 exposure, a concentration of oxidant that may be encountered in severe episodes of smog, we undertook a study to examine the effects of lower levels of O_3. Rats were exposed to either 0.2, 0.5 or 0.8 ppm O_3 for 7 days, and effects in the lung were compared by measuring selected biochemical parameters. As shown in Figure 6.16, the activities of various marker enzymes in lung tissue—mitochondrial succinate-cytochrome *c* reductase, microsomal NADPH-cytochrome *c* reductase and cytosolic glucose-6-phosphate dehydrogenase and glutathione peroxidase—were augmented fairly in proportion to the O_3 concentrations to which the animals were exposed.

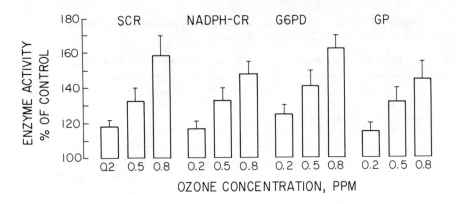

Figure 6.16 Effect of varying concentrations of ozone exposure on marker enzyme
activities in lung tissue. Control values were as shown in legends to
Figures 6.3, 6.7 and 6.11.

Results presented thus far are from studies involving continuous exposure of animals to oxidant. In order to simulate ambient conditions, in
which the human population may receive variable or brief periods of daily
exposure, rats were exposed to O_3 intermittently. The exposures were at
two levels of O_3—0.5 ppm and 0.8 ppm—for 2, 4, 6, 8 and 24 hr per
day for one week. At the end of the exposures rats from both control
and exposed groups were killed and the lungs analyzed for changes in
marker enzyme activities.

Typical results are described for succinate oxidase activity in lung
homogenate. As shown for 0.8 ppm O_3 exposure (Figure 6.17), the
changes, which were maximum for continuous exposure (24 hr daily),
were significant down to a 4-hr exposure per day. It may be noted that
the changes due to 24-hr daily exposure were only slightly greater than
those due to 8-hr daily exposure, although in the former instance the
duration of exposure was three times longer. For 0.5 ppm O_3 exposure
(Figure 6.17), the significant changes were observed down to a 6-hr
daily exposure. Here, too, the difference in changes due to 24-hr and
8-hr daily exposure was small.

Other enzyme activities assayed were 2-oxoglutarate oxidase in lung
homogenate and glucose-6-phosphate dehydrogenase, glutathione reductase
and glutathione peroxidase in lung cytosol. The changes observed for
these enzyme activities were essentially the same as those illustrated for
succinate oxidase activity. The results suggest that the biochemical
changes in the lung were fairly dependent upon the length of daily exposure to O_3, and that for 24-hr and 8-hr daily exposures the differences

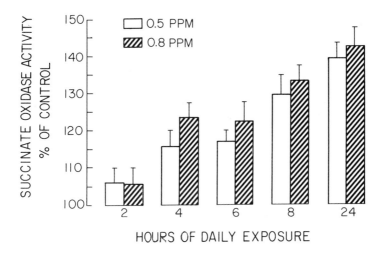

Figure 6.17 Effect of continuous *vs.* intermittent ozone exposure on succinate oxidase activity in lung homogenate. Control value was 650 ± 72 nmol O_2/min · lung.

in changes were much smaller than would be expected normally. These observations are in agreement with the recent morphological findings.[71]

Biochemical Changes due to Inflammatory Cells

Inflammatory cells or alveolar free cells are known to increase in number in the lung after pulmonary injury. In this study an assessment was made of the contribution of alveolar free cells to overall augmentation of lung enzymatic activities.

Alveolar free cells, as obtained by lavaging the lungs of control and O_3-exposed rats, were 90% alveolar macrophages and the rest polymorphonuclear leukocytes and small monocytes. The rate of oxygen consumption for oxidation of succinate in homogenates of alveolar free cells was 7.5 ± 1.1 nmol O_2/min x mg protein. This rate was not different for cell homogenates from control and exposed rat lung, and was approximately the same as in lung homogenate of control rats. Similarly the activity of glucose-6-phosphate dehydrogenase was measured in alveolar free cells, and no difference was observed for control and exposed rat lungs. However, the yield of alveolar free cells, which was approximately a million from each control lung (equivalent to 1 mg of protein), was 50-100% greater from exposed lungs. Alveolar free cells, therefore, might have a minor contribution to overall augmentation of enzymatic activities in O_3-exposed rat lungs.

Recovery from Oxidant Exposure

Having observed that oxidant exposures elicit biochemical changes in the lung, the questions came as to the duration of these changes and recovery of animals. Therefore the following studies were carried out in order to provide answers to some of these questions.

In one set of experiments rats were exposed to 3 ppm O_3 for 4 hr and then allowed to recover in room air. Although no animals died during exposure, 20-25% of them died within 12 hr after exposure, but not thereafter. Acute respiratory failure was the apparent cause of death, and such postexposure death signified that O_3 exposure caused severe lung injury. As judged from the activities of various marker enzymes—succinate oxidase and glucose-6-phosphate dehydrogenase (Figure 6.18) the biochemical changes in the lungs of exposed rats exhibited at least three different phases. Immediately after the exposure (*i.e.,* at 0 hour of recovery) there was a decrease in enzyme activities (20-25% relative to control, $p < 0.05$). Thereafter, the enzyme activities began to increase, attaining a peak (45-100% over control, $p < 0.001$) between 3 and 4 days, but then began to decline approaching the control values after 21 days of recovery.

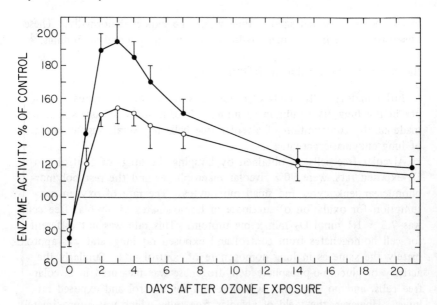

Figure 6.18   Marker enzyme activities in lung tissue of animals recovering from a 3 ppm ozone exposure for 4 hr. Control values were: 650 ± 72 nmol O_2/min · lung for succinate oxidase (O - O) in homogenate, and 2198 ± 190 nmol NADPH formed/min · lung for glucose-6-phosphate dehydrogenase (● - ●) in cytosol.

In another set of experiments rats were continuously exposed to 0.8 ppm O_3 for 3 days and then allowed to recover in room air. As judged from the activities of a series of marker enzymes—succinate oxidase (Figure 6.19), glucose-6-phosphate dehydrogenase (Figure 6.20) and amino acid incorporation into proteins (Figure 6.21)—the biochemical parameters, which increased 30-60% over control ($p < 0.01$) after 3 days of exposure, declined sharply after cessation of the exposure and returned to control values in approximately 7 days. These observations were in sharp contrast to those shown in Figure 6.2 which showed that the biochemical parameters maintained an elevated level if exposure to 0.8 ppm O_3 continued beyond a 3-day period (*e.g.*, for up to 7 or 30 days). If the recovered animals were reexposed to the same dosage of O_3 (0.8 ppm for 3 days) the metabolic changes again increased to levels (Figures 6.19, 6.20 and 6.21) comparable to the initial exposure.

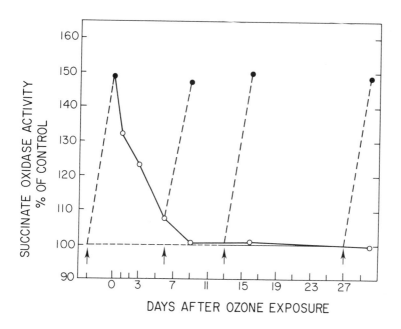

Figure 6.19   Succinate oxidase activity in lung tissue of animals recovering from 0.8 ppm ozone exposure for 3 days. After the initial exposure (indicated by arrow on the left-hand side) animals were allowed to recover. After recovery for various periods of time the animals were reexposed (as shown by arrows). The rise in enzyme activity due to exposure is shown by broken lines, and the decline of activity during recovery is shown by solid line.

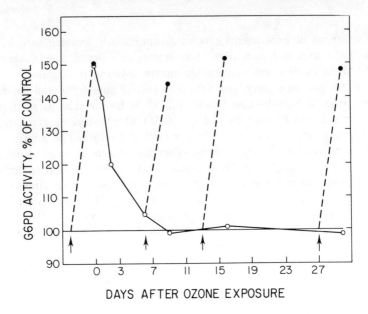

Figure 6.20   Glucose-6-phosphate dehydrogenase (G6PD) activity in lung tissue of animals recovering from 0.8 ppm ozone exposure for 3 days. Conventions are as described in legend to Figure 6.19.

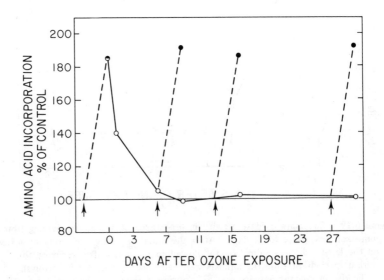

Figure 6.21   Amino acid incorporation into lung tissue proteins of animals recovering from 0.8 ppm ozone exposure for 3 days. Conventions are as described in legend to Figure 6.19.

The results from these two sets of experiments demonstrate that animals that sustain lung injury from oxidant exposures undergo a recovery that can be followed by monitoring the changes in lung metabolism. The rate and the length of recovery seems to depend upon the degree of initial lung injury. The period of recovery required after exposure to 0.8 ppm O_3 was one week, whereas more than three weeks were needed for recovery after exposure to 3 ppm O_3. These results also demonstrate that biochemical changes resulting from the oxidant exposures conducted in this study are not permanent. As shown for low-level exposure (0.8 ppm O_3), these changes disappear with the termination of exposure and reappear with recurrence of exposure.

GENERAL DISCUSSION AND CONCLUSIONS

The results of this study, which encompasses a series of exposure conditions and a profile of metabolic activities in lung tissue, demonstrate that O_3 and NO_2 cause alterations of lung metabolism in experimental animals. The overall observations are depression of lung metabolism after high-level exposures (*e.g.*, 2-4 ppm O_3 for hours); elevation of metabolic activities after low-level exposures (*e.g.*, 0.2-0.8 ppm O_3 or 5-15 ppm NO_2 for days) or during recovery from high-level exposures; and development of adaptation or tolerance against a continued low-level exposure. The biochemical bases for the observed metabolic alterations, their correlation with morphologic changes, and their possible physiologic consequence or environmental health significance will be discussed.

The biochemical mechanisms for O_3 and NO_2 effects in the lung have been of major interest to researchers. The basic mechanisms for lung injury and metabolic perturbations caused by O_3 and NO_2 seem to be coincident with the oxidizing and radiomimetic properties of these two gases. Thus, oxidation of functional groups such as –SH, –NH_2, –CHO and phenolic –OH and peroxidation of unsaturated lipids either directly or via free radical-mediated reactions have been considered. Although these reactions of O_3 and NO_2 with plant or animal tissues, including lung tissue, under *in vitro* conditions have been amply documented,[6,17,32-34,63,72,73] their occurrence under *in vivo* conditions has not been proven with a high degree of certainty. To date, the oxidative loss of –SH groups has been demonstrated but only after a high-level, short-term O_3 exposure.[6,10,24] In low-level oxidant exposures, which may be of relevance to a smog-polluted environment, the oxidation products of –SH do not seem to accumulate. Since low concentrations of O_3 or NO_2 are thought to react with lung tissue in focal areas, it is possible that –SH oxidation (*e.g.*, mixed disulfide formation) in focal areas may remain undetected due to averaging of healthy and injured tissues during homogenization. It is also possible that normal (or augmented) enzymatic pathways that favor disulfide reduction are able to restore −SH groups under conditions of low-level exposure.

Likewise the occurrence of lipid peroxidation and the accumulation of lipid peroxidation products such as malonaldehyde or conjugated dienes in lung tissue during low-level exposures have been investigated. Although two laboratories have reported evidence for the occurrence of lipid peroxidation *in vivo,*[7,26,74] no confirmation of these observations has been achieved by other laboratories, including ours. Since enzymatic or other mechanisms are known to exist in lung and other tissues for destruction of lipid peroxides,[7,9,21] it is possible that lipid peroxidation products do not accumulate in lung tissue during oxidant exposure. Nonetheless, the concept of lipid peroxidation in the lung due to O_3 or NO_2 exposure will persist.

Two other mechanisms that have been considered are: loss of activities of enzymes dependent upon −SH group or membrane structure for their function, and an alteration of membrane permeability and loss of functions of intracellular organelles, *e.g.,* mitochondria. Although these mechanisms leading to metabolic perturbations in the lung have been shown in relatively high-level exposures (2-4 ppm O_3 for hours), they may indeed represent important indices of lung cellular injury, inasmuch as only focal areas of the lung (*e.g.,* centriacinar regions) possibly bear the brunt of oxidant interaction.

The augmentation of lung metabolism in low-level exposures or during recovery from a high-level exposure possibly represents a response of lung tissue to injury. The magnitude of increases in various metabolic parameters observed may be a measure of lung tissue injury caused by oxidant exposures, and appears to be fairly proportional to oxidant concentration in the inspired air. The augmentation of metabolic parameters suggests that repair processes may occur in injured lung tissue, and that renewal and/or proliferation of cells and synthesis of cellular components may all be contributory to the overall augmentation.

From the morphological point of view, the pulmonary lesions resulting from low-level oxidant exposures appear to be an initial damage to the bronchiolar epithelial cells and the Type 1 epithelial cells of the adjacent alveoli, followed by a replacement of damaged cells via proliferation of bronchiolar cuboidal cells and alveolar Type 2 cells, respectively.[4,5,13,71] Of particular importance are the alveolar Type 2 cells, which normally comprise perhaps 10% of the overall lung cellular population, contain abundant mitochondria and other organelles, and exhibit high metabolic activity. A proliferation of this cell type following lung injury may significantly elevate metabolic activities, such as in the lungs of oxidant-exposed animals.[4,5,15,45] Likewise, the proliferative response of cuboidal epithelial cells of the bronchioles, and possibly other cell types in the alveolar interstitium or the parenchymal tissue, may be involved in the enhancement of lung metabolism after oxidant exposure.

The biochemical changes, which reach the maximal increase approximately 3 days after oxidant exposure, seem to follow a time-course similar to the morphological changes, *i.e.*, the cellular proliferation in the lung during low-level exposure also occurs in 3 days.[4,5,13,71] The biochemical and morphological changes evoked during the first few days of oxidant exposure possibly bring about a state of adaptation whereby a continued exposure results in little or no net damage to lung tissue. Hence, the metabolic activities or morphological changes reach a plateau. The return of metabolic activities in lung tissue toward control values a few days after the termination of oxidant exposure may be ascribed to a cessation of injury and a relative completion of repair processes. The recurrence of biochemical changes after reexposure of animals may reflect a reinitiation of injury and repair processes in the lung. The biochemical changes in the lung resulting from oxidant exposures are, therefore, reversible.

Health effects of environmental oxidants should be of concern to the human population. Significant concentrations of O_3 appear in airplane cabins at altitudes greater than 30,000 feet, and in the vicinity of high voltage electric equipment during operation.[75,76] Likewise, NO_2 in large concentrations may arise from auto exhaust and stacked hay in silos.[2] While the human exposure to high concentrations of O_3 or NO_2 may be accidental, low-level exposure may result from the photochemical smog that contains both O_3 and NO_2. In the air basin of southern California the yearly average for oxidant concentration is 0.1-0.2 ppm, but in severe episodes of smog the oxidant concentration may become as high as 0.9 ppm.[77] The data presented in this paper and also those reported by others[4,5,7,9,78-80] testify that exposure to low-level oxidants (0.2-0.9 ppm O_3 or 5-15 ppm NO_2) may cause significant biochemical and morphological lesions in the lung.

Finally, a low-level oxidant exposure seems to act as an inducer of biochemical and morphological changes. These changes are transient, and, on a short-term basis, may have a physiologic significance in that they confer a resistance against further lung injury in an oxidant environment. However, the long-term effects of these changes resulting from a continued exposure are yet to be determined. Whether or not low-level oxidant exposures can lead to an enhanced aging, or a development of chronic bronchitis or pulmonary carcinoma, fibrosis or emphysema in experimental animals should be determined by conducting long-term exposure studies. Such studies may help assess the true health consequences of environmental oxidants in humans exposed to photochemical smog.

ACKNOWLEDGMENTS

This study was supported in part by USEPA contract 68-03-2221 and USPHS-NIH grants HL 17719 and HL 19668, and Research Career Development Award 1 KO4 HL 00301 (to M.G.M.).

REFERENCES

1. Jaffe, L. S. "The Biological Effects of Ozone on Man and Animals," *Amer. Ind. Hyg. Assoc. J.* 28:268 (1967).
2. Stokinger, H. E. and D. L. Coffin. "Biological Effects of Air Pollutants," In: *Air Pollution*, 3rd ed. A. C. Stern, Ed. (New York: Academic Press, Inc., 1968), p. 445.
3. Cross, C. E., A. J. DeLucia, A. K. Reddy, M. Z. Hussain, C. K. Chow and M. G. Mustafa. "Ozone Interaction with Lung Tissue: Biochemical Approaches," *Amer. J. Med.* 60:929 (1976).
4. Evans, M. J., L. J. Cabral, R. J. Stephens and G. Freeman. "Renewal of Alveolar Epithelium in the Rat Following Exposure to NO_2," *Amer. J. Pathol.* 70:175 (1973).
5. Stephens, R. J., M. F. Sloan, M. J. Evans and G. Freeman. "Early Response of Lung to Low Levels of Ozone," *Amer. J. Pathol.* 74:31 (1974).
6. DeLucia, A. J., P. M. Hoque, M. G. Mustafa and C. E. Cross. "Ozone Interaction with Rodent Lung. I. Effect on Sulfhydryls and Sulfhydryl-Containing Enzyme Activities," *J. Lab. Clin. Med.* 80:559 (1972).
7. Chow, C. K. and A. L. Tappel. "An Enzymatic Protective Mechanism Against Lipid Peroxidation Damage to Lungs of Ozone-Exposed Rats," *Lipids* 7:518 (1972).
8. Mustafa, M. G., A. J. DeLucia, G. K. York, C. Arth and C. E. Cross. "Ozone Interaction with Rodent Lung. II. Effects on Oxygen Consumption of Mitochondria," *J. Lab. Clin. Med.* 82:357 (1973).
9. Chow, C. K. and A. L. Tappel. "Activities of Pentose Shunt and Glycolytic Enzymes in Lungs of Ozone-Exposed Rats," *Arch. Environ. Health* 26:205 (1973).
10. DeLucia, A. J., M. G. Mustafa, C. E. Cross, C. G. Plopper, D. L. Dungworth and W. S. Tyler. "Biochemical and Morphological Alterations in the Lung Following Ozone Exposure," *Amer. Inst. Chem. Eng. Symp. Ser.* 71:93 (1975).
11. Mustafa, M. G. "Influence of Dietary Vitamin E on Lung Cellular Sensitivity to Ozone in Rats," *Nutr. Reports Int.* 11:473 (1975).
12. Chow, C. K., M. G. Mustafa, C. E. Cross and B. K. Tarkington. "Effects of Ozone Exposure on the Lungs and the Erythrocytes of Rats and Monkeys: Relative Biochemical Changes," *Environ. Physiol.* 5:142 (1975).

13. Dungworth, D. L., W. L. Castleman, C. K. Chow, P. W. Mellick, M. G. Mustafa, B. K. Tarkington and W. S. Tyler. "Effect of Ambient Levels of Ozone on Monkeys," *Fed. Proc.* 34:1970 (1975).

14. Mustafa, M. G. and S. D. Lee. "Pulmonary Biochemical Alterations Resulting from Ozone Exposure," *Ann. Occup. Hyg.* 19:17 (1976).

15. Mustafa, M. G. "Augmentation of Mitochondrial Oxidative Metabolism in Lung Tissue During Recovery of Animals from Acute Ozone Exposure," *Arch. Biochem. Biophys.* 165:531 (1974).

16. Fisher, A. B., A. Scarpa, K. F. LaNoue, D. Bassett and J. R. Williamson. "Respiration of Rat Lung Mitochondria and the Influence of Ca^{2+} on Substrate Utilization," *Biochem.* 12:1438 (1973).

17. Mustafa, M. G. and C. E. Cross. "Effects of Short-Term Ozone Exposure on Lung Mitochondrial Oxidative and Energy Metabolism," *Arch. Biochem. Biophys.* 162:585 (1974).

18. Bucher, T., R. Czok, W. Lamprecht and E. Latzko. "Pyruvate," In: *Methods of Enzymatic Analysis,* H. U. Bergmeyer, Ed. (New York: Academic Press, Inc., 1965), p. 253.

19. Hohorst, H. J. "L-Lactate Determination with Lactic Dehydrogenase and DPN," In: *Methods of Enzymatic Analysis,* H. U. Bergmeyer, Ed. (New York: Academic Press, Inc., 1975), p. 266.

20. Tietze, F. "Disulfide Reduction in Rat Liver," *Arch. Biochem. Biophys.* 138:177 (1970).

21. Little, C. and P. J. O'Brien. "An Intracellular GSH Peroxidase with a Lipid Peroxide Substrate," *Biochem. Biophys. Res. Commun.* 31:145 (1968).

22. Massaro, D., H. Weiss and M. R. Simon. "Protein Synthesis and Secretion by Lung," *Amer. Rev. Resp. Dis.* 101:198 (1970).

23. Sedlak, J. and R. H. Lindsay. "Estimation of Total, Protein-Bound and Nonprotein Sulfhydryl Groups in Tissue with Ellman's Reagent," *Anal. Biochem.* 25:192 (1968).

24. DeLucia, A. J., M. G. Mustafa, M. Z. Hussain and C. E. Cross. "Ozone Interaction with Rodent Lung. III. Oxidation of Reduced Glutathione and Formation of Mixed Disulfides Between Protein and Nonprotein Sulfhydryls," *J. Clin. Invest.* 55:794 (1975).

25. Klotsch, H. and H. U. Bergmeyer. "Glutathione," In: *Methods of Enzymatic Analysis,* H. U. Bergmeyer, Ed. (New York: Academic Press, 1965), p. 363.

26. Fletcher, B. L. and A. L. Tappel. "Protective Effects of Dietary Alpha-Tocopherol in Rats Exposed to Toxic Levels of Ozone and Nitrogen Dioxide," *Environ. Res.* 6:165 (1973).

27. Hartree, E. F. "Determination of Protein: A Modification of the Lowry Method that Gives a Linear Photometric Response," *Anal. Biochem.* 48:422 (1972).

28. Michaelis, L. and S. Granick. "The Polymerization of the Free Radicals of the Wurster Dye Type: The Dimeric Resonance Bond," *J. Amer. Chem. Soc.* 65:1747 (1943).

29. Ou, L. C. and S. M. Tenney. "Properties of Mitochondria from Hearts of Cattle Acclimatized to High Altitude," *Resp. Physiol.* 8:151 (1970).

30. Ascenbrenner, V., R. Zak, A. F. Cutilleta and M. Rabinowitz.

"Effect of Hypoxia on Degradation of Mitochondrial Components in Rat Cardiac Muscle," *Amer. J. Physiol.* 221:1418 (1971).

31. Shertzer, H. G. and J. Cascarano. "Mitochondrial Alterations in Heart, Liver and Kidney of Altitude-Acclimated Rats," *Amer. J. Physiol.* 223:632 (1972).

32. Thompson, W. W., W. M. Dugger, Jr. and R. L. Palmer. "Effects of Ozone on the Fine Structure of the Palisade Parenchyma Cells of Bean Leaves," *Can. J. Bot.* 44:1677 (1966).

33. Mudd, J. B., T. T. McManus, A. Ongrin and T. E. McCullough. "Inhibition of Glycolipid Biosynthesis in Chloroplasts by Ozone and Sulfhydryl Reagents," *Plant Physiol.* 48:335 (1971).

34. Wong, C. W. "Effect of Ozone on Sulfhydryl Groups of Ribosomes in Pinto Bean Leaves. Relationship with Ribosome Dissociation," *Biochem. Biophys. Res. Commun.* 44:1429 (1971).

35. Nobel, P. S. and C. Wong. "Ozone Increases the Permeability of Isolated Pea Chloroplasts," *Arch. Biochem. Biophys.* 157:388 (1973).

36. Mustafa, M. G., A. J. DeLucia, C. E. Cross, G. K. York and D. L. Dungworth. "Effect of Ozone Exposure on Lung Mitochondrial Oxidative Metabolism," *Chest (Suppl.)* 66:16S (1974).

37. Segal, W. "Enhancement of Succinate Oxidation in Lung and Liver Mitochondria of Tuberculous Mice," *Arch. Biochem. Biophys.* 113:750 (1966).

38. Kilroe-Smith, T. A. and M. G. Breyer. "Changes in Activities of Respiratory Enzymes in Lungs of Guinea-Pigs Exposed to Silica Dust," *Brit. J. Ind. Med.* 20:243 (1963).

39. Breyer, M. G., T. A. Kilroe-Smith and H. Prinsloo. "Changes in Activities of Respiratory Enzymes in Lungs of Guinea-Pigs Exposed to Silica Dust. II. Comparison of the Effects of Quartz Dust and Lampblack on the Siccinate Oxidase System," *Brit. J. Ind. Med.* 21:32 (1964).

40. Fritts, H. W., Jr., B. Strauss, W. Wichern, Jr. and A. Courand. "Utilization of Oxygen in Lung of Patients with Diffuse, Nonobstructive Pulmonary Disease," *Trans. Assoc. Amer. Phys.* 76:302 (1963).

41. Strauss, B. "*In Vitro* Respiration of Normal and Pathologic Human Lung," *J. Appl. Physiol.* 19:503 (1964).

42. Oberling, C. "The Structure of Cytoplasm," *Int'l. Rev. Cytol.* 8:1 (1959).

43. Muscatello, U. and I. P. Ronchetti. "The Relation Between Structure and Function in Mitochondria. Its Relevance in Pathology," In: *Pathobiology Annual*, Vol. 2, H. L. Ioachim, Ed. (New York: Appleton-Century-Crofts, 1972), p. 1.

44. Bowden, D. H. and J. P. Wyatt. "Lung Injury and Repair: A Contemporary View," In: *Pathology Annual*, Vol. 5, S. C. Somers, Ed. (New York: Appleton-Century-Crofts, 1970), p. 279.

45. Adamson, I. Y. R. and D. H. Bowden. "The Type 2 Cell as Progenitor of Alveolar Epithelial Regeneration. A Cytodynamic Study on Mice After Exposure to Oxygen," *Lab Invest.* 30:35 (1974).

46. Kapanci, Y., E. R. Weibel, H. P. Kaplan and F. R. Robinson. "Pathogenesis and Reversibility of the Pulmonary Lesions of Oxygen Toxicity in Monkeys. II. Ultrastructural and Morphometric Studies," *Lab. Invest.* 20:101 (1969).
47. Gould, V. E., R. Tosco, R. F. Wheelis, N. S. Gould and Y. Kapanci. "Oxygen Pneumonitis in Man. Ultrastructural Observations on the Development of Alveolar Lesions," *Lab. Invest.* 26:499 (1972).
48. Tierney, D. F. "Lactate Metabolism in Rat Lung Tissue," *Arch. Intern. Med.* 127:858 (1971).
49. Ayers, L. and D. F. Tierney. "Pentose Pathway: A Possible Metabolic Mechanism to Protect the Lung from High PO_2," *Amer. Rev. Resp. Dis.* 103:906 (1971).
50. Wallace, H. W., T. P. Stein and E. M. Liquori. "Lactate and Lung Metabolism," *J. Thorac. Cardiovas. Sur.* 68:810 (1974).
51. Young, S. L. and J. H. Knelson. "Increased Glucose Uptake by Rat Lung with Onset of Edema," *Physiologist* 16:494 (1973).
52. Gassenheimer, L. N. and R. A. Rhoades. "Influence of Forced Ventilation on Substrate Metabolism in the Perfused Rat Lung," *J. Appl. Physiol.* 37:224 (1974).
53. Chvapil, M. and Y. M. Peng. "Oxygen and Lung Fibrosis," *Arch. Environ. Health* 30:528 (1975).
54. Braasch, W., S. Gudbjarnason, P. S. Puri, K. G. Ravens and R. J. Bing. "Early Changes in Energy Metabolism in the Myocardium Following Acute Coronary Artery Occlusion in Anesthetized Dogs," *Circ. Res.* 23:429 (1968).
55. Vorne, M. and P. Arvela. "Effect of Carbon Tetrachloride-Induced Progressive Liver Damage on Drug Metabolizing Enzymes and Cytochrome P-450 in Rat Liver," *Acta Pharmacol. Toxicol.* 29:417 (1971).
56. Beaconsfield, P. and A. Capri. "Localization of an Infectious Lesion and Glucose Metabolism Via the Pentose Phosphate Pathway," *Nature* 201:825 (1964).
57. Kimball, R. E., K. Reddy, T. H. Peirce, L. W. Schwartz, M. G. Mustafa and C. E. Cross. "Oxygen Toxicity: Augmentation of Antioxidant Defense Mechanisms in Rat Lung," *Amer. J. Physiol.* 230:1425 (1976).
58. Witschi, H. P. and S. Kacew. "Studies on the Pathological Biochemistry of Lung Parenchyma in Acute Parquat Poisoning," *Med. Biol.* 52:104 (1974).
59. McCord, J. M., C. O. Beauchamp, S. Gioscin, H. P. Misra and I. Fridovich. "Superoxide and Superoxide Dismuase," In: *Oxidases and Related Redox Systems,* T. E. King, H. S. Mason and M. Morrison, Eds. (Baltimore: University Park, 1973), p. 51.
60. Crapo, J. D. and D. F. Tierney. "Superoxide Dismutase and Pulmonary Oxygen Toxicity," *Amer. J. Physiol.* 226:1401 (1974).
61. Menzel, D. B. "Toxicity of Ozone, Oxygen and Radiation," *Ann. Rev. Pharmacol.* 10:379 (1970).
62. Dugger, W. M. and I. P. Ting. "Air Pollutant Oxidant: Their Effects on Metabolic Processes in Plants," *Rev. Plant Physiol. Ann.* 21:215 (1970).

63. Nasr. A. N. M. "Biochemical Aspects of Ozone Intoxication," *J. Occup. Med.* 9:589 (1967).

64. Clark, J. M. and C. J. Lambertson. "Pulmonary Oxygen Toxicity: A Review," *Pharmacol. Rev.* 23:37 (1971).

65. Fairchild, E. J. "Tolerance Mechanisms: Determinants of Lung Responses to Injurious Agents," *Arch. Environ. Health* 14:111 (1967).

66. Davies, H. C. and R. E. Davies. "Biochemical Aspects of Oxygen Poisoning," *Handb. Physiol.* 2:1047 (1965).

67. Mountain, J. T. "Detecting Hypersensitivity to Toxic Substances," *Arch. Environ. Health* 6:357 (1963).

68. King, M. E. *Biochemical Effects of Ozone.* Doctoral dissertation. Illinois Institute of Technology (1961).

69. Hussain, M. Z., M. G. Mustafa, C. K. Chow and C. E. Cross. "Ozone-Inducing Increase of Lung Proline Hydroxylase Activity and Hydroxyproline Content," *Chest* (Suppl.) 69:273 (1976).

70. Hussain, M. Z., C. E. Cross, M. G. Mustafa and R. S. Bhatnagar. "Collagen Synthesis in Lungs of Rats Exposed to Low Levels of Ozone," *Life Sci.* 18:897 (1976).

71. Schwartz, L. W., D. L. Dungworth, M. G. Mustafa, B. K. Tarkington and W. S. Tyler, "Pulmonary Response of Rats to Ambient Levels of Ozone: Effects of a 7-Day Intermittent or Continuous Exposure," *Lab. Invest.* 34:565 (1976).

72. Mudd, J. B., R. Leavitt, A. Ongun and T. T. McManus. "Reaction of Ozone with Amino Acids and Proteins," *Atmos. Environ.* 3: 669 (1969).

73. Little, C. and P. J. O'Brien. "The Effectiveness of a Lipid Peroxide in Oxidizing Protein and Nonprotein Thiols," *Biochem. J.* 106:419 (1968).

74. Thomas, H. V., P. K. Mueller and R. L. Lyman. "Lipoperoxidation of Lung Lipids in Rats Exposed to Nitrogen Dioxide," *Science* 159:532 (1968).

75. Bennett, G. "Ozone Contamination of High Altitude Aircraft Cabins," *Aerospace Med.* 33:969 (1962).

76. Stokinger, H. E. "Ozone Toxicology: A Review of Research and Industrial Experience, 1954-1964," *Arch. Environ. Health* 10:719 (1965).

77. *Ten-Year Summary of California Air Quality Data, 1963-1972.* State of California Air Resources Board, Sacramento (1974).

78. Werthamer, S., P. D. Penha and L. Amaral. "Pulmonary Lesions Induced by Chronic Exposure to Ozone," *Arch. Environ. Health* 29:164 (1974).

79. Penha, P. D. and S. Werthamer. "Pulmonary Lesions Induced by Long-Term Exposure to Ozone," *Arch. Environ. Health* 29:282 (1974).

80. Yuen, T. G. and R. P. Sherwin. "Hyperplasia of Type 2 Pneumocytes and Nitrogen Dioxide (10 ppm) Exposure," *Arch. Environ. Health* 22:178 (1971).

CHAPTER 7

REACTION OF OZONE WITH BIOLOGICAL MEMBRANES

J. B. Mudd and B. A. Freeman

Department of Biochemistry
University of California
Riverside, California 92502

INTRODUCTION

The effects of ozone on plants are easily visible to the naked eye. At concentrations well below those experienced in polluted air there is first a darkening of the green color of the leaves, and subsequently dead cells, usually white in appearance, can be seen on the upper surface. The dead cells are typically in the palisade parenchyma. Damage is prevented under conditions that result in the closure of the leaf stomates, thus preventing access of gases to the susceptible cells.

The effects of ozone on animals are not so obvious. There is no eye irritating effect, and subjective responses such as headache, nausea and choking sensation in the upper respiratory tract cannot be specifically related to ozone. As one might expect, the lung is a primary point of attack by ozone. The consequences of this attack, at concentrations actually experienced in polluted air, cannot be seen by the naked eye on autopsy of experimental animals. However, scanning electron microscopy and transmission electron microscopy demonstrate damage in the region of the terminal and/or respiratory bronchioles. The Type I epithelial cells are particularly susceptible to damage.[1]

Both in the leaves and in the lungs, specific cell types are affected. One may ask whether this specificity is a reflection of special properties of the cellular membrane or the metabolic capability of the cytoplasmic contents of the cell. It has been frequently argued that since ozone is a very reactive gas and since in biological systems the plasma membrane is one of the first points of contact, we need look no further than the membrane to understand the basis for toxicity. However, there are many examples indicating effects of ozone distant from the membrane. In plants, degradation of chloroplast polysomes is an early event in the toxicity of ozone.[2,3] In animals the increase in sleeping time of phenobarbital-treated mice can be attributed to effects of ozone on the drug metabolism machinery of the liver.[4] Such observations can be countered by the proposal that ozone can react with components of the membrane that are then released into the cytoplasm (and in the case of animals eventually into the blood stream) where secondary events can occur. Proponents of the cytoplasm as the primary point of attack can equally well claim that cytoplasmic effects change the energy balance of the cell and that this change is manifested as an effect on membrane permeability.

These arguments have been expressed in the ozone literature for some time. It does not seem that they can be resolved with the intact biological system because one can never be sure that the effect observed is the very first. It therefore seems appropriate to study and understand simple model systems before we can approach again the living cell with knowledge that can guide our experiments. We have reviewed the literature concerning the effects of ozone on (1) proteins and (2) lipids, and attempted to apply this information to an understanding of the effects of ozone in biological membranes. We would like to know whether ozone has its primary effect at the plasma membrane, or whether ozone can penetrate the plasma membrane without affecting it and then damage the contents of the cell, or even cells beyond those first contacted.

REACTION WITH PROTEINS

Pure Amino Acids

Previero, Scoffone and co-workers examined the reaction of ozone with pure amino acids dissolved in anhydrous formic acid.[5,6] They found that cysteine was converted to cysteic acid, methionine to methionine sulfone, tryptophan to kynurenine and tyrosine to aspartic acid and oxalic acid. All other amino acids were resistant to ozone. In the reaction of ozone with tryptophan, the recovery as kynurenine was solvent-dependent, being 72% in formic acid, 52% in acetic acid, and zero in dimethylformamide. Likewise, the stability of kynurenine exposed to ozone was greatest in formic acid and least in dimethyl formamide. Further work from the same laboratory showed that the ozonization of tryptophan in simple peptides followed the same reaction, and that cystine in peptides could be oxidized to cysteic acid.[5,7]

Studies of reactions of ozone with amino acids in aqueous buffered solutions showed results comparable to those of Scoffone and co-workers. Notable differences were that under aqueous conditions histidine was oxidizable, methionine was converted to methionine sulfoxide, and tyrosine was converted to products that included 2,4-dihydroxyphenyl alanine but not aspartic acid.[8] Of the indole compounds, Ordin and Propst noted that indole acetic acid is oxidized.[9] Other indole derivatives such as 5-hydroxy-tryptophan, 5-hydroxy-tryptamine and 5-hydroxy-indoleacetic acid are also susceptible to oxidation by ozone.[10] The order of reactivity of amino acids in aqueous solution is cysteine > tryptophan = methionine > tyrosine > histidine > cystine = phenylalanine.[8] Previero and Bordignon gave the order of reactivity in anhydrous formic acid as tryptophan > methionine ≫ cystine > tyrosine.[11] The oxidation of thiol groups has also been reported by Menzel.[12]

In mixtures of amino acids the degree of oxidation of amino acids is predictable on the basis of the reaction of single amino acids.[8] In other cases, however, there is a preference in the substances oxidized by ozone. For example in roughly equal mixtures of NADH and tryptophan, or NADH and methionine, there is clearly a preferential oxidation of NADH.[13] In mixtures of GSH and NADH, however, there is some protection of NADH by GSH, but this effect is concentration-dependent; at low concentrations GSH is not oxidized until the NADH oxidation is complete.[13]

Pure Proteins

Giese et al.[14] noted that ozone altered the absorbance spectrum of tryptophan and tyrosine; these changes, they found, were also apparent in ozone-treated serum albumin. Similar results were obtained with gelatin and egg albumin. Previero and Bordignon measured the effects of ozone on globulin, trypsin, lysozyme and gramicidin and found that the tryptophan residues were 63-89% converted to N-formyl kynurenine.[11]

The decrease in enzyme activity of catalase, peroxidase, papain and urease after treatment with ozone was measured by Todd.[15] He found that the amount of ozone required to cause 50% inhibition was two orders of magnitude less for papain than for the other three enzymes. He also compared the effects of ozone and hydrogen peroxide and found that for papain ten times more hydrogen peroxide was required for 50% inhibition. Therefore the effects of ozone could not be attributed to generation of hydrogen peroxide.

Ribonuclease was inhibited by ozone, although 15-fold molar excesses were needed for 50% inhibition.[8][*] The inhibition was compared with the amino acid analysis and it was found that inhibition correlated with decreases: tyrosine > histidine > cystine.

Since avidin was known to require tryptophan for its activity in binding biotin,[8] it was suitable for checking inactivation of protein properties by oxidation of the tryptophan residues. The binding of biotin was prevented by the ozone treatment of avidin and this was accompanied by spectral changes characteristic of the oxidation of tryptophan. Previous binding of biotin to avidin prevented the oxidation of the tryptophan residues by ozone.

Menzel[12] has reported the inactivation of SH-requiring enzymes papain and glyceraldehyde-3-phosphate dehydrogenase. These enzymes could be partially reactivated by cysteine, indicating that at least part of the oxidized –SH was converted to –S–S–.

The inactivation of lysozyme by ozone has been observed a number of times. Previero et al.[16] found that tryptophan residues 108 and 111 were selectively converted to N-formyl kynurenine derivatives, but there was no loss in enzymic activity. Imoto et al.[17] found this result to be inexplicable because other cases of oxidation of tryptophan 108 led to inactivation. Leh and Mudd[18] investigated lysozyme inactivation by ozone in aqueous media. The enzyme was 95% inactivated by a two-fold molar excess of ozone over enzyme. Tryptophan residues 108 and 111 were oxidized, and in addition there was oxidation of methionine 105 and tyrosine 23. The inactivation by ozone is consistent with other findings using other reagents such as iodine and N-bromosuccinimide. Kuroda et al.[19] have also studied the inactivation of lysozyme by ozonization in aqueous media. These experiments were conducted at pH 5.0 and the analyses made of enzyme 80% inactivated. (Leh and Mudd analyzed lysozyme inactivated 95% by ozonization at pH 7.0.[18]) The results of Kuroda et al.[19] and Leh and Mudd[18] agree that tryptophan, methionine, cysteine and tyrosine are oxidized, but they differ in that Kuroda et al.[19] concluded that the tryptophan residue preferentially oxidized is 62. The difference is due possibly to the different pH of the reaction mixtures. Kuroda et al.[19] and Leh and Mudd[18] agree that lysozyme is sensitive to ozone, in contrast to the report by Previero et al.[16]

In Vivo and In Vitro Systems Related to Protein Oxidation

One may question the physiological relevance of results obtained from the reaction of ozone with pure amino acids and pure proteins. Are

*The reference cited here erroneously describes reaction of ozone with 5 μg ribonuclease. The amount was 5 mg ribonuclease.

these reactions relevant in the living cell?   Results from the well-defined system should be consistent with results obtained *in vivo* and with isolated tissues, cells or subcellular organelles.   The trouble with the latter systems is that they are capable of adjustment, so one event sets a cascade of secondary events in motion and it is then difficult to interpret the measured changes.

Lysozyme presents an illustrative case.   We know that lysozyme reacts rather readily with ozone.[18,19]   Consistent with this result is the observation that the lysozyme in tears of individuals exposed to smog is 60% less than normal.[20]   It is also known that the lysozyme (as well as β-glucuronidase and acid phosphatase) of alveolar lavage of rabbits exposed to ozone is 40-60% less than the control.[21,22]   This result was somewhat complicated by the observation that whereas the control animals retained the lysosomal enzymes in the pellet sedimented at 15,000 x g, the enzyme from the treated animals was found partially in the supernatant.   Thus the enzyme inactivation was compounded by increased fragility of the alveolar macrophage and the subcellular organelles.   An even greater complication is present in the results of Chow *et al.*[23] who found an increase in the lysozyme activity in lung washings from animals exposed to ozone.   This result can be rationalized on the grounds that heterophiles are found in the alveolar sacs after ozone exposure and contribute to the lysozyme content of the lung washings.[24,25]

There are several other cases of increases in enzyme activity after exposure to ozone.   Chow and Tappel[23,26,27] have demonstrated increases in the activity of GSH peroxidase, GSH reductase and G6P dehydrogenase. They view these increases as a response to the formation of lipid peroxide:

$$\text{lipid (RH)} \xrightarrow{O_3} \text{peroxidized lipid (ROOH)}$$

$$\text{ROOH} + 2\text{GSH} \xrightarrow[\text{peroxidase}]{\text{glutathione}} \text{ROH} + H_2O + \text{GSSG}$$

$$\text{GSSG} + \text{NADPH} + H + \xrightarrow[\text{reductase}]{\text{glutathione}} 2 \text{ GSH} + \text{NADP}^+$$

$$\text{NADP}^+ + \text{G6P} \xrightarrow{\text{G6P dehydrogenase}} \text{NADPH} + H^+ + \text{6P-gluconate}$$

Since G6P dehydrogenase is a known −SH requiring enzyme, one might have expected it to be inactivated by ozone.   If this is the case it is clear that this decrease is overshadowed by the increase in response to stress. Recovery from ozone stress can overshoot the normal level when the stress is removed: a case in point is the increase in nonprotein SH in rat lungs.[28]   The work of DeLucia *et al.*[29] also shows that acute exposures (2 ppm O_3, 4-8 hr) lower the activity of G6P dehydrogenase.   This may be interpreted as both direct inactivation and inhibition of the compensatory response.

Goldstein *et al.*[30] have noted that the red blood cells of mice exposed to ozone have less acetylcholineesterase activity and less glutathione. The same result was obtained by Buckley *et al.*[31] from the blood of human volunteers exposed to ozone. Goldstein and McDonagh[32] examined the effect of ozone on membranes of isolated human red cells and again observed the decrease in acetylcholineesterase and thiol, but they also found a large decrease in the fluorescence due to tryptophan. However, the total tryptophan was little changed. It appears that the small population of tryptophan residues in a hydrophilic environment are readily accessible to ozone attack while those in a hydrophobic environment neither fluoresce nor are accessible to ozone.

In the study of Buckley *et al.*[31] the level of G6PD rose in the red cells as it had in lungs of rats exposed to ozone. It should be remembered that decrease in GSH and increase in the hexose monophosphate pathway specific activity in red cells is a general response to oxidative stress and is not restricted to ozone.[33]

Summary: Proteins and Amino Acids

The effects of ozone on proteins and amino acids are most easily detected as changes in enzymic activities. Direct effects lower the activities of various enzymes depending on their reliance on amino acids susceptible to oxidation by ozone. Indirect effects can cause increases in enzymic activity because of the response of the system to ozone. For example, exposure of lungs to ozone causes a change in cell type of the epithelium. It is to be expected that the new distribution of cell type will exhibit a different spectrum of enzyme activities.

Research with pure proteins has shown the variation in susceptibility. Lysozyme is very susceptible to inactivation by ozone whereas urease is very resistant. The results obtained with pure proteins must be followed by investigations of the relevance in biological systems at ozone concentrations experienced in polluted atmospheres. The susceptibility of lysozyme is in good agreement with the decrease in the tears of people exposed to polluted air. On the other hand, the finding of susceptibility of a purified blood serum protein may well be irrelevant either because (1) very little ozone reaches the blood or (2) ozone reaching the blood reacts mostly with the predominant protein, serum albumin.

REACTIONS WITH LIPIDS

Comparison of Ozonolysis and Lipid Peroxidation

In the biological literature there has been a predeliction to consider ozonization and peroxidation as synonymous. They are not.

Peroxidation

The reaction scheme is shown in Figure 7.1. Features of this system are that the product is indeed a lipid peroxide (which may be converted to the corresponding hydroxide in biological systems), that the product has conjugated double bonds that can be detected by absorbance at 233 nm, and that fatty acids with three or more double bands yield malonaldehyde as a minor reaction product.[34,35]   Malonaldehyde is frequently measured after reaction with thiobarbituric acid, but it can also be detected because of the absorbance of the enol form above pH 7 at 267 nm.[36]

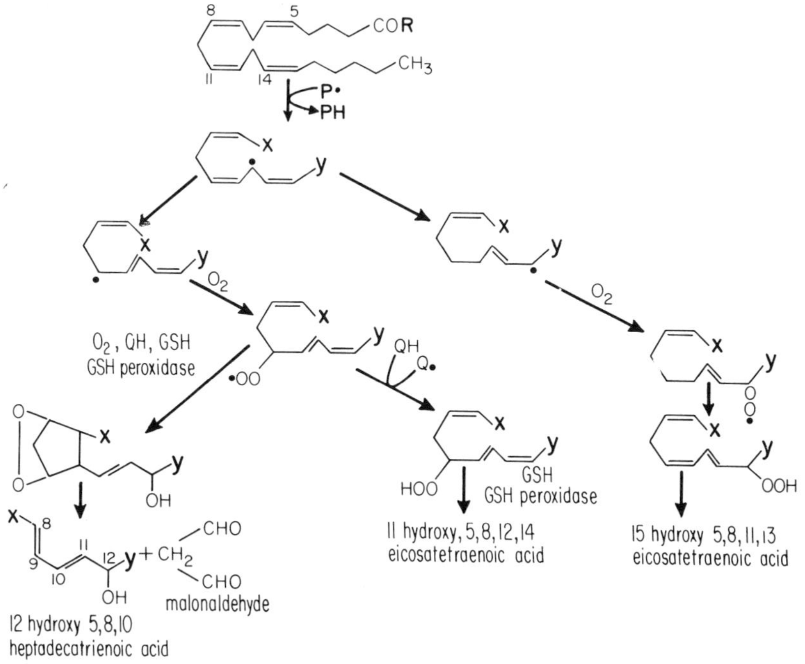

Figure 7.1   Schematic representation of lipid peroxidation.

Ozonization

There is no reason to believe that ozonization in biological materials proceeds any differently than in chemical systems.[37] Figure 7.2 shows reaction schemes for monoenoic and polyenoic systems ozonized in water. If the compound ozonized is a methylene-interrupted double bond system, malonaldehyde can be produced directly. Hydrogen peroxide is formed if the ozonolysis is conducted in aqueous mixtures. In contrast to lipid peroxidation, there are no radical intermediates, there is no lipid peroxide, and there is no conjugation of double bonds. The only point in common with peroxidation is malonaldehyde production, and unfortunately this is usually measured as an index of lipid peroxidation in ozone treated systems.

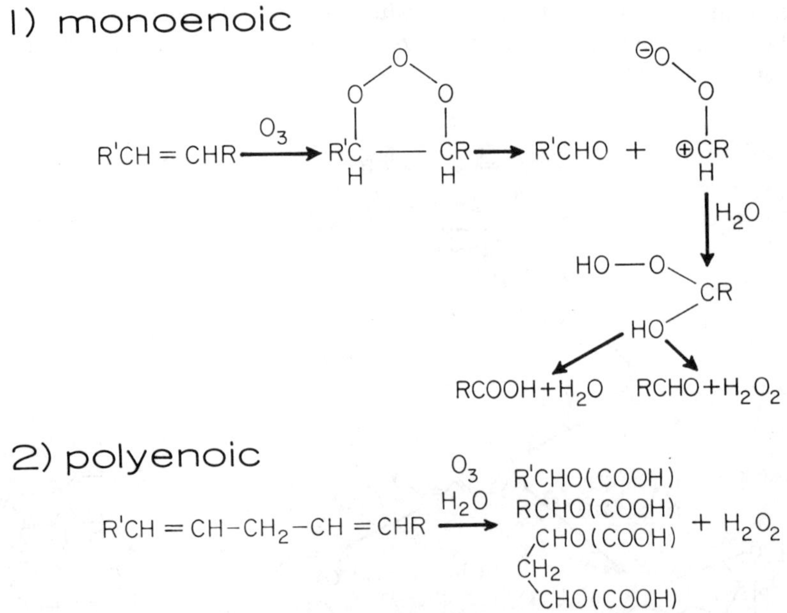

Figure 7.2 Schematic representation of ozone reaction with monoenoic and polyenoic fatty acids.

It is possible that the hydrogen peroxide or the hydroxyhydroperoxide could initiate radical reactions giving rise to lipid peroxidation, but this should be considered a side reaction. Bailey *et al.*[38] have presented evidence for free radical formation during ozonization of trimesitylvinyl alcohol, a highly hindered olefin, but they state ". . . no radical has heretofore been characterized or observed, to our knowledge, as a primary product of ozonization of an olefin." If lipid peroxidation does take place in biological systems exposed to ozone, we view this as a secondary action, comparable to the initiation of lipid peroxidation by chaotropic reagents.[39,40]

Pure Fatty Acids

Reaction of ozone with unsaturated fatty acids in aqueous media yields a mixture of products. Pryde *et al.*[41] found that at pH 6.7 and 2 hr reaction at 100°C there was about half as much carboxylic acid produced as carbonyl compounds. Hydrogen peroxide is produced when the reaction is conducted above neutral pH. It is noteworthy that ozonization in aqueous alkaline hydrogen peroxide diverts primary ozonization products to carboxylic acids.[42] Therefore, it is possible that hydrogen peroxide produced during ozonolysis may be utilized in secondary reactions.

Mudd *et al.*[43] treated oleate and linoleate with ozone in phosphate buffer in the presence or absence of glutathione. In both cases the yield of hydrogen peroxide was 40-50% of the ozone introduced when glutathione was absent. In the presence of glutathione approximately 2 moles SH were oxidized per mole of ozone and no hydrogen peroxide was detected. No malonaldehyde was detected in the case of oleate. The yield of malonaldehyde from linoleate was 2% of the ozone input and this was not changed by the presence or absence of glutathione. This malonaldehyde could only come from direct ozonolysis since peroxidation of linoleate does not produce malonaldehyde.[34] Malonaldehyde is derived in lipid peroxidation by way of a cyclic peroxide.[34,35] Baker and Wilson[44] examined the toxic effect of ozonized fatty acids on glycolysis of Ehrlich ascites cells. The inhibitory property was traced to the hydrogen peroxide produced in the breakdown of the ozonide. Malonaldehyde was eliminated from consideration as the toxic substance.

Roehm *et al.*[45] have compared the effects of ozone and nitrogen dioxide on fatty acids. They found that nitrogen dioxide stimulated production of malonaldehyde and conjugation of double bonds as would be expected from a peroxidation mechanism. These reactions were inhibited by antioxidants much as vitamin E, BHT and BHA. In contrast, films of unsaturated fatty acids exposed to ozone did not show double bond conjugation, but malonaldehyde was produced. This oxidation was unaffected by antioxidants. In aqueous suspensions of unsaturated fatty acids ozone caused some double bond conjugation, and the reaction was partially prevented by antioxidants. In this case there was a mixture of direct ozonolysis and peroxidation. Pryor and Stanley[46] have stated that peroxidation of methyl linoleate can be initiated by ozone.

Goldstein et al.[47] have examined ozone-treated linoleic acid for the production of free radicals. Spin resonance signals were observed, but only after prolonged treatment with ozone and "only while ozonizing." The ozonolysis was done in an aqueous medium and one signal was characteristic of peroxyl, peroxy or hydroxyl free radicals. The other two were attributed to organic radicals.

Pure Phospholipids

Mudd et al.[48] examined the effect of ozone on liposomes prepared from egg yolk lecithin. Since these liposomes formed as lipid bilayers, they have been considered as models of the biological membrane. In the absence of glutathione, hydrogen peroxide was produced to the extent of 15% of the ozone introduced and malonaldehyde to the extent of 0.8%. In the presence of glutathione, —SH was oxidized, no hydrogen peroxide was detected and the malonaldehyde was lowered to 0.4%. By comparison with free fatty acids, the liposomes were more resistant and better protected by glutathione.

Teige et al.[49] studied the reaction of ozone on phospholipid liposomes and on red blood cells. The red blood cells were remarkably resistant to lysis, but the cells were rapidly lysed by the ozonized lipid. This was taken to mean that the lipids in the red cell were very resistant to oxidation by ozone. The ozone-treated liposomes leaked previously trapped glucose. Fatty acid analysis showed that all unsaturated acids were oxidized, and that one mole of hydrogen peroxide was produced for each double bond broken. Malonaldehyde was produced to the extent of 1-2% of the ozone reacted. The ultraviolet absorbance spectrum showed no double bond conjugation, but a new peak at 265 nm was characteristic of the enol of malonaldehyde.[36] Examination of products by GLC/MS revealed the presence of azelaic acid and 9-al-nonanoic acid, the expected products of ozonolysis. Thus in these experiments a classical ozonolysis pathway was preponderant, and no evidence at all was found of lipid peroxidation.

In Vivo and *In Vitro* **Systems**
Related to Lipid Oxidation

Red Blood Cells

Goldstein and Balchum[50] exposed human red blood cells to ozone and found an increase in malonaldehyde. When the treated cells were washed, most of the malonaldehyde was found in the supernatant. Balchum *et al.*[51] using the same system (20 ml of a 1/5 suspension of red blood cells exposed to 40 ppm ozone flowing at 10 ml/min for 2 hr) found a dramatic decrease in the unsaturated fatty acids. Evidence has been presented that hydrogen peroxide is produced in red cells of mice exposed to ozone.[52] This hydrogen peroxide could be attributed to ozonization of double bonds of lipids or other compounds.

Lungs

Goldstein *et al.*[53] reported that a lipid extract from lungs of mice (exposed to 0.4-0.7 ppm for 4 hr) showed an absorbance peak at 233 nm, characteristic of peroxidized lipid. It is noteworthy that rats exposed to 1 ppm NO_2 for 4 hr developed conjugated dienes in the extracted lung lipids only after 16 hr.[60] According to the results of Roehm *et al.*[45] nitrogen dioxide is more likely to initiate peroxidation than is ozone.

Menzel *et al.*[54] found that the fatty acid composition of lung tissue of rats exposed to 1 ppm O_3 for 9 days showed a decline in oleic acid and linoleic acid but a significant increase in arachidonic acid. This increase in arachidonic acid has also been found in lung washings of rats exposed to 1.1 ppm O_3 for 5-7 days (1.3 to 15.6%).[55] There were also increases in linoleic acid (10.3 to 13.1%). These results can not be explained as part of an oxidation scheme but rather must be involved in degradation of complex lipids, infiltration of abnormal materials, or altered metabolic pathways. On longer exposures to ozone (6 weeks at 0.5 ppm ozone) the increase in arachidonic acid was only minor.[56] In contrast to these results Huber *et al.*[57] found no significant change in the fatty acid composition of lung tissue or lung lavage of rabbits exposed to 5 ppm ozone for 3 hr. Dowell *et al.*[58] found that the macrophage lavaged from the lungs of rabbits exposed to ozone were more susceptible to osmotic lysis, but no evidence was found for lipid peroxidation by measuring either double bond conjugation or malonaldehyde. Changes in lipid metabolism in the lung of ozone-treated animals have been indicated by the results of Kyei-Aboagye *et al.*[59] There was decreased incorporation of fatty acids into lecithin but an increased specific activity of lipids found in the lung washings.

Chow and Tappel[23,26,27] have proposed that glutathione peroxidase, glutathione reductase and G6P dehydrogenase are increased in activity in rat lungs in response to the formation of lipid peroxide after exposure to ozone. Lipid peroxide was estimated by measuring malonaldehyde, which could have been formed by alternative pathways (see page 9). Each enzyme rises in response to an imbalance of concentrations of substrates. It should be noted that these substrates include GSH and

NADPH, both of which are readily oxidizable by ozone. The initial stimulation of glutathione peroxidase could also be a response to the formation of hydrogen peroxide rather than lipid peroxide. Chow *et al.*[23] have also noted that in lungs exposed to nitrogen dioxide there were increases in glutathione reductase and glucose-6-phosphate dehydrogenase but not in glutathione peroxidase. This result does not fit well with the hypothesis of detoxification since nitrogen dioxide is known to generate lipid peroxide both *in vitro*[45] and *in vivo*.[60]

Privett and co-workers[61-64] have studied toxic effects of ozonides and lipid peroxides injected into the blood stream of experimental animals. The rationale for these experiments was that ozone could create fatty acid ozonides and peroxides and they were responsible for the toxic effect. The ozonides and peroxides did have a dramatic effect on the lung, comparable to the effect of ozone,[55] but it is not conclusive that this result justifies the rationale. The result testifies to the fragility of the lung. Both hydroperoxide and ozonide increased arachidonate and decreased oleate in the lung lipid (as did ozone). But the compounds also caused edema and it is notable that the lipid analyses of the affected lungs tend towards those of the serum.

Plants

Tomlinson and Rich[65] have analyzed the fatty acids of tobacco leaves exposed to ozone (1 ppm, 30-60 min). The largest decrease was in palmitic acid, and the unsaturated fatty acids were little affected. This result was largely corroborated by Swanson *et al.*[66] who treated tobacco plants for 2 hr with 0.3 ppm ozone. Changes in fatty acid composition were within experimental error. Thin-layer chromatography of the intact lipids also failed to show major changes. Tomlinson and Rich[67] have reported an increase in the sterol derivatives after exposure of tobacco leaves to ozone. Frederick and Heath[68] have exposed *Chlorella* cells to ozone and measured changes in viability, content of malonaldehyde, and fatty acid composition. There was a reciprocal relationship between viability and malonaldehyde, and slight decreases in the unsaturated fatty acids. These experiments were conducted at a flow rate of 2.6 μmol/min and an approximate ozone concentration of 160 ppm, much higher than the previously cited studies on plants. The formation of malonaldehyde was also studied by Tomlinson and Rich.[69] They exposed pinto beans (*Phaseolus vulgaris* L.) to 0.25 ppm ozone for 3 hr, and analyzed the plants 1, 3 and 18 hr after exposure for fatty acid composition and malonaldehyde content. The fatty acid composition was unchanged and malonaldehyde was found only in leaves that had visible symptoms. It was concluded that lipid peroxidation was a consequence of this initial damage caused by the ozone.

Verkroost[70] examined the effect of ozone on *Scenedesmus obtusiusculus.* He passed a gas stream containing 150 ppm ozone at a flow rate of 120 ml/min through 80 ml of culture for 4 hr. After this, photosynthesis was inhibited by 75.6% and there was a decrease in lipid content of 66.7%. However, the fatty acid composition was almost the same as the control, and no malonaldehyde could be detected.

Summary

The reaction of ozone with lipids in model systems indicates that the predominant course of reaction is classical ozonolysis of double bonds. In the presence of water, short chain aldehydes and hydrogen peroxide are major products. In model systems there is little evidence for lipid peroxidation, and inhibitors of free radical reactions have little effect on the oxidation. Ozone increases the permeability of model membrane systems composed of purified phospholipids, concomitant with fatty acid ozonolysis.

In biological systems the importance of the above reactions is questionable. Integral proteins of the biological membrane are exposed and it is conceivable that ozone reacts preferentially with these proteins rather than the lipid of the membrane. There is also evidence that ozone can pass through the cytoplasmic membrane without causing damage, and have its effects inside the cell.

In vivo the changes in lipid components may be secondary events. For example, the increase in arachidonic acid in lungs of exposed animals can hardly be attributed to a direct effect of ozone. Changes in lipid synthetic activity may also be in response to the initial degradative effects of ozone. The type II alveolar epithelial cells that become predominant after ozone exposure have special properties in the synthesis of lung surfactant. The malonaldehyde that is sometimes measured in tissues after ozone exposure may be derived by direct ozonolysis of polyenoic structures or by initiation of lipid peroxidation. In the latter case, we view this as a secondary process in the succession of responses to ozone, cellular disruption similar to that caused by many chaotropic reagents and not specific for ozone.

REACTIONS WITH BIOLOGICAL SYSTEMS

For humans who breathe polluted air, the dosages received can be calculated when the pollutant concentration is known. For example, at

1 ppm and normal temperature and pressure 22.4 liters of inhaled air at 1 ppm pollutant concentration would contain 22.4 μl, *i.e.,* 1μmol of the pollutant. The alveolar ventilation in an average human at rest is 315 liters/hr.[71] Therefore the intake of pollutant in 1 hr breathing 1 ppm O_3 in air would be 14 μmol. (Values for other concentrations and times can easily be calculated.)

If the alveolar surface area is taken as 100 m^2 and the thickness of the cell layer between the alveolar space and the blood in the capillary is taken as 0.5 μm,[71] the volume occupied by this layer is 50 ml. Thus the dosage to the lungs of a person breathing 1 ppm O_3 for 1 hr is 14 μmol/50 ml or 280 μmol/l. The area of the lung actually affected by ozone is in the terminal and respiratory bronchiole region. If this is in the range of 5-10% of the total surface for gas exchange, the dosage in this region may be 2800-5600 μmol/l, and if only the alveolar epithelium is affected, this dosage will increase again by a factor of approximately two.

At the opposite extreme, we can calculate dosage to the blood assuming that inhaled ozone (or any other pollutant) can pass the alveolar epithelium, the basement membrane, and the capillary wall (as oxygen does). If we take the blood volume as 5.0 liters, the dosage for a person breathing 1 ppm for 1 hr would be 2.8 μmol/l. This is at least 100 times less than the lung dosage and maybe 4000 times less.

In plants, the gas exchange depends on the aperture of the stomates. The internal area of the leaf where the gas exchange takes place is 6 to 31 times as large as the surface area of the leaf.[72] Plants are clearly capable of assimilating the carbon dioxide present in the atmosphere at 300 ppm, since all of life depends on photosynthesis. The uptake of gases is proportional to water solubility except in cases where the dissolved gas is rapidly converted, such as CO_2, or reacted, such as O_3.[73] The uptake of gases from the atmosphere by plants is affected by wind velocity below 3 miles/hr. Above 3 miles/hr it was found that the uptake of ozone by alfalfa leaves was 10 μl/min/m^2 leaf area/pphm. The air was being circulated at 6.8 million liters/hr or 30,000 μmol/hr at 0.1 ppm. The uptake under these conditions was 270 μmol/in.^{2} leaf surface. Since the vegetation exposed had a leaf surface of approximately 14 m^2, the total uptake was 3,800 μmol of ozone. Therefore the uptake of ozone was only a fraction of that to which the plants were exposed. This uptake in plants is passive and depends on diffusion, whereas uptake in mammals combines an active intake with a phase limited by diffusion.

The Biological Membrane

The biological membrane serves as a physicochemical interface between two distinct environments. Since there are compositional differences between the cytoplasm and the cell surroundings, an asymmetry between the outer and inner halves of the plasma membrane can be expected and has been observed. Membranes serve as osmotic regulators, are capable of the energy-mediated active transport of molecules against a concentration gradient, maintain an organized and discrete biochemical environment so that biochemical reactions may proceed in an efficient fashion, and provide a scaffolding for many of the enzymes involved in metabolic processes. Membranes found within the cell which make up the endomembrane system also perform similar functions for the mitochondria, endoplasmic reticulum, chloroplasts, lysosomes and microsomes. Although these organelles differ from the plasma membrane in many functions, they also possess structural and chemical similarities.

Proteins are the major component of nearly all cell membranes, from 50 to 70% by weight. The remainder is made up of phospholipids, glycolipids, glycerides and cholesterol. The lipids exist in a bilayer with the polar portions oriented towards the cytoplasm and extracellular regions, while the apolar regions of the lipids such as the phospholipid acyl chains and cholesterol are oriented inwards away from the aqueous environment (Figure 7.3). Extrinsic proteins (Type 2, Figure 7.3) are usually folded in order to internalize apolar amino acids away from the aqueous environment, thus allowing the protein to interact with the cell membrane and its environment via ionic interactions. Partially buried proteins and transmembrane proteins (Type 1, Figure 7.3) are amphipathic, allowing stabilizing interactions with both the polar and nonpolar regions of the membrane lipid phase.[74]   These proteins can in some cases aggregate with themselves and other proteins to form intramembranous particles, the small "bumps" seen on the membrane freeze-etch fracture face of many cell types.

Membrane lipids have characteristic melting points affected by the chain length of fatty acyl moieties, the number of double bonds in these fatty acids, and the relative mol% of cholesterol in the membrane. A membrane having short chain fatty acids containing numerous double bonds will tend to be very fluid. Cholesterol causes phospholipids to pack closer and eliminates the calorimetrically observable lipid fluid to solid phase transitions. Extensive reviews have been published on the fluid nature of the cell membrane.[75,76]

Most membrane components are capable of lateral mobility in the plane of the membrane, with the rate of lateral movement depending on

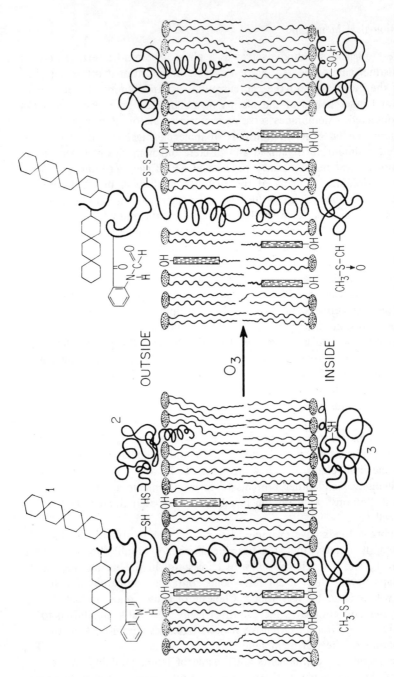

Figure 7.3 Schematic representation of ozone reaction with membrane proteins. Type 2 protein is associated with outer side of membrane, Type 1 protein is transmembranous, and Type 3 protein is associated with inner side of membrane.

the size of the component and the viscosity of the membrane. Membranes are not completely randomized; there is evidence for proteins associating with specific lipid species[77] and for certain lipid species self-associating in heterogeneous areas of the membrane.[78] There is also extensive evidence for cytoplasmic skeletal components mediating the distribution and lateral movement of integral proteins and their sometimes tightly associated lipids.[79] This skeletal network includes the microfilaments and microtubules seen to occur in the alveolar macrophage, and the contractile protein spectrin, which is associated with the human erythrocyte membrane.[80] Hence membrane fluidity and the resulting lateral mobility of membrane components appear to be generally and functionally important phenomena while at the same time there is clear evidence that fluidity and mobility is restricted in certain membranes or regions of membranes under particular conditions.

The distribution of proteins and lipids within most cell membranes is asymmetric. The sugar residues of glycoproteins and most glycolipids are exposed on only the outer face of the membrane.[81] There are enzymes that are characteristic of only the outer half of membranes, while others serve as markers for the cytoplasmic half of the membrane. The human erythrocyte membrane has been seen to have an asymmetric distribution of phospholipids, with the outer half of the bilayer consisting of 100% of the total sphingomyelin and 75% of the total phosphatidyl choline. The inner half of the bilayer contains 100% of the total phosphatidyl serine and 80% of the total membrane phosphatidyl ethanolamine.[82] This phospholipid asymmetry is also maintained in the presence of slow rates of transmembrane "flip-flop" or transposition, a phenomenon not seen with glycoproteins or glycolipids but sometimes seen with cholesterol. Phospholipid transposition has been demonstrated using liposomes bearing spin labels attached to polar phospholipid head groups or by using a purified phospholipid exchange protein to remove ^{32}P-labeled outer bilayer phospholipids. A recent investigation using spin-labeled phosphatidyl choline in intact human erythrocytes reported a transposition $t_{1/2}$ of 7 hr.[83]

The fact that erythrocytes can carry vast amounts of O_2 implies that cell membranes are freely permeable to nonreactive dissolved gases. Evidence to be presented in subsequent sections will also implicate the passage of ozone across cell membranes. Ozone is 10 times more soluble in aqueous systems than oxygen, while oxygen is more soluble in media of lower polarity. A problem in elucidating the effects of ozone on cell membranes and cytoplasmic contents lies in determining whether ozone itself or some product released after the reaction of ozone with cellular constituents (such as H_2O_2, aldehydic compounds, free radicals, hydroperoxides) can be held responsible for the toxic effects. It remains to be seen if ozone reacts in the apolar hydrocarbon region of the membrane with the same efficacy it does in aqueous systems.

Lungs

Extensive ozone inhalation studies using rodents and primates have demonstrated that the lung is the major site of toxicity, with the terminal and/or respiratory bronchiole region and the type I pneumocytes especially susceptible to damage. This quality has made the lung an area of extensive toxicological study. These studies are hampered and sometimes confused by the structural complexity of the lung and by adaptive responses resulting from ozone exposure. There are many distinctive cell types in pulmonary tissue, some of which are unique to the lungs but most of which resemble cells of other organs. Most of these cells are difficult to fractionate, and although they have dissimilar metabolic processes, it would be unreasonable at present to assign biochemical markers to assess the effects of ozone on specific cell types. This becomes especially important when lung responses to ozone exposure are considered, such as the infiltration of serum, the activation and infiltration of polymorphonuclear leucocytes and proliferation of specific undamaged pulmonary cells and organelles. Therefore, microscopy and histochemical techniques have become valuable in determining the effects of ozone on the lung.

Other reported gross changes in lung morphology following exposure to ozone include lesions in the bronchiolar region, shifts from one cell type to another, alterations in the alveolar basement membrane and engorged capillaries adjacent to alveoli. Functional alterations induced by ozone include a decrease in tidal volume and an increase in respiratory rate, both of which can be ascribed to secondary effects of edema. There is also a decrease in airway caliber accompanied by an increase in respiratory flow resistance, possibly occurring as a result of bronchoconstriction caused by histamine released from damaged pulmonary mast cells,[84] or the observed thickening of bronchiolar walls.[85] Increases in lung volume and decreases in lung elasticity have been measured after exposure of animals to ozone. Buell *et al.* suggested that aldehydic compounds produced by ozone oxidation of lung proteins served to cross-link lung material, thereby reducing elasticity.[86]

This section concerns the deleterious effects of ozone on complexes of pulmonary cells that make up functional units, particular cell types, and subcellular organelles of the lung. Some correlations can be made between the biochemical level which are ultimately expressed at the structural-functional level in the lungs.

Alveoli

The alveoli are separated from erythrocytes by only 0.5 μm. The squamous epithelial cells (Type I) overlay most of the alveolar gas exchange surface, and the cuboidal epithelial cells (Type II) can most frequently be seen in the alveolar corners. Type II cells are the site of dipalmitoyl phosphatidylcholine synthesis. This is the principal component of the pulmonary surfactant that lowers the surface tension of the alveoli and allows inflation of alveoli of different diameters with relatively low pressures.

The first observable effects of low ambient ozone concentrations (0.2-0.4 ppm for a few hours) is desquamation and loss of ciliated cells from the trachea, large bronchioles and terminal bronchioles. Type I cells are also lost from alveoli closest to the terminal bronchioles, many times leaving a denuded alveolar basement wall. The number of cells destroyed and the distance of the alveoli from the terminal bronchioles that are affected both seem to be a function of the concentration of ozone the animals are exposed to, rather than the length of the exposure.[87] The Type II pneumocytes are seen to be resistant to the effects of ozone. Stephens[88] saw the Type I cell disappearance as beginning with mitochondrial swelling, followed by a pulling away of the cell from the basement lamina, blebbing of the cell membrane, and eventual plasma membrane disruption, which spews cytosol into the alveolar cavity. Sometimes even the denuded basement lamina disrupts, allowing serum, erythrocytes, and leucocytes responding to tissue damage to enter, resulting in mild edema. All of these observations suggest that ozone is affecting the cell membrane, the contents of the cell and the metabolism of the cell, with cell destruction resulting from one or more of these effects.

Adamson demonstrated that in the developing rat lung, Type II cells divide and generate Type I cells.[89] This process seems to be the mode of alveolar repair in rat lungs after about 24 hr of exposure to 0.5 ppm ozone.[1] The alveoli remain lined with the resistant Type II progenitor cells until cessation of ozone exposure allows the return of Type I cells.

Evans[90] measured ^{3}H-thymidine incorporation into alveolar cells after ozone exposure. Immediately after exposure, the rate of DNA synthesis in the alveolar epithelial cells decreased below control levels. About 24-48 hours after cessation of ozone exposure, the number of cells synthesizing DNA increased up to and above control levels. The intensity of this repair process increased as the concentration of ozone was increased during the exposure period. The increases in DNA synthesis can be ascribed to a replacement of alveolar Type I cells and a proliferation of alveolar

macrophages. The initial decreases in DNA synthesis are probably due
to the disruption of enzymes involved in DNA synthesis and cell division.

Using electron microscopy and histochemical techniques, Castleman *et
al.* have seen changes in the activities of several alveolar enzymes.[91] The
enzymes most affected were those along the walls of the terminal bronchioles and along the interalveolar septa. After rats were exposed to
0.8 ppm for 7 days, ATPase increased, which appeared to be an adaptation phenomenon rather than an increase in alveolar cell number. Infiltration of leucocytes increased the ATPase activity of the alveoli. The
exposed lungs also had decreased NADH and NADPH diaphorase activities
in the ozone-infiltrated areas, suggesting that these intramitochondrial
enzymes are either being inhibited by ozone or that the epithelial cells
that these mitochondria reside in are being destroyed. Decreases in mitochondrial cytochrome oxidase were not seen even though the diaphorases
were inhibited, suggesting that ozone is capable of passing into the
alveoli, crossing the epithelial cell membranes, entering the mitochondria,
and inhibiting the activities of more sensitive enzymes before cell destruction occurs. Zones of alveoli closest to the terminal bronchioles had the
most pronounced changes in enzyme activities, suggesting that most ozone
reacts in these areas with less ozone reaching deeper alveoli.

Alveolar Macrophage

The alveolar macrophage is a bone marrow-derived phagocytic cell
capable of independent division that is found in pulmonary alveolar septa
and air spaces. Macrophages are integral components in the pulmonary
defense system against both living and inert particulates, being able to
sterilize alveoli by ingesting inhaled bacteria. The phagocytic process, reviewed by Stossel,[92] consists of four basic events. There is (1) a chemo-
tactically induced motile response of the macrophage towards the invaded
site, (2) the macrophage selectively recognizes what to attack via endo-
cytosis by determining the surface characteristics of the invading particle,
(3) engulfment, an ATP-dependent process, occurs and oxidative phosphorylation is concurrently stimulated, and (4) engulfment forms a
vacuole termed a phagosome and enzymes are delivered to this opera-
tional site via a fusion process called degranulation. Some of the enzymes
delivered to the phagosome are acid hydrolases, including acid phosphatase,
β-glucuronidase and lysozyme. Changes in the levels and distribution of
these enzymes have been studied after ozone exposure.

Freeman *et al.*[85] observed the number of macrophages recovered from
ozone-exposed dog lungs to increase with the degree of ozone exposure.
Concentration of ozone seemed to be more critical than time of exposure,

i.e., more macrophages were recovered when dogs were exposed to 3 ppm O_3 for 8 hr, as contrasted to a 1 ppm O_3 exposure for 24 hr. Dowell *et al.*[58] exposed rabbits to 10 ppm O_3 for 3 hr and obtained fewer recoverable macrophages by lavage than in controls. When lower ozone concentrations were used (0.5 or 2.0 ppm, 8 hr/day for 7 days) almost twice the control number of macrophages were recovered by lavage. Greater numbers of polymorphonuclear leucocytes and erythrocytes were also seen in the ozone-exposed animals. A loss of viability in isolated macrophages when exposed to as little as 0.06 ppm O_3 for an hour was seen by Weissbecker *et al.*,[93] when measured by the trypan blue exclusion method. It is difficult to reconcile these seemingly conflicting results unless one assumes the isolation of macrophages affects their viability after exposure to low ozone concentration, and that very high ozone concentrations destroy macrophages that might otherwise increase in number.

Alveolar macrophages purified from ozone-exposed rabbits by Dowell *et al.*[70] were seen to be more susceptible to osmotic lysis as ozone exposure increased. This osmotic fragility increase was believed to occur in the absence of lipid peroxidation since there was an absence of thiobarbituric acid-measurable material and there was no evidence of conjugated dienes when the UV absorbance in the 235-238 nm range was measured.

Histochemical investigations by Castleman *et al.*[94] demonstrate an effect of ozone on one of the alveolar macrophage acid hydrolases, acid phosphatase. This enzyme, normally lysosomally localized in the macrophage, was seen to have both a vacuolar and cytoplasmic localization after ozone exposure. Dillard *et al.*[24] obtained biochemical evidence for similar cytoplasmic increases in the lysosomal hydrolases acid phosphatase, cathepsins A, B, C and D, β-N-acetylglucosaminidase, and benzoylarginine-β-napthylamide amidohydrolase when rats were exposed to a concentration of ozone similar to that of Castleman (0.7 ppm for 7 days). The lung lysosomal fraction was seen to lose hydrolytic activity as the cytoplasmic fraction gained activity. Hurst *et al.*[22] also saw this rearrangement phenomenon. These investigators observed an overall depression in hydrolytic activities after their short (3 hr) exposures; activities returned to 90% of control levels 24 hr after cessation of exposure.

The inhibition of the hydrolases was prevented when macrophages exposed to ozone *in vitro* contained GSH in their media,[95] implying that ozone damage is mediated by damage to sulfhydryls, GSH consumes introduced ozone, or that GSH detoxifies ozone-derived substances. Thus it appears that ozone exposure initially depresses lysosomal hydrolase activity in the alveolar macrophage while a concommitant hydrolase subcellular relocalization occurs. Longer exposures to ozone result in an increase in hydrolase activities, which can be ascribed to increased macrophage number. These results also suggest that ozone can cross the macrophage plasma membrane and labilize the lysosomal membrane. Since there is a close association between lysosomal damage and subsequent cell destruction,[96] it appears that the ozone damage to macrophages can be potentiated by the ozone-related release of lysosomal hydrolases into the alveolar macrophage cytoplasm, which could then proceed to break down membrane components.

Investigations by several groups have demonstrated convincingly that ozone has detrimental effects on pulmonary phagocytes (primarily the macrophage), which can reduce their bactericidal activity and increase the susceptibility of organisms to bacterial infection. The experiments of Warshauer *et al.*[97] and Goldstein *et al.*[98] have demonstrated that a 4-hr exposure of rats to 0.5 ppm ozone is the minimum that will cause measurable impairment of pulmonary bactericidal function. Vitamin E deficiency did not affect this threshold dose but vitamin E did protect against longer and more acute exposures. Goldstein *et al.*[99] infected rat lungs with a finely dispersed aerosol of *Staphylococcus aureus,* which became evenly distributed throughout the lung. Unexposed rats were able to phagocytose 90% of the bacteria after 3 hr, with 23% of all bacteria in the lung still viable (*i.e.,* there was a 77% clearance rate). After 2.5 ppm ozone exposure for 4 hr, the rats were able to phagocytose 79% of the bacteria, but there was a negative clearance rate (bacteria were multiplying in the lung). It therefore appears that ozone can cause a minor impairment in the bacterial ingestion properties of macrophages, while at the same time inducing a major impairment in the phagosomal killing mechanisms of the macrophage.

Experiments of Coffin *et al.*[25] indicate that bacterial ingestion by rabbit lung macrophages is inhibited by ozone. These results demonstrate that ozone most likely inhibits the activity of the macrophage hydrolases rather than causing a deleterious effect on the cell membrane or a related contractile system involved in phagocytosis, ultimately resulting in the observed increase in respiratory infections after exposure to ozone. Some of these deleterious effects may be offset by the increases in numbers of alveolar macrophages and the leucocyte infiltration seen in ozone-exposed lungs. Care must also be taken in interpreting biochemical and histochemical results obtained after ozone exposures because the data may reflect cell population or enzyme distribution shifts rather than initial biochemical changes.

Microsomes

When cells are disrupted by certain methods, the endoplasmic reticulum (ER) buds off into small vesicles termed microsomes, which can be either smooth or rough depending on whether the microsomes were derived from ribosome-containing rough ER or smooth ER. Microsomes are bounded by an intact membrane and retain the ability to transport ions, synthesize proteins, metabolize lipids and perform a multitude of other biochemical functions. Microsomes are also extremely rich in a cytoplasmic mixed function oxidase system termed the cytochrome P-450 system, which is an integral part of the systemic armament to oxidize drugs and aromatic hydrocarbons.

Palmer *et al.*[100] have reported decreases in the cytochrome P-450 requiring benz-(a)-pyrene hydroxylase after exposing hamsters to ozone. The effect of ozone on this enzyme may either be a direct effect on the enzyme or on a cofactor required for the reaction such as the cytochrome P-450 system. Goldstein[101] has seen rabbit lung cytochrome P-450 levels decrease 60% 3.5 days after exposure to 1 ppm ozone for 1.5 hr. Palmer *et al.* later measured the effect of ozone on lung bronchial mucosa, which is where most human and benz-(a)-pyrene-induced cancers arise[102] rather than the lung parenchymal tissue previously measured. A 53% decrease in benz-(a)-pyrene hydroxylase resulted from exposure to 0.75 ppm ozone for 3 hr. The levels of this soluble microsomal enzyme returned to normal within 1 day after exposure. These results all imply that ozone may pass at least two barrier membranes to damage cytoplasmic contents, resulting in a possible increased susceptibility to environmental carcinogens. The mechanism of the microsomal enzyme damage is still unclear.

Mitochondria

Investigators have noted that one of the first indicators of cell damage by ozone is a swelling of mitochondria within the cell and a swelling and displacement of cristae.[87] This phenomenon has been seen in both Type II cells and macrophages.[88]

When Rhesus monkeys were exposed to 0.2-0.8 ppm ozone 8 hr a day for 7 days, the mitochondrial enzyme succinate oxidase was seen to increase 20-40% in lung homogenates.[103] Mustafa *et al.* have investigated some of the interactions of ozone with lung mitochondria. Rats exposed to 2 ppm ozone for 8 hr were seen to have a 25% decrease in O_2 consumption (succinate oxidation), which was accompanied by a 25% decrease in tissue SH. There was also no observable evidence of lipid peroxidation as measured by malonyldialdehyde production or the UV absorbance of conjugated dienes.[104]   In this same report, Mustafa observed that a longer exposure period of 0.8 ppm ozone for 15 days stimulated mitochondrial O_2 consumption as much as 45%. Succinate oxidase specific activity was stimulated by only 15%, suggesting that there was proliferation of mitochondria after certain lengths of ozone exposure. This result can probably be correlated with the proliferation of ozone-resistant and mitochondria-rich Type II cells, since increases were seen in both Type II cells and mitochondria recovered from lung homogenates. In addition, an infiltration of mitochondria-containing macrophages and polymorphonuclear leucocytes could increase O_2 consumption in lung homogenates and increase the number of isolatable mitochondria from these homogenates.

Mitochondrial oxidative metabolism in cells recovering from 3 ppm ozone exposure for 4 hr was examined.[105]   Initially O_2 consumption decreased 20% below controls. Twelve hours after cessation of exposure, the control rate of O_2 consumption was reached again. Then, O_2 consumption was 55% over controls 2 days after exposure cessation, and 21 days later the O_2 consumption was still 15% over the control rate. No increases in the number of mitochondria per pulmonary cell were seen, but there was Type II cell proliferation. Total lung mitochondria increased 30% after 4 days of recovery, while there was a concurrent 20% increase in O_2 consumption per milligram mitochondrial protein. These results confirm that ozone exposure initially depresses mitochondrial oxidative metabolism and then results in oxidative metabolism increases during a recovery period, increases due to cell proliferation and increases in oxidative metabolism specific activity. The increase in specific activity could be due to increased work demands or hyperplasia.

Isolated mitochondria from ozone-exposed animals are seen to become more permeable to the entry of NADH across the membrane.[106]   There was also a 20% decrease in mitochondrial protein sulfhydryls and an absence of detectable lipid peroxidation. GSH, α-tocopherol and ascorbate were all unable to afford protection during in vivo ozone exposures, and were unable to reverse ozone-inhibited mitochondrial functions. In ozone-exposed rats and monkeys, there were decreases in substrate utilization, coupled phosphorylation, and respiratory control. Respiratory inhibition can occur when ozone interacts with the respiratory chain at the level of the dehydrogenases, which have SH group functional sites.

Haugaard[107] has demonstrated the importance of SH groups in oxidative phosphorylation by showing that DTNB [5,5'-dithiobis-(2-nitrobenzoic acid)] prevents substrate phosphorylation. The DTNB treatment implied that SH groups were important in the activity of dehydrogenases and P_i entrance into the mitochondria. These observations become more significant for ozone-damaged mitochondria since Freebairn[108] has shown that ozone-exposed suspensions of plant and animal mitochondria can have a reversal in the inhibition of O_2 consumption by the reducing agents GSH and ascorbate.

From the information presently available, it is difficult to assess the mode of ozone interaction with pulmonary mitochondria. It is known that ozone exposure results in an initial swelling and O_2 consumption-inhibition in a single mitochondrion. It is not known whether the subsequent increases in the specific activity of certain mitochondrial enzymes are due to more active unexposed mitochondria from proliferating cells or an alteration in the oxidative metabolism of the exposed mitochondria after recovery. Hackenbrock has observed swelling, cristae deformation and other ultrastructural differences in mitochondria as the metabolic state and rate of electron transport changes.[109,110] Recently, it has also been seen that osmotic swelling of mitochondria can inhibit respiration, probably by disorganizing the putative complex of Krebs cycle enzymes on the inner surface of the inner mitochondrial membrane.[111] It then becomes evident that the ozone-induced alterations in mitochondrial metabolism and morphology can be due to a myriad of possible factors such as a direct effect on membrane lipids allowing permeability changes, inhibition of proteins involved in active transport, and inhibition of cytochromes and dehydrogenases within the mitochondria membrane proteins.

Red Blood Cells

Red blood cells are useful for studying the effects of ozone on cell membranes and cytoplasm since they are metabolically and structurally uncomplicated. Mammalian erythrocytes are not capable of protein synthesis after enucleation and are only able to metabolize sugars using glycolytic and hexose monophosphate pathway enzymes. Therefore, ozone-induced alterations in red cell proteins and lipids *in vitro* should be uncomplicated by adaptive processes.

Ozone has been shown to be responsible for various extrapulmonary effects. Some of these investigations used above-ambient ozone concentrations for short periods of time, which probably does not simulate longer exposure periods at ambient concentrations. Goldstein *et al.*[30] observed decreases in the acetylcholinesterase (AChE) activity of mice breathing 8 ppm ozone for four hours. AChE is an enzyme found partially buried in the lipid portion of the erythrocyte with the catalytic site exposed only on the outside of the cell (Type I, Figure 7.3).

O'Malley *et al.*[112] have shown erythrocyte AChE to be sensitive to H_2O_2 and lipid peroxide *in vitro*. In mice inhaling 0.2 ppm ozone for 2 hr Veninga[113] has observed an increase in serum glutamic-pyruvic-transaminase, an enzyme that indicates liver damage. This investigation and others[114],[115] in which hamsters breathed 0.2 ppm ozone for 5 hr, showed an increased frequency of lymphocyte chromosomal aberrations, with the lymphocytes either binucleated or with broken chromosomes. Exposure of rats and mice to 5 to 7 ppm ozone for 90 min resulted in an increase in the H_2O_2 in circulating erythrocytes.[52] Exposure of the animals to lower levels of ozone did not reveal the presence of H_2O_2. This could be a result of undetectable or no effects of ozone on erythrocyte H_2O_2 levels at low ozone concentrations or the preferential elimination of low concentrations of erythrocyte cytoplasmic H_2O_2 by glutathione peroxidase.[116]

Buckley et al.[117] observed that human volunteers had increased erythrocyte osmotic fragility, glucose-6-phosphate dehydrogenase (G6PD) activity and lactic dehydrogenase (LDH) activity while erythrocyte AChE activity and GSH level decreased after breathing 0.5 ppm ozone for 3 hr. How many of these changes are due to removal of cells from circulation remains to be seen, since it is known that ozone causes sphering of erythrocytes,[117] resulting in an increased rate of splenic sequestration of these misshapen or fragile cells.[40]   Older cells, which are more susceptible to oxidant damage, could then be selectively filtered out of the systemic circulation, effectively resulting in a lowering of the mean age of the remaining cells.   Younger cells are known to have higher ATP levels, more resistance to osmotic lysis,[118] greater G6PD activity[119] and possibly greater LDH activity. If oxidative stress causes any decrease in intracellular ATP or NADPH levels, the activity of the G6PD will increase correspondingly.[120]   Therefore it is difficult to ascribe some of the ozone-related alterations in enzyme activities seen in vivo to adaptational phenomenon when they could be due to changes in mean cell age or an impairment of an unrelated metabolic process. The circulatory alterations observed by the aforementioned investigators are still important because they demonstrate that short exposures to ambient ozone concentrations can cause damage beyond the initial pulmonary site of injury.

In vitro experiments with red cells have shown that ozone is capable of effecting damage to both the inside and the outside of the cell before cell lysis occurs. Goldstein has seen ozone exposure to lower neuraminic acid levels on cell glycoproteins, rendering the erythrocytes more sensitive to complement-mediated antibody damage.[121] The same group has observed oxidation of ozone-susceptible amino acids in exposed membrane proteins.[32] P'an and Jegier[122] observed ozone-inhibition of the activities of outer membrane-bound enzymes.

Goldstein has seen decreases in unsaturated fatty acid levels of erythrocytes exposed to ozone,[51] increases in cellular osmotic fragility and the production of thiobarbituric acid positive materials indicative of lipid peroxidation.[50] Results from our laboratory using approximately four times greater ozone concentration reacting per exposed cell gave different results. No changes in overall phospholipid composition, fatty acid composition and TBA positive material were seen. A 22% decrease in AChE activity and a 30% activity decrease in the electrostatically membrane-bound cytoplasmic enzyme glyceraldehyde-3-phosphate dehydrogenase (GAPD) (Type 3, Figure 7.3) was observed in the presence of 12% hemolysis. GAPD has ozone-sensitive cysteine and tryptophan residues required for catalysis.[123] These results suggested that ozone is capable of passing through the apolar regions of cell membranes without affecting lipids and eventually causing damage to cellular contents.

Menzel et al.[124,125] observed formation of Heinz bodies (irregularly shaped intracellular bodies staining with reducing dyes for light microscopy) after treating erythrocytes with fatty acid ozonides and after exposure of mice to 0.85 ppm ozone for 48 hr. In vitro exposures of human erythrocytes did not result in Heinz bodies when in the absence of ozonides or ozonide sources. Heinz bodies are believed to be a disulfide-linked polymer of methemoglobin sometimes covalently linked to the erythrocyte membrane via a disulfide bridge. These results imply that ozonides produced by the reaction of ozone with lung or serum lipids can have their effects expressed within the erythrocyte.

Shimasaki and Privett[119] incubated red cells with fatty acid hydroperoxides and saw losses in phosphatidylethanolamine, unsaturated fatty acids and α-tocopherol with concomitant increases in fluorescent products and TBA positive materials. The fatty acid hydroperoxides probably oxidized membrane fatty acids, and produced malonyldialdehyde, which is capable of cross-linking amino-containing lipids and producing Schiff's-base fluorophores,[126,127] which would effectively eliminate PE from resolution by TLC. It remains to be seen whether ozone acts by intermediates such as hydroperoxides, since no losses in red cell PE or PS have been observed after ozone exposures.

Plant Cell Membranes

Changes in the permeability of plant cells after exposure to ozone have been reported for 20 years.[128,129,130] Some authors have concluded that there is a direct effect of ozone on membrane function and that the cell membranes are primary sites for ozone attack.[130,131] On the other hand Evans and Ting[132] have reported that ozone and dinitrophenol inhibit potassium transport in a similar manner and have concluded that ozone decreased the energy sources. This observation indicates that the effect of ozone on membrane permeability may be a consequence of an effect on energy metabolism, *i.e.*, an attack on the same site, oxidative phosphorylation, attacked by dinitrophenol. Chimklis and Heath[133] have reported the effect of ozone on potassium efflux from *Chlorella sorokiniana*. They noted that the stimulation of potassium efflux occurred 5-15 seconds after exposure to ozone and concluded that the effect was a primary one. It may be noted that the studies of Jeanjean *et al.*[134] on the effects of N-ethylmaleimide on phosphate uptake by *Chlorella pyrenoidosa* showed that this effect was also very rapid. If the first effect of ozone is on the plasmalemma of plant cells, we are still left with the problem of whether the protein or the lipid component is affected first. The above comments indicate that sulfhydryl oxidation may be a factor.

Hill and Littlefield[135] measured the inhibition of photosynthesis by low concentrations of ozone. Concentrations of 0.6 ppm for 45 min inhibited CO_2 uptake by about 50%. Recovery to control rates took about 2 hr. It was significant that transpiration of water was similarly affected, suggesting an effect on stomates. This was measured and the effects of ozone on photosynthesis and transpiration correlated closely with changes in stomatal aperature. Stomatal closure is associated with large amounts of K^+ efflux from the guard cells.[136] Thus the effect of ozone could be visualized as an effect on permeability. However, several physiological factors affect guard cell turgor and the possibility can not be eliminated that the effect of ozone is on the intracellular mechanism that regulates potassium content. Indeed, the recovery of guard cells when ozone exposure ceases argues against irreparable membrane damage. Thus the effects of ozone on cytoplasmic membrane permeability are almost completely enigmatic in molecular terms.

Bacteria

Relatively little is known about the interactions of ozone with the membranes of microorganisms. Investigations by Hamelin and Chung[137,138] suggest that ozone is capable of crossing the cell wall and membrane because ozone exposure causes *Escherichia coli* mutagenesis, DNA single strand breakage and a detrimental effect on DNA repair enzymes used for recovery from UV light exposure. Scott and Lesher[139] believed that ozone did not enter *E. coli* since a 40-fold excess of ozone over intracellular GSH did not oxidize all of the GSH to GSSG. This is not unreasonable, considering ozone has been seen to react with many more cell components other than sulfhydryls. Therefore, ozone may be able to enter the bacteria. Although there were no substantiating GLC results, bacterial lysis from ozone was felt to be a result of membrane fatty acid oxidation.

Summary

Ozone is seen to have far-reaching effects on cells and their membranes, ranging from oxidation of amino acid residues on exposed cell surface proteins to the inhibition of mitochondrial enzymes necessary for energy metabolism, which are present within the double membrane-containing subcellular organelle. The cellular damage caused by ozone *in vivo* seems to be a function of ozone concentration rather than the duration of exposure, suggesting that the depth of reactive gas infiltration is concentration dependent. It appears that a certain number of cell sites need to become oxidized before necrosis will occur. Longer exposures at low ozone concentration place an oxidative stress on cells and multicellular organelles, which induces tolerance and protective mechanisms. All of these biological responses imply that ozone is affecting all aspects of cellular existence—the synthesis of cell components, the energy metabolism of the cell, the transport of molecules across the cell membrane, cell membrane integrity, and cell reproduction. Experimental evidence has been presented for all of these effects. It now remains to be seen what sequence and relative importance each of these factors have in cell toxicity and damage to whole organisms when exposed to ozone.

ACKNOWLEDGMENT

The authors' research has been supported by Research Grant ES00917 from the National Institute of Environmental Health Sciences.

REFERENCES

1. Stephens, R. J., M. F. Sloan, M. J. Evans, and G. Freeman. "Alveolar Type I Cell Response to Exposure to 0.5 ppm Ozone for Short Periods," *Environ. Mol. Pathol.* 20:11 (1974).
2. Chang, C. W. "Effect of Ozone on Ribosomes in Pinto Bean Leaves," *Phytochem.* 10:2863 (1971).
3. Chang, C. W. "Effect of Ozone on Sulfhydryl Groups of Ribosomes in Pinto Bean Leaves. Relationship with Ribosome Dissociation," *Biochem. Biophys. Res. Commun.* 44:1429 (1971).
4. Gardner, D. E., J. W. Illing, F. J. Miller and D. L. Coffin. "The Effect of Ozone on Pentobarbital Sleeping Time in Mice," *Res. Commun. Chem. Pathol. Pharm.* 9:689 (1974).
5. Previero, A., E. Scoffone, P. Pajetta, and C. A. Benassi. "Indagini della Struttura delle Proteine X Comportamento degli Amminoacidi di Fronte all'Ozono," *Gazz. Chim. Italiana* 93:841 (1963).
6. Previero, A., E. Scoffone, C. A. Benassi, and P. Pajetta. "Indagini sulla Struttura delle Proteine XI Modificazioni del Residuo del Triptofano in Catena Peptidica," *Gazz. Chim. Italiana* 93:850 (1963).

7. Previero, A. and E. Scoffone. "Indagini sulla Struttura della Proteine XII Ossidazione dei Legami desolfuro con Ozono in Peptidi della Cistina," *Gazz. Chim. Italiana* 93:859 (1963).
8. Mudd, J. B., R. Leavitt, A. Ongun and T. T. McManus. "Reaction of Ozone with Amino Acids and Proteins," *Atmos. Environ.* 3:669 (1969).
9. Ordin, L. and B. Propst. "Effect of Airborne Oxidants on Biological Activity of Indoleacetic Acid," *Botan. Gas.* 123:170 (1962).
10. Meiners, B. A. "The Effects of Ozone on Serotonin and Monoamine Oxidase in Rat Lung," Master's Thesis, University of California, Riverside (1974).
11. Previero, A. and E. Bordignon. "Modifica Controllata di Triptofano, metionina, Cistina e Tirosina in Peptidi Naturali e Proteine," *Gazz. Chim. Italiana* 94:630 (1964).
12. Menzel, D. B. "Oxidation of Biologically Active Reducing Substances by Ozone," *Arch. Environ. Hlth.* 23:149 (1971).
13. Mudd, J. B., F. Leh and T. T. McManus. "Reaction of Ozone with Nicotinamide and Its Derivatives," *Arch. Biochem. Biophys.* 161:408 (1974).
14. Giese, A. C., M. L. Leighton and R. Bailey. "Changes in the Absorption Spectra of Proteins and Representative Amino Acids Induced by Ultraviolet Radiations and Ozone," *Arch. Biochem. Biophys.* 40:71 (1952).
15. Todd, G. W. "Effect of Low Concentrations of Ozone on the Enzymes Catalase, Peroxidase, Papain and Urease," *Physiol. Plantanum* 11:457 (1958).
16. Previero, A., M.-A. Coeetti-Previero and P. Jolles. "Localization of Nonessential Tryptophan Residues for the Biological Activity of Lysozyme," *J. Mol. Biol.* 24:261 (1967).
17. Imoto, T., L. N. Johnson, A. C. T. North, D. C. Phillips and J. A. Rupley. In *The Enzymes* VII, P. D. Boyer, Ed. (New York and London: Academic Press, 1972), p. 665.
18. Leh, F. and J. B. Mudd. "Reaction of Ozone with Lysozyme," *Amer. Chem. Soc. Symp. Series* 3:22 (1974).
19. Kuroda, M., F. Sakiyama and K. Narita. "Oxidation of Tryptophan in Lysozyme by Ozone in Aqueous Solution," *J. Biochem.* 78:641 (1975).
20. Sapse, A. T., B. Bonavida, W. Stone and E. E. Sercarz. "Human Tear Lysozyme, III. Preliminary Study on Lysozyme Levels in Subjects with Smog Eye Invitation," *Am. J. Oph.* 66:76 (1968).
21. Holzman, R. S., D. E. Gardner and D. L. Coffin. "*In Vivo* Inactivation of Lysozyme by Ozone," *J. Bacteriol.* 96:1562 (1968).
22. Hurst, D. J., D. E. Gardner and D. L. Coffin. "Effect of Ozone on Acid Hydrolases of the Pulmonary Alveolar Macrophage," *J. Retic. Soc.* 8:288 (1970).
23. Chow, C. K., C. J. Dillard and A. L. Tappel. "Glutathione Peroxidase System and Lysozyme in Rats Exposed to Ozone or Nitrogen Dioxide," *Environ. Res.* 7:311 (1974).
24. Dillard, C. J., N. Urribarri, K. Reddy, B. Fletcher, S. Taylor, B. de Lumen, S. Langberg and A. L. Tappel, "Increased Lysosomal

Enzymes in Lungs of Ozone-Exposed Rats," *Arch. Environ. Hlth.* 25:426 (1972).

25. Coffin, D. L., D. E. Gardner, R. S. Holzman and F. J. Wolock. "Influence of Ozone on Pulmonary Cells," *Arch. Environ. Hlth.* 16:633 (1968).

26. Chow, C. K. and A. L. Tappel. "An Enzymatic Protective Mechanism Against Lipid Peroxidation Damage to Lungs of Ozone-Exposed Rats," *Lipids* 7:518 (1972).

27. Chow, C. K. and A. L. Tappel. "Activities of Pentose Shunt and Glycolytic Enzymes in Lungs," *Arch. Environ. Hlth.* 26:205 (1973).

28. DeLucia, A. J., M. G. Mustafa, M. Z. Hussain and C. E. Cross. "Ozone Interaction with Rodent Lung. III. Oxidation of Reduced Glutathione and Formation of Mixed Disulfides Between Protein and Nonprotein Sulfhydryls," *J. Clin. Invest.* 55:794 (1975).

29. DeLucia, A. J., P. M. Hoque, M. G. Mustafa and C. E. Cross. "Ozone Interaction with Rodent Lung: Effect on Sulfhydryls and Sulfhydryl-Containing Enzyme Activities," *J. Lab. Clin. Med.* 80: 559 (1972).

30. Goldstein, B. P., B. Pearson, C. Lodi, R. D. Buckley and O. J. Balchum. "The Effect of Ozone on Mouse Blood *In Vivo*," *Arch. Environ. Hlth.* 16:648 (1968).

31. Buckley, R. D., J. D. Hackney, K. Clark and C. Posin. "Ozone and Human Blood," *Arch. Environ. Hlth.* 30:40 (1975).

32. Goldstein, B. D. and E. M. McDonagh. "Effect of Ozone on Cell Membrane Protein Fluorescence. I. *In Vitro* Studies Utilizing the Red Cell Membrane," *Environ. Res.* 9:179 (1975).

33. Gaetani, G. D., J. C. Parker and H. N. Kirkman. "Intracellular Restraint: A New Basis for the Limitation in Response to Oxidative Stress in Human Erythrocytes Containing Low-Activity Variants of Glucose-6-Phosphate Dehydrogenase," *Proc. Natl. Acad. Sci.* 71:358 (1974).

34. Dahle, L. K., E. G. Hill and R. T. Holman. "The Thiobarbituric Acid Reaction and the Autoxidations of Polyunsaturated Fatty Acid Methyl Esters," *Arch. Biochem. Biophys.* 98:253 (1974).

35. Niehaus, W. G. and B. Samuelsson. "Formation of Malonaldehyde from Phospholipid Arachidonate During Microsomal Lipid Peroxidation," *Eur. J. Biochem.* 6:126 (1968).

36. Kwon, T.-W. and B. M. Watts. "Determination of Malonaldehyde by Ultraviolet Spectrophotometry," *J. Food Sci.* 28:627 (1973).

37. Bailey, P. S. "The Reactions of Ozone with Organic Compounds," *Chem. Revs.* 58:925 (1958).

38. Bailey, P. S., F. E. Potts and J. W. Ward. "Fre Radical Formation During Organization of a Hindered Olefin," *J. Amer. Chem. Soc.* 92:230 (1970).

39. Hatefi, Y. and W. G. Hanstein. "Lipid Oxidation in Biological Membranes. I. Lipid Oxidation in Submitochondrial Particles and Microsomes Induced by Chaotropic Agents," *Arch. Biochem. Biophys.* 138:73 (1970).

40. Walls, R., S. K. Kumar and P. Hochstein. "Aging of Human Erythrocytes. Differential Sensitivity of Young and Old Erythrocytes

to Hemolysis Induced by Peroxide in the Presence of Thyroxine,"
Arch. Biochem. Biophys. 174:463 (1976).

41. Pryde, E. H., D. J. Moore and J. C. Cowan. "Hydrolytic, Reductive and Pyrolytic Decomposition of Selected Ozonolysis Products. Water as an Ozonization Medium," *J. Am. Oil Chem. Soc.* 45:888 (1968).

42. Fremery, M. I. and E. K. Fields. "Emulsion Ozonization of Cyclo-olefins in Aqueous Alkaline Hydrogen Peroxide," *J. Org. Chem.* 28:2537 (1963).

43. Mudd, J. B., T. T. McManus and A. Ongun. In *Proceedings 2nd International Clean Air Congress,* Inhibition of Lipid Metabolism in Chloroplasts by Ozone. (New York: Academic Press, 1971), p. 256.

44. Baker, N. and L. Wilson. "Inhibition of Tumor Glycolysis by Hydrogen Peroxide Formed from Autoxidation of Unsaturated Fatty Acids," *Biochem. Biophys. Res. Commun.* 11:60 (1963).

45. Roehm, J. N., J. G. Hadley and D. B. Menzel. "Antioxidants *vs.* Lung Disease," *Arch. Int. Med.* 128:88 (1971).

46. Pryor, W. A. and J. B. Stanley. "A Suggested Mechanism for the Production of Malonaldehyde During the Autoxidation of Polyunsaturated Fatty Acids. Nonenzymatic Production of Prostaglandin Endoperoxides During Autoxidation," *J. Org. Chem.* 40:3615 (1975).

47. Goldstein, B. D., O. J. Balchum, H. B. Demopoulos and P. S. Duke. "Free Radicals Associated with Ozonization of Linoleic Acid," *Arch. Environ. Hlth.* 17:46 (1968).

48. Mudd, J. B., T. T. McManus, A. Ongun and T. E. McCullough. "Inhibition of Glycolipid Biosynthesis in Chloroplasts by Ozone and Sulfhydryl Reagents," *Plant Physiol.* 48:336 (1971).

49. Teige, B., T. T. McManus and J. B. Mudd. "Reaction of Ozone with Phosphatidylcholine Liposomes and the Lytic Effect of Products on Red Blood Cells," *Chem. Phys. Lipids* 12:153 (1976).

50. Goldstein, B. D. and O. J. Balchum. "Effect of Ozone on Lipid Peroxidation in the Red Blood Cell," *Proc. Soc. Exp. Biol. Med.* 126:356 (1967).

51. Balchum, O. J., J. S. O'Brien and B. D. Goldstein. "Ozone and Unsaturated Fatty Acids," *Arch. Environ. Hlth.* 22:32 (1971).

52. Goldstein, B. D. "Hydrogen Peroxide in Erythrocytes. Detection in Rats and Mice Inhaling Ozone," *Arch. Environ. Hlth.* 26:279 (1973).

53. Goldstein, B. D., C. Lodi, C. Collinson and O. J. Balchum. "Ozone and Lipid Peroxidation," *Arch. Environ. Hlth.* 18:631 (1969).

54. Menzel, D. B., J. N. Roehm and S. D. Lee. "Vitamin E: The Biological and Environmental Antioxidant," *J. Agr. Food Chem.* 20:481 (1972).

55. Shimasaki, H., T. Takatori, W. R. Anderson, H. L. Horten and O. S. Privett. "Alteration of Lung Lipids in Ozone Exposed Rats," *Biochem. Biophys. Res. Commun.* 68:1256 (1976).

56. Roehm, J. N., J. G. Hadley and D. B. Menzel. "The Influence of Vitamin E on the Lung Fatty Acids of Rats Exposed to Ozone," *Arch. Environ. Hlth.* 24:237 (1972).

57. Huber, G. L., R. J. Mason, M. LaForce, N. J. Spencer, D. E. Gardner and D. L. Coffin. "Alterations in the Lung Following the Administration of Ozone," *Arch. Int. Med.* 128:81 (1971).
58. Dowell, A. R., L. A. Lohrbauer, D. Hurst and S. L. Lee. "Rabbit Alveolar Macrophage Damage Caused by *In Vivo* Ozone Inhalation," *Arch. Environ. Hlth.* 21:121 (1970).
59. Kyei-Aboagye, K., M. Hazucha, I. Wyszogrodski, D. Rubinstein and M. E. Avery. "The Effect of Ozone Exposure *In Vivo* on the Appearance of Lung Tissue Lipids in the Endobronchial Lavage of Rabbits," *Biochem. Biophys. Res. Commun.* 54:907 (1973).
60. Thomas, H. V., P. K. Mueller and R. L. Lyman. "Lipoperoxidation of Lung Lipids in Rats Exposed to Nitrogen Dioxide," *Science* 159:532 (1968).
61. Cortesi, R. and O. S. Privett. "Toxicity of Fatty Ozonides and Peroxides," *Lipids* 7:715 (1972).
62. Privett, O. S. and R. Cortesi. "Observations on the Role of Vitamin E in the Toxicity of Oxidized Fats," *Lipids* 7:780 (1972).
63. Takatori, T. and O. S. Privett. "Studies of Serum Lecithin-Cholesterol Acyl Transferase Activity in Rat: Effect of Vitamin E Deficiency, Oxidized Dietary Fat, or Intravenous Administration of Ozonides or Hydroperoxides," *Lipids* 9:1018 (1974).
64. Tan, W. C., R. Cortesi and O. S. Privett. "Lipid Peroxide and Lung Prostaglandins," *Arch. Environ. Hlth.* 28:82 (1974).
65. Tomlinson, H. and S. Rich. "Relating Lipid Content and Fatty Acid Synthesis to Ozone Injury of Tobacco Leaves," *Phytopath.* 59:1284 (1969).
66. Swanson, E. S., W. W. Thomson and J. B. Mudd. "The Effect of Ozone on Leaf Cell Membranes," *Can. J. Botany* 51:1213 (1973).
67. Tomlinson, H. and S. Rich. "Effect of Ozone on Sterols and Sterol Derivatives in Bean Leaves," *Phytopath.* 61:1404 (1971).
68. Frederick, P. E. and R. L. Health. "Ozone-Induced Fatty Acid and Viability Changes in *Chlorella*," *Plant Physiol.* 55:15 (1975).
69. Tomlinson, H. and S. Rich. "Lipid Peroxidation, a Result of Injury in Bean Leaves Exposed to Ozone," *Phytopath.* 60:1531 (1970).
70. Verkroost, M. "The Effect of Ozone on Photosynthesis and Respiration of *Scenedesmus obtusiusculus*CHOD," *Meded. Landbouwhogeschool Wageningen* 74:19 (1974).
71. West, J. B. *Respiratory Physiology—The Essentials.* (Baltimore: Williams and Wilkins, 1974), p. 185.
72. Turrell, F. M. "The Area of the Internal Exposed Surface of Dicotyledon Leaves," *Am. J. Bot.* 23:255 (1936).
73. Hill, A. C. "Vegetation: A Sink for Atmospheric Pollutants," *J. Air Pollution Contr. Assoc.* 21:341 (1971).
74. Marchesi, V. T., T. W. Tillack, R. L. Jackson, J. P. Segrest, and R. E. Scott. "Chemical Characterization and Surface Orientation of the Major Glycoprotein of the Human Erythrocyte Membrane," *Proc. Nat. Acad. Sci. U.S.A.* 69:1445 (1972).
75. Singer, S. J. and G. Nicolson. "The Fluid Mosaic Model of the Structure of Cell Membranes," *Science* 175:720 (1972).

76. Singer, S. J. "The Molecular Organization of Membranes," *Ann. Rev. Biochem.* 43:805 (1974).
77. Kleeman, W. and H. McConnell. "Interactions of Proteins and Cholesterol with Lipids in Bilayer Membranes," *Biochim. Biophys. Acta* 419:206 (1976).
78. DeKruyff, B., P. Van Dyck, R. Demel, A. Schiujiff, F. Brants and L. L. M. Van Deenen. "Nonrandom Distribution of Cholesterol in PC Bilayers," *Biochim. Biophys. Acta* 356:1 (1974).
79. Nicolson, G. L. "Transmembrane Control of the Receptors on Normal and Tumor Cells. I. Cytoplasmic Influence over Cell Surface Components," *Biochim. Biophys. Acta* 457:57 (1976).
80. Elgsaeter, A., D. M. Shatton and D. Branton. "Intramembrane Particle Aggregation in Erythrocyte Ghosts. II. The Influence of Spectrin Aggregation," *Biochim. Biophys. Acta* 426:101 (1976).
81. Nicolson, G. L. and S. J. Singer. "The Distribution and Asymmetry of Mammalian Cell Surface Saccharides Utilizing Ferritin-Conjugated Plant Agglutinins as Specific Saccharide Stains," *J. Cell. Biol.* 60: 236 (1974).
82. Zwaal, R. F. A., B. Roelofsen, P. Comfurius, and L. L. M. Van Deenen. "Organization of Phospholipids in Human Red Cell Membranes as Detected by the Action of Various Purified Phospholipases," *Biochim. Biophys. Acta* 406:83 (1975).
83. Rousselet, A., C. Guthmann, J. Matricon, A. Bienvenue and P. Devaux. "Study of the Transverse Diffusion of Spin Labeled Phospholipids in Biological Membranes. I. Human Red Blood Cells," *Biochim. Biophys. Acta* 426:357 (1976).
84. Easton, R. E. and S. D. Murphy. "Experimental Ozone Preexposure and Histamine Effect on the Acute Toxicity and Respiratory Function Effects of Histamine in Guinea Pigs," *Arch. Environ. Hlth.* 15: 160 (1967).
85. Freeman, G., R. J. Stephens, D. L. Coffin and J. F. Stara. "Changes in Dogs' Lungs after Long-Term Exposure to Ozone. Light and Electron Microscopy," *Arch. Environ. Hlth.* 26:209 (1973).
86. Buell, G. C., Y. Tokiwa and P. K. Mueller. "Potential Cross-Linking Agents in Lung Tissue. Formation and Isolation After *In Vivo* Exposure to Ozone," *Arch. Environ. Hlth.* 10:213 (1965).
87. Boatman, E. S., S. Sato and R. Frank. "Acute Effects of Ozone on Cat Lungs. II. Structural," *Am. Rev. Resp. Dis.* 110:157 (1974).
88. Stephens, R. J., M. F. Sloan, M. J. Evans and G. Freeman. "Early Response of Lung to Low Levels of Ozone," *Am. J. Pathol.* 74:31 (1974).
89. Adamson, I. and D. H. Bowden. "Derivation of Type 1 Epithelium from Type 2 Cells in the Developing Rat Lung," *Lab Invest.* 32:736 (1975).
90. Evans, M. J., W. Mayr, R. F. Bils and C. G. Loosli. "Effects of Ozone on Cell Renewal in Pulmonary Alveoli of Aging Mice," *Arch. Environ. Hlth.* 22:450 (1971).
91. Castleman, W., D. L. Dungworth and W. S. Tyler. "Histochemically Detected Enzymatic Alterations in Rat Lung Exposed to Ozone," *Exp. Mol. Pathol.* 19:402 (1973).

92. Stossel, T. P. "Phagocytosis," *New Eng. J. Med.* 290:717,774,833 (1974).

93. Weissbecker, L., R. D. Carpenter, P. C. Luchsinger and T. S. Osdene. "*In Vitro* Alveolar Macrophage Viability. Effect of Gases," *Arch. Environ. Hlth.* 18:756 (1969).

94. Castleman, W., D. L. Dungworth and W. S. Tyler. "Cytochemically Detected Alterations of Lung Acid Phosphatase Reactivity Following Ozone Exposure," *Lab. Invest.* 29:310 (1973).

95. Hurst, D. J. and D. L. Coffin. "Ozone Effect on Lysosomal Hydrolases of Alveolar Macrophages *In Vitro*," *Arch. Int. Med.* 9:125 (1971).

96. Slater, T. F. "Lysosomes and Experimentally Induced Tissue Injury," In *Lysosomes in Biology and Pathology*, J. T. Dingle and H. B. Fell, Eds. (Amsterdam: North-Holland Publishing Co., 1969), Vol. 1, p. 469.

97. Warshauer, D., E. Goldstein, P. D. Hoeprich and W. Lippert. "Effects of Vitamin E and Ozone on the Pulmonary Antibacterial Defense System," *J. Lab. Clin. Med.* 83:228 (1974).

98. Goldstein, E., W. S. Tyler and P. D. Hoeprich. "Adverse Influence of Ozone on Pulmonary Bactericidal Activity of Murine Lung," *Nature* 229:262 (1971).

99. Goldstein, E., W. Lippert and D. Warshauer. "Pulmonary Alveolar Macrophage Defense Against Bacterial Infection of the Lung," *J. Clin. Invest.* 54:519 (1974).

100. Palmer, M. S., D. Swanson and D. Coffin. "Effect of Ozone on Benzpyrene Hydroxylase Activity in the Syrian Golden Hamster," *Cancer Res.* 31:730 (1971).

101. Goldstein, B. D., S. Solomon, B. S. Pasternak and D. R. Bickers. "Decrease in Rabbit Lung Microsomal Cytochrome P-450 Levels Following O_3 Exposure," *Res. Commun. Chem. Pathol. Pharmacol.* 10:759 (1975).

102. Palmer, M. S., R. Exley and D. Coffin. "Influence of Pollutant Gases on Benzpyrene Hydroxylase Activity," *Arch. Environ. Hlth.* 25:439 (1972).

103. Dungworth, D. L., W. L. Castleman, G. K. Chow, P. W. Mellick, M. G. Mustafa, B. Tarkington and W. S. Tyler. "Effect of Ambient Levels of Ozone on Monkeys," *Fed. Proc.* 34:1670 (1975).

104. Mustafa, M. G., A. DeLucia, G. K. York, C. Arth and C. E. Cross. "Ozone Interaction with Rodent Lung. II. Effects on Oxygen Consumption of Mitochondria," *J. Lab. Clin. Med.* 82:357 (1973).

105. Mustafa, M. G. "Augmentation of Mitochondrial Oxidative Metabolism in Lung Tissue During Recovery of Animals from Acute Ozone Exposure," *Arch. Biochem. Biophys.* 165:531 (1974).

106. Mustafa, M. G. and C. E. Cross. "Effects of Short-Term Ozone Exposure on Lung Mitochondrial Oxidative and Energy Metabolism," *Arch. Biochem. Biophys.* 162:585 (1974).

107. Haugaard, N., N. H. Lee, R. Kostrzewa, R. S. Horn and E. Haugaard. "The Role of Sulfhydryl Groups in Oxidative Phosphorylation and Mitochondria," *Biochim. Biophys. Acta* 172:198 (1969).

108. Freebairn, H. T. "Reversal of Inhibitory Effects of Ozone on Oxygen Uptake of Mitochondria," *Science* 126:303 (1957).
109. Hackenbrock, C. R. "Ultrastructural Bases for Metabolically Linked Mechanical Activity in Mitochondria. I. Reversible Ultrastructural Changes with Change in Metabolic Steady State in Isolated Liver Mitochondria," *J. Cell. Biol.* 30:269 (1966).
110. Hackenbrock, C. R. "Ultrastructural Bases for Metabolically Linked Mechanical Activity in Mitochondria. II. Electron Transport-Linked Ultrastructural Transofmration in Mitochondria," *J. Cell. Biol.* 37: 345 (1968).
111. Abdul Matlib, M. and P. A. Srere. "Oxidative Properties of Swollen Rat Liver Mitochondria," *Arch. Biochem. Biophys.* 174:705 (1976).
112. O'Malley, B., C. Mengel, W. Merriwether and L. Zirkle. "Inhibition of Erythrocyte Acetylcholinesterase by Peroxides," *Biochem.* 5:40 (1966).
113. Veninga, T. "Ozone-Induced Alterations in Murine Blood and Liver," Preprint 2nd International Clean Air Congress, New York (1970).
114. Zelac, R. and H. Bevis. "Inhaled O_3 as a Mutagen. I. Chromosome Aberrations Induced in Chinese Hamster Lymphocytes," *Environ. Res.* 4:262 (1971).
115. Zelac, H. and H. Bevis. "Inhaled O_3 as a Mutagen. II. Effect on the Frequency of Chromosome Aberrations Observed in Irradiated Chinese Hamsters," *Environ. Res.* 4:325 (1971).
116. Cohen, G. and P. Hochstein. "Glutathione Peroxidase: The Primary Agent for the Elimination of H_2O_2 in Erythrocytes," *Biochem.* 2: 1420 (1965).
117. Lamberts, H., R. Brinkman and T. Veninga. "Radiomimetric Toxicity of Ozonised Air," *Lancet* (January 18, 1964), p. 133.
118. Cohen, N. S., J. E. Ekholm, M. G. Luthra and D. J. Hanahan. "Biochemical Characterization of Density-Separated Human Erythrocytes," *Biochim. Biophys. Acta* 419:229 (1976).
119. Shimasaki, H. and O. Privett. "Studies on Role of Vitamin E in the Oxidation of Blood Components by Fatty Hydroperoxides," *Arch. Biochem. Biophys.* 169:506 (1975).
120. Yoshida, A. "Hemolytic Anemia and G6PD Deficiency," *Science* 179:532 (1973).
121. Goldstein, B. D., L. Lai and R. Cuzzi-Spada. "Potentiation of Complement-Dependent Membrane Damage by Ozone," *Arch. Environ. Hlth.* 28:40 (1974).
122. P'an, A. Y. S. and Z. Jegier. "The Effect of Sulfur Dioxide and Ozone on Acetylcholinesterase," *Arch. Environ. Hlth.* 21:498 (1970).
123. Heilmann, H. D. and G. Pfleiderer. "On the Role of Tryptophan Residues in the Mechanism of Action of Glyceraldehyde-3-Phosphate Dehydrogenase as Tested by Specific Modification," *Biochim. Biophys. Acta* 384:331 (1975).
124. Menzel, D. B., R. J. Slaughter, A. M. Bryant and H. O. Jauregui. "Prevention of Ozonide-Induced Heinz Bodies in Human Erythrocytes by Vitamin E," *Arch. Environ. Hlth.* 30:234 (1975).
125. Menzel, D. B., R. J. Slaughter, A. M. Bryant and H. O. Jauregui. "Heinz Bodies Formed in Erythrocytes by Fatty Acid Ozonides

and Ozone," *Arch. Environ. Hlth.* 30:296 (1975).
126. Trombly, R. and A. L. Tappel. "Fractionation and Analysis of Fluorescent Products of Lipid Peroxidation," *Lipids* 10:441 (1975).
127. Trombly, R., A. L. Tappel, J. G. Coniglio, W. M. Grogan and R. K. Rhamy. "Fluorescent Products and Polyunsaturated Fatty Acids of Human Testes," *Lipids* 10:591 (1975).
128. Erickson, L. C. and R. T. Wedding. "Effects of Ozonated Hexene on Photosynthesis and Respiration of *Lemma minor*," *Amer. J. Bot.* 43:32 (1956).
129. McFarlane, J. C. and I. McNulty. "The Effect of Ozone on Cell Permeability," *Proc. Utah Acad. Sci.* 43:54 (1966).
130. Evans, L. S. and I. P. Ting. "Ozone-Induced Membrane Permeability Changes," *Amer. J. Bot.* 60:155 (1973).
131. Perchorowicz, J. T. and I. P. Ting. "Ozone Effects on Plant Cell Permeability," *Amer. J. Bot.* 61:787 (1974).
132. Evans, L. S. and I. P. Ting. "Effect of Ozone on [86] Rb-Labeled Potassium Transport in Leaves of *Phaseolus vulgaris* L.," *Phytochem.* 8:855 (1974).
133. Chimiklis, P. E. and R. L. Health. "Ozone-Induced Loss of Intracellular Potassium Ion from *Chlorella sorokiniana*," *Plant Physiol.* 56:723 (1975).
134. Jeanjean, R., A. Hourmant and G. Ducet. "Effect des Inhibiteurs de Groupes SH sur le Transport du Phosphate chez *Chlorella pyrenoidasa*," *Biochimie* 57:383 (1975).
135. Hill, A. C. and N. Littlefield, "Ozone Effect on Apparent Photosynthesis, Rate of Transpiration and Stomatal Closure in Plants," *Environ. Sci. Technol.* 3:52 (1969).
136. Raschke, K. "Stomatal Action," *Ann. Rev. Plant Physiol.* 26:309 (1975).
137. Hamelin, C. and Y. S. Chung. "Resistance a lozone chez *Escherichia coli.* II. Relations avec certains mecanismes de reparation de l'ADN," *Molec. Gen. Genet.* 129:177 (1974).
138. Hamelin, C. and Y. S. Chung. "Characterization of Mucoid Mutants of *Escherichia coli* K-12 Isolated After Exposure to Ozone," *J. Bacteriol.* 122:19 (1975).
139. Scott, D., B. McNair and E. C. Lesher. "Effect of Ozone on Survival and Permeability of *Escherichia coli*," *J. Bacteriol.* 85:567 (1963).

CHAPTER 8

AIRWAY HYPERIRRITABILITY INDUCED BY OZONE

J. A. Nadel and L.-Y. Lee

Cardiovascular Research Institute and
Departments of Medicine and Physiology
University of California San Francisco Medical Center
San Francisco, California

Asthma is a disease characterized by recurrent attacks of bronchoconstriction, due in large part to contraction of airway smooth muscle. Classically, asthmatic bronchospasm has been thought to be due to the direct effects on airway smooth muscle of mediators such as histamine released as a result of the reaction of inhaled antigens with specific antibodies fixed to sensitized mast cells. However, this simple explanation of asthma does not adequately explain several facts: First, in healthy individuals, delivery of mediators (*e.g.*, histamine, prostaglandins, serotonin) does not result in asthmatic-type bronchoconstriction. The response to bronchoactive drugs is small in healthy individuals and in no way mimics a clinical attack of asthma. Second, patients with atopic rhinitis may respond with bronchoconstriction to inhaled aerosols of specific antigen but do not have clinical evidence of asthma. Third, in many patients with atopy and asthma, clinical attacks may be precipitated by non-antigenic stimuli, such as cold air, inhalation of irritating chemicals and dusts, respiratory maneuvers (such as hyperventilation, laughing and coughing).

The tendency of patients with asthma to develop bronchoconstriction to a greater extent in response to smaller doses of various stimuli than do healthy individuals appears to be an important characteristic of all asthmatic patients, regardless of the presence or absence of evidence of atopy.[1] The fact that the increased responsiveness to histamine,[1] aerosols of citric acid,[1] aerosols of propellant and surfactant,[2] cold air,[1] and respiratory maneuvers[1] is abolished by atropine suggests that parasympathetic pathways are involved, and we have suggested that an exaggerated vagal reflex response could be a cause of hyperreactivity.[1,3] The stimuli that cause an increased bronchomotor response (e.g., histamine, chemical and mechanical irritants, airway deformation) have one feature in common: They stimulate the rapidly adapting receptors in the airway epithelium. Because stimulation of these receptors results in reflex bronchoconstriction in animals and in healthy humans, we have suggested that damage to the airway epithelium could sensitize the airway epithelial receptors, causing increased bronchoconstriction via a vagal reflex.[3,4] In asthmatic patients, damage to the airway epithelium might be due to inflammatory changes secondary to the immunologic response or could be due to damage by other mechanisms (e.g., respiratory viruses; inhaled pollutants).[5,6]

The study of hyperreactivity in asthmatic patients is complicated by hypertrophy and hyperplasia of airway smooth muscle, the presence of variable degrees of airway obstruction, treatment with drugs, and the occurrence of IgE—mediated antigen—antibody reactions. Therefore, we have turned our attention to healthy subjects who might be expected to have transient damage of the airway epithelium but who are otherwise normal. Our hypothesis is that these individuals will have normal bronchomotor tone (since they will not be releasing mediators), but that they will have an increased response to mediators (e.g., histamine) because of sensitization of vagal epithelial receptors and subsequent reflex bronchoconstriction.

Because viral respiratory tract infections cause transient damage to the airway epithelium,[7] we studied the effect of inhalation of histamine diphosphate aerosol (1.6%, 10 breaths) delivered from a nebulizer (De Vilbiss No. 40) on airway resistance in otherwise healthy subjects with colds.[5] Baseline airway resistance was not significantly different in 16 normal subjects with colds compared with eleven healthy control subjects. However, inhalation of histamine aerosol produced a greater ($218\pm54.6\%$, mean $\pm$ S.E.) increase in airway resistance in the subjects with colds compared with the control group ($30.5\pm5.5\%$ increase; $P<0.01$). Atropine sulfate aerosol (0.2%; 20 breaths) reversed and prevented the exaggerated bronchomotor response in the subjects with colds, indicating that postganglionic cholinergic pathways were involved in the mechanism.

The hyperreactivity was transient and returned to normal in 2-6 weeks. The threshold concentration of citric acid aerosol that produced cough in seven subjects with colds was significantly lower than that in control subjects or in the seven subjects after recovery ($P<0.05$), suggesting that the exaggerated cholinergic response was due to a decreased threshold for stimulation of the rapidly adapting sensory receptors in the airways.

Damage to the airway epithelium can also be produced by ozone.[8,9] If our hypothesis that damage to the airway epithelium is a cause of hyperirritability, then low doses of ozone should cause exaggerated broncho-motor responses to histamine, and these exaggerated responses should be abolished by atropine sulfate or by blocking conduction in the vagus nerves. To study the effect of ozone on the bronchomotor response to histamine in five dogs, we generated ozone by passing a constant flow of filtered dry air into a commercial ozonator (Ozone Research and Equipment, Inc. Model 03VI) and diluted it with clean air in a glass mixing chamber. We monitored the concentration of ozone with a chemilumenescent ozone analyzer (Monitor Lab, Inc. Model 8410) and adjusted the concentration to produce levels between 0.7 and 1.2 ppm by weight. Dogs were exposed during anesthesia (sodium pentobarbital, 25-30 mg/kg, iv). Administration of 2% histamine aerosol (DeVilbiss Nebulizer, No. 40; 5 breaths) increased total pulmonary resistance (R_L) reproducibly in each dog (mean increase, 5.1 cm $H_2O/l/s$). On the day of ozone exposure the increase of R_L after histamine was unchanged. Twenty-four hours after ozone exposure, the baseline R_L was unchanged compared to the control state before ozone, but the increase of R_L caused by histamine (mean, 10.7 cm $H_2O/l/s$) was greater than in the control state. This transient state of bronchial hyperreactivity was maximal twenty-four hours after exposure to ozone and returned to control levels gradually over 7-28 days.

To test our hypothesis that cholinergic postganglionic pathways were involved in the increased responsiveness of the airways to inhaled histamine aerosol, we pretreated the dogs with atropine sulfate aerosol (1.5% solution; 10 breaths). Atropine did not affect the baseline R_L significantly, either before or after ozone, indicating that little baseline "cholinergic tone" existed in the airways. Before ozone, atropine diminished the peak increase of R_L caused by histamine from 5.4 to 3.8 cm $H_2O/l/s$. After ozone, atropine diminished the peak increase of R_L after histamine from 9.7 to 4.5 cm $H_2O/l/s$. After atropine, the bronchomotor response to histamine after ozone was not significantly different from pre-ozone controls, implicating postganglionic cholinergic pathways in the increased response to histamine after ozone. Since the vagus nerves provide the cholinergic innervation of the airway smooth muscle, we studied the effect of blocking conduction in the cervical vagus nerves. Cooling the vagus nerves did not affect baseline R_L significantly, before or after ozone, confirming our impression that little cholinergic tone existed. Before ozone, vagal cooling diminished the peak increase of R_L after histamine from 4.8 to 3.9 cm $H_2O/l/s$. After ozone, vagal cooling diminished the peak increase of R_L after histamine from 9.4 to 4.4 cm $H_2O/l/s$. Thus, during vagal cooling the bronchomotor response to histamine before and after ozone was not significantly different.

These studies indicate that short term exposure to low concentrations of ozone causes a marked increase of bronchial reactivity to inhaled histamine in otherwise healthy dogs. Histamine can act locally on airway smooth muscle, and it can also stimulate vagal sensory receptors in the airways and cause reflex bronchoconstriction. These two effects may occur in varying degrees under varying conditions. The fact that atropine or cooling of the vagus nerves abolished the increased response to histamine implicates the cholinergic vagal pathways. Ozone at low concentrations causes airway epithelial damage, and we propose that this damage "sensitizes" the vagal sensory receptors and increases the reflex response when they are stimulated (*e.g.*, by histamine). The rapid, shallow breathing pattern observed after inhalation of ozone[10] may also be explained by oxidant damage to the airway epithelium with subsequent effects on vagal nerve endings and reflex stimulation of ventilation.

Ozone concentrations in ambient atmospheres may approach the concentrations used in this study. Consequent airway epithelial damage may increase the bronchial reactivity, especially in patients with pulmonary diseases (*e.g.*, asthma).

ACKNOWLEDGMENTS

Supported in part by: U.S. Public Health Service Program Project Grant HL-06285 and Pulmonary SCOR Grant HL-14201 and HL-19156. Studies of viruses performed in conjunction with D. W. Empey, L. A. Laitinen, L. Jacobs and W. M. Gold. Studies of ozone performed in conjunction with E. R. Bleecker.

REFERENCES

1. Simonsson, B. G. "Clinical and Physiological Studies on Chronic Bronchitis. III. Bronchial Reactivity to Inhaled Acetylcholine," *Acta Allergol.* 20:325 (1965).
2. Sterling, G. M. and J. C. Batten. "Effect of Aerosol Propellants and Surfactants on Airway Resistance," *Thorax* 24:228 (1969).
3. Nadel, J. A. "Structure-Function Relationships in the Airways: Bronchoconstriction Mediated Via Vagus Nerves or Bronchial Arteries; Peripheral Lung Constriction Mediated Via Pulmonary Arteries," *Med. Thorac.* 22:231 (1965).
4. Simonsson, B. G., F. M. Jacobs and J. A. Nadel. "Role of Autonomic Nervous System and the Cough Reflex in the Increased Responsiveness of Airways in Patients with Obstructive Airway Disease," *J. Clin. Invest.* 46:1812 (1967).
5. Empey, D. M., L. A. Laitinen, L. Jacobs, W. M. Gold and J. A. Nadel. "Mechanisms of Bronchial Hyperreactivity in Normal Subjects After Upper Respiratory Tract Infection," *Amer. Rev. Respir. Dis.* 113:131 (1976).

6. Nadel, J. A. "Airways: Autonomic Regulation and Airway Responsiveness," In: *Bronchial Asthma: Mechanisms and Therapeutics.* E. B. Weiss and M. S. Segal, Eds. (Boston: Little Brown & Co., 1976), pp. 155-162.
7. Hers, J. F. Ph. and J. Mulder. "Broad Aspects of the Pathology and Pathogenesis of Human Influenza," *Amer. Rev. Respir. Dis.* 83(2, pt 2):84 (1961).
8. Boatman, E. S., S. Sato and R. Frank. "Acute Effects of Ozone on Cat Lungs. II. Structural," *Amer. Rev. Respir. Dis.* 110:157 (1974).
9. Scheel, L. D., O. J. Dobrogorski, J. T. Mountain, J. L. Svirbely and H. E. Stokinger. "Physiologic, Biochemical, Immunologic and Pathologic Changes Following Ozone Exposure," *J. Appl. Physiol.* 14:67 (1959).
10. Folinsbee, L. J., F. Silverman and R. J. Shephard. "Exercise Responses Following Ozone Exposure," *J. Appl. Physiol.* 38:996 (1975).
11. Bleecker, E. R., D. J. Cotton, S. P. Fischer, P. D. Graf, W. M. Gold and J. A. Nadel. "The Mechanism of Rapid, Shallow Breathing After Inhaling Histamine Aerosol in Exercising Dogs," *Amer. Rev. Respir. Dis.* 114:909 (1976).

CHAPTER 9

PACKING OF LIPIDS IN CELL MEMBRANES, ENTRANCE OF FOREIGN MOLECULES, MEMBRANE STRUCTURE AND MEMBRANE FUNCTION

G. Rouser

> Division of Neurosciences
> City of Hope National Medical Center
> Duarte, California 91010

with the assistance of
R. C. Aloia

> Departments of Anesthesiology and Biochemistry
> Loma Linda University
> Loma Linda, California 92354

BULK-PHASE PROPERTIES OF LIPIDS IN MEMBRANES

Lipids in cell membranes are associated with protein. It has been shown that although some molecules of lipid interact with protein, most of the lipid molecules pack next to other lipid molecules to form a bulk phase that retains the properties native to the pure lipid. The close similarity of the properties of lipids in membranes to the lipid extracted from the membranes was first recognized by differential scanning calorimetry of bacterial whole cells and lipids extracted from them.[1] In the study, calorimetry was used as a means to detect phase transitions as a function of temperature. Subsequent work has extended the findings to other bacteria, fungi, protozoa, plants and animal cell membranes.[2-21] Phase transitions largely dependent upon lipids were defined by the use of spin-labeled molecules, X-ray diffraction, force–area relationships of lipid monolayers, measurement of the activities of various enzymes and the rate of transport of various substances, as well as calorimetry. In addition to the studies in which lipid in membranes was compared with extracted lipid, there is a

141

sizable volume of literature relating the activities of enzymes and transport rates to differences in the fatty acid composition of membrane lipids.

The close similarity of phase transitions of pure lipids and lipids in membranes is observable only when the lipids are hydrated as in mono-layers over water or bilayer vesicles. Since anhydrous lipids have very high melting points, it is apparent that the polar groups of lipids in membranes are hydrated. Also, since the phase transitions of a molecular species of a phospholipid are not in general obscured by mixing other species, it appears that lipid molecules in general show a high preference for packing in domains composed of the same molecular species.

Each method used to detect phase transitions has certain limitations. Thus, an enzyme or transport system may not be associated with all of the lipids in a membrane, and thus may not show all of the transitions dis-closed by other methods. There are two different types of phase transi-tions (see next section). This was first clearly recognized when a spin label was used to detect phase transitions of dioleoyl phosphatidyl choline.[19] Differential scanning calorimetry had been used to show that the transition to the solid state begins at -20°C. The spin label method showed another transition at +29°C. The failure of calorimetry to detect some transitions is attributable to a canceling effect caused by balancing endothermic and exothermic processes. Thus, when transitions involve both acyl chain orientations and a change in the degree of hydration of polar groups, calorimetry may not show a peak. In addition, some spin labels do not appear to enter all lipid compartments since they do not show all of the transitions disclosed by other spin labels. Also, X-ray diffraction is generally used to detect transition to the solid state by the appearance of the characteristic 4.2-Å spacing. Thus, the method will not define the other type of phase transition noted above.

ENTRY OF FOREIGN MOLECULES INTO MEMBRANES

Spin label studies have shown that a variety of molecular sizes and shapes can be accommodated in membranes. Many spin labels are lipophilic, but one, Tempo, is a small molecule with appreciable water solubility that enters both polar and hydrocarbon regions of membranes. Thus, it appears that exclusion from this space is largely based upon molecular size, and the presence of ionic groups.

The hydrocarbon free space can be considered as a vibrational space. Entry of a foreign molecule would thus decrease acyl chain conformational changes. Also, when a sufficient amount of the foreign molecule enters, the increase in disorder of packing can cause a lowering of the typical transition temperature as shown for yeast grown in the presence of adamantane[12] and growth of bacterial cells that do not normally contain cholesterol in a cholesterol supplemented medium.[6] Since adamantane lowered the transition by about 5°C and cholesterol by 6°C, and the latter was incorporated to about 9-12% by weight, it appears that foreign molecules may occupy up to 12% of the total lipid space or up to about 18% of the total hydrocarbon space. The latter figure is probably somewhat higher than the true vibrational space since it includes some stretching that results in alteration of membrane permeability, and causes such phenomena as a doubling of oxygen consumption by adamantane-grown yeast.

Two striking examples of the effects of the entry of foreign molecules on membranes are the hemolysis of red blood cells by retinal[24] and the inactivation of lipid-containing viruses by butylated hydroxy toluene.[25] Red cell hemolysis by retinal is related to a lipid-phase transition at about 22°C since entry of retinal and hemolysis are blocked below 20-22°C. Entry into membranes of other types of cells is also related to the general toxicity at high vitamin A intake levels. The inactivation of lipid-containing viruses by BHT is a clear indication of the effects of a commonly ingested substance upon a membrane. The lipid viruses are composed of a membrane surrounding a nucleic acid core. The viruses are formed by insertion of virus protein into the host cell plasma membrane followed by approach of the core to the membrane surface and budding off of the virus particle.

The examples given above show the extensive implications of the entry of foreign molecules into membranes for environmental pollutant effects, general membrane structure-function relationships, virology, immunology, cancer research etc. Entrance of anesthetic molecules is considered in a later section of this chapter. Results of systematic studies of foreign molecule entry and effects are not available. Thus, it is clear that a systematic investigation beginning with individual molecular species available by chemical synthesis combined with studies of isolated membranes and whole animal effects is of great importance. These investigations will involve detailed definitions of how membrane lipids pack. Recent advances in this area are considered in the following sections.

THE PHYSICAL STATES OF LIPIDS AND DEFINITION OF TRANSITION FROM ONE STATE TO ANOTHER BY GRAPHIC METHODS

Lipid molecules show a marked tendency to associate. Although single-chain lipids such as hydrocarbons and alcohols can be heated to a temperature that will produce a free-flowing (nonviscous) liquid as can mono-, di-, and triglycerides, phospholipids in the anhydrous state have melting points that are very high, with some being well above 100°C and independent of the nature of the acyl chains. When transitions are determined for hydrated phospholipids as bilayer vesicles or monolayers, they are much lower and match those found for lipids in membranes as noted previously. Even when hydrated, it appears from physical measurements that phospholipids do not exist as free-flowing liquids. Polar lipids in general appear to have two characteristic phase transitions and thus appear to exist in three states that can be designated: viscous liquid (VL); soft solid (SS); solid (S). Each transition represents a change to a more highly associated, ordered state. Although the transitions for individual molecular species of polar lipids have a fairly abrupt onset, they extend over a range of $5.5^{\circ}C$ to $16.5^{\circ}C$. The range is observed by differential scanning calorimetry and spin label data plotted arithmetically. However, when the proper plot of spin label motion vs $1/K^{\circ}$ is used, only the high-temperature side of the transition makes an appreciable alteration in the slope of the line. Thus, definition of transitions is preferable in general from the high-temperature side. The transitions can be designated: VL→SS and SS→S. In addition to these general transitions, some lipids show a second solid-state change that has been referred to as the pretransition. This transition appears to be the result of a shift from tilted packing of molecules in the solid phase at lower temperatures to vertical packing at higher temperatures. This difference in packing appears to explain the difference between melting points of lipids with an even number vs an odd number of carbon atoms. This transition can be designated, ST→SVt (solid tilted to solid vertical).

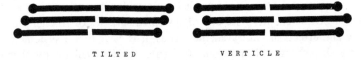

TILTED   VERTICLE

Diagram 1

Although the conformation of carbon chains has generally been assumed always to be the fully extended, zig-zag arrangement, this appears to be incorrect. Measurement of carbon-carbon distances of various acyl chains in urea and thiourea adducts disclosed two conformations.[26] One was the traditional zig-zag with a carbon to carbon distance of 1.260 Å and the other a curled or twisted conformation with a carbon-carbon distance of 1.100 Å. It was subsequently shown[27] that the twisted, 1.100 Å conformation is characteristic of acyl chains in the liquid state, or what is termed here the viscous liquid state. The twisted conformation was shown to be the only one compatible with density and volume data. As will be shown below, a third, shorter (more twisted) conformation is characteristic of the solid state.

Although most of the data for spin label motion was presented in the literature as log motion vs $1/°K$, graphic analysis shows the correct function to be Motion vs $1/°K$, for the ratio hydrocarbon to polar component. When the correct plot is used for spin label motion in lipid vesicles, the relationship is similar to that seen on the log vs $1/°K$ plot, but phase transition points can be fixed more accurately. A dramatic difference is noted, however, with data for spin label motion in some membranes. Thus, data presented as log motion vs $1/°K$ for 5N10 in LM cell plasma membrane vesicles shows a series of straight lines with distinct slope changes,[21] whereas the correct plot, motion vs $1/°K$, gives a single line with only small deviations upward at phase transitions, and returns to the general line over a small temperature range (compensation). In contrast, lipid extracted from the membranes shows permanent slope changes, and motion goes down at phase transitions. Lipid extracted from membranes gives the result expected from studies of individual molecular species. Since lipid-protein interaction does not prevent the lipids from undergoing phase transitions, the difference between lipid alone and lipid in membranes appears to be the orientation of the bilayer. Since lipid bilayers orient perpendicular to the plane of the vesicle, it appears that bilayers in the membrane are parallel to the plane of the vesicle. This orientation causes lipid polar groups to face each other, and compensation at phase transitions is explainable as expansion of the molecules that have not undergone a phase transition into the space made available as a result of the phase transition with volume reduction of the molecules they face. This expansion can account for the temporary increase of motion since the space made available as a result of expansion more than compensates for the decrease in motion in the hydrocarbon region of the other species. The return to the general line is a reversal of the expansion effect that is attributable to an increase in hydration of lipid polar groups that reduces the space available for lipid molecules.

Other spin label motion data are in keeping with the interpretation for compensation. Since compensation is not possible with a single molecular species, spin label motion in a membrane reconstituted with a single molecular species of lipid should be the same as motion in pure lipid vesicles. This has been shown to be the case for the Ca^{++} pump as its native lipid does not show compensation of phase transitions. This correlates well with its lipid composition since it is composed of 64-69% phosphotidyl choline that has two major molecular species (with closely similar phase transitions) that can face each other.

The three general types of plots presented in the literature for spin label motion and enzyme and transport process activity illustrated in

Figure 9.1 can be explained as follows: Plots of spin label motion showing only small temporary departures from a general line (no major slope

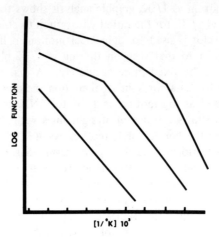

Figure 9.1 Schematic representation of the three general types of Arrhenius plots found in the literature. See text for discussion.

change) arise from the use of the proper plot (motion or log motion vs $1/^{\circ}K$) and compensation, whereas incorrect plots may show one or more slope changes, or, when properly plotted from lack of compensation. The plots of enzyme activity and transport process rates (log vs $1/^{\circ}K$) are attributable to compensation, partial compensation, or the absence of compensation.

Spin label data have been presented mostly as values for the hydrocarbon region, but some data are available for the ratio of the hydrocarbon to polar components. For the ratio to be reliable, phase transitions of water must be excluded as a factor. The method of graphic analysis described in the final section of this chapter was applied to the density and vapor pressure of water. The correct function appears to be log vs $1/^{\circ}K$ for vapor pressure (Figure 9.3). This is readily apparent since a line without slope change over a wide range is obtained. The plot is the compensated type since there is no change at the two transitions visible to the eye (melting and boiling points). In contrast, the function is log density vs $^{\circ}C$, and there are many discontinuities that cannot be fixed accurately with values at intervals of $1^{\circ}C$. Previous studies of the change of properties of water at solid surfaces disclosed transitions at $14\text{-}16^{\circ}$, $29\text{-}32^{\circ}$, $44\text{-}46^{\circ}$ and $59\text{-}62^{\circ}$,[68] that were interpreted as phase transitions, although some authors[69]

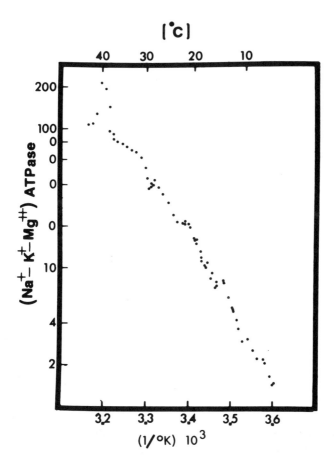

Figure 9.2 Arrhenius plot of aminobutyric acid transport to illustrate the compensated type plot discussed in the text. Redrawn from Reference 21.

attributed similar discontinuities to capillary wall effects. The numerous phase transitions apparent for water indicate that the ratio of hydrocarbon to polar components of spin label motion must be used with caution. It appears that the compensated type of plot obtained for membranes and the vapor pressure of water has not been recognized previously because a small number of widely spaced values were used, and values that deviated more than others from the general line were attributed to error (see page 281 of reference 88).

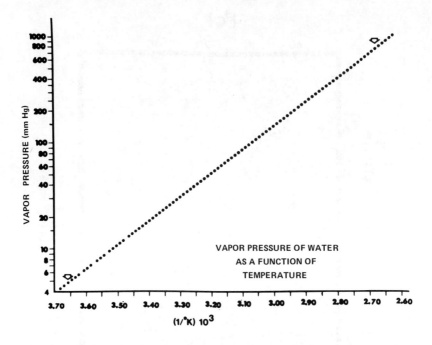

Figure 9.3 Arrhenius plot of the vapor pressure of water as a function of temperature. This is a typical compensated plot that does not show irregularities at known phase transitions (0°C = 3.66 and 100°C = 2.68).

QUALITATIVE AND QUANTITATIVE VARIATIONS IN LIPID COMPOSITION, AND THEIR RELATIONSHIP TO ACYL CHAIN AND MOLECULAR CONFORMATIONS

Lipid classes may be divided into four general groups. The first group consists of lipids that occur largely, if not in most cells entirely, as droplets. This includes triglycerides and cholesterol esters in animals. Because packing of molecules is not under a space-filling regulation as it is in membranes, this type of lipid varies more in fatty acid composition as a function of diet. Plants may utilize other types of long-chain fatty acid esters such as those of long-chain alcohols for storage purposes.

The other three groups of lipids occur in membranes. Each group occupies a separate space that cannot be filled by members of the other groups. Members of one group, the gangliosides and ceramide polyexosides have several carbohydrate residues. It is not surprising that these long, highly polar molecules should occupy a separate space. Evidence that gangliosides are a separate group comes from studies of brain lipids that show large changes with age. Although extensive replacement of one type of ganglioside by another is observed,[28] no replacements are observed between gangliosides and cholesterol, phospholipids, cerebroside or sulfatide.[29] Immunological data for the human red blood cell show clearly that the polar groups of various types of gangliosides and the related ceramide polyhexosides are exposed at the surface and are thus available for interaction with antibodies and/or enzymes such as galactose oxidase. These glycolipids thus appear to insert into the membrane with their polar groups projecting outward from its surface.

Cholesterol is the only member of a separate lipid packing class in animal cell membranes. That it occupies a space not entered by other types of lipids is shown by the failure to find any indication of replacement of cholesterol by other lipids. In addition, after compilation of the data from the literature that included values for cholesterol, phospholipid classes and, in some cases, fatty acids of phospholipid classes, no packing principle for cholesterol with any particular class of phospholipid or particular molecular species of phospholipid was found. This search for correlations showed that there was no way that cholesterol could pack with phospholipids. This subject is considered in more detail in the next section of this chapter.

The fourth group of lipids that can occupy the same type of space are the polar lipids that include phospholipids; phosphatidyl choline (PC), phosphatidyl ethanolamine (PE), phosphatidyl serine (PS), phosphatidyl inositol (PI), phosphatidyl glycerol (PG), diphosphatidyl glycerol (DPG), phosphatidic acid (PA), sphingomyelin (Sph) and ceramide aminoethylphosphonate (CAEP): and the glycolipids; cerebroside (Cer) and sulfatide (Sulf) in animals, and in addition mono- and diglycosyl diglycerides (MGDG and DGDG) in plants and some microorganisms, and the plant sulfolipid (SL). The remarkable feature of polar lipid distribution is its uniformity. The fact that even a one carbon deviation in length is not allowable (*e.g.* propanolamine for ethanolamine, threonine for serine, etc.) shows that polar lipid packing is highly restrained (see later sections). Although animals do not utilize MGDG or DGDG and microorganisms most commonly do not utilize PC, Sph or PS, and some use only acidic phospholipids, these replacements are for length and volume equivalents. Thus, glucose, galactose and inositol are each about the size of a phosphate group or choline and serine moieties when a part of a polar lipid.

The next step in understanding lipid packing principles is the evaluation of quantitative variations of lipid class composition. Although different membranes from the same cell, different organs and different organisms may show large quantitative differences,[30] the composition of each membrane is both characteristic and reproducible. Thus, mitochondria from of all organs are characterized by high DPG, Sph and cholesterol compared to other membranes of the cell. The relative amounts of the lipid classes of mitochondria from different organs differs, but the characteristic features are preserved, and in each organ, quantitative values are very reproducible. Plasma membranes in general have characteristically a lipid class distribution that is the opposite of mitochondrial distribution. Thus, DPG is absent or present in trace amounts, and Sph, PS and cholesterol are higher than in other membranes. These differences do not arise from differences in metabolic production since phospholipids other than DPG and cholesterol are synthesized in the endoplasmic reticulum, and it is characteristically different from other membranes.

Thus, the general picture is one of a highly ordered and reproducible set of lipid class compartments in animal cell membranes. This ordered state is related to the specificity of lipid protein interactions controlled in part by a protein conformation charge code that specifies a particular lipid class. In contrast, in plants that can adapt to lower environmental temperatures, there is extensive replacement among polar lipid classes, and the composition is determined by temperature.[31] The degree of unsaturation of carbon chains required to prevent the formation of too much solid lipid causes lipid class replacement based upon metabolic production of the proper molecular species of each lipid class. Such plants have clearly dropped the charge codes for lipid classes, and thus, in general, molecules of the same length can replace each other. It is to be noted that animals such as the California ground squirrel that adapts for hibernation and can then reduce its body temperature to 1-2°C do not show such lipid class changes. This animal has a polar group charge code and adapts largely by changing fatty acid composition. It is to be noted that a study of lipid requirements for various lipid-dependent enzymes has disclosed a high degree of specificity for lipid-protein interaction. Thus, as an example, β-hydroxybutyric acid dehydrogenase has a high specificity for binding and activation by phosphatidyl choline.

The next step in understanding the principles of membrane polar lipid class packing is to examine and explain the variations in acyl chain composition. The comparison of animals with plants discloses a pattern similar to that noted for phospholipid class composition. Animal cell membranes appear in general to be coded for lipid classes with specific acyl chains. This is shown very clearly by the composition data for linoleic acid ($18^2\Delta^{9,12}$) and arachidonic acid ($20^4\Delta^{5,8,11,14}$) that are derived from linoleic acid. The standard designation for fatty acids is used here. Thus, 18^2 designates an 18 carbon acid with 2 double bonds, and $\Delta^{9,12}$ specifies that the bonds are between carbons 9 and 10 and 12 and 13 counting from the carboxyl group. Molecular species are designated as *e.g.,* $18^0 18^2$, with the acid in position 1 of the molecule given first. Animals cannot synthesize linoleic acid and thus when this acid is excluded from the diet the amounts of linoleic and arachidonic acids in polar lipids are reduced. In response to these deficiencies, $20^3 (\Delta^{5,8,11})$ derived from oleic acid $(18^1 \Delta^9)$ appears in large amount on a fat-free diet. This replacement has been reported in many different studies, and is very widely appreciated. Supplementation of a fat-free diet with linolenic acid $(18^3 \Delta^{9,12,15})$ causes [32] replacement of 20^3 by 20^5 $(\Delta^{5,8,11,14,17})$. It is thus apparent that a code exists from the carboxyl end of the acyl chain, and that the best fit next to 20^4 is 20^5 that has an additional double bond after the four of arachidonic acid. The next best fit is 20^3 that retains the first three double bonds of 20^4.

Replacement of linoleic acid follows a similar pattern in that 18^2 $(\Delta^{9,12})$ is replaced by $18^1 (\Delta^9)$. Thus $18^0 18^2$ is replaced by $18^0 18^1$ and $18^1 18^1$ and $16^0 18^2$ by $16^0 18^1$. There is no $18^2 \Delta^{6,9}$ produced from oleic acid. Thus retention of the first double-bond position from the carboxyl end is of primary importance. Linolenic acid does not replace linoleic acid because it is a shorter molecule (see later sections of this chapter).

Some membranes such as those of the retina have characteristically high $22^6 (\Delta^{4,7,10,13,16,19})$ whose sole precursor is linolenic acid. Although data for a fat-free diet supplemented with linoleic acid do not appear to be available for evaluation of replacements for 22^6, ordinary diets fed to animals and consumed by man are a reasonable approximation of the fat-free plus linoleic acid diet since they have little or no linolenic acid, and the only source of 22^6 is the relatively small amount of 22^6 in the diet. Many membrane analyses do show the presence of high 22^6 along with significant amounts of 22^5, and, in general (as expected), the isomer derived from linoleic acid that retains the first five double bonds of 22^6 is usually larger in amount. The data suggest a somewhat less rigid specificity for 22^6 replacement by 22^5 than replacement of 20^4 by 20^3 or 20^5.

In the nervous system, linoleic acid is a very minor component. Although this is probably due to the presence of a code for 18^1 and the absence of a code for 18^2, it is probably also partly due to the failure of metabolic production of 18^2 molecular species since some bulk-phase (central core) replacement is to be expected (see later sections).

It thus appears that membrane protein can code for saturated acyl chains as well as those with 1,2,4,5, and 6 double bonds. The general absence of 18^3 indicates that there is no code for this fatty acid. In agreement with this is the occurrence of 18^3 in large amounts in bacteria, fungi and plants where acyl chain coding appears to be absent.

Although some analyses of animal membrane phospholipids show the presence of 20^5 (and in some cases without the presence of 20^4), there is no evidence for a code for 20^5.

There are three main features to note about the occurrence of saturated fatty acids in the polar lipids of animals. The first is that odd–carbon fatty acids occur in trace amounts only except for 23^0 and 25^0 in sphingomyelin. Thus, it appears that there is some factor that excludes odd–carbon fatty acids. The chain length range for even carbon saturated acids in animal cells is 14 and 18 carbons, and, in plants, 12^0 can also be present in a significant amount. Animals use longer chain acids (22-26 carbons) in sphingolipids only, whereas some plants use fatty acids with 20-28 carbons in glycerolphospholipids. The natural distribution of the fatty acids correlates quite well with acyl chain conformational differences disclosed by plotting melting point vs 1/# carbon atoms (Figures 9.4-9.6). Data for saturated hydrocarbons, odd–and even–numbered

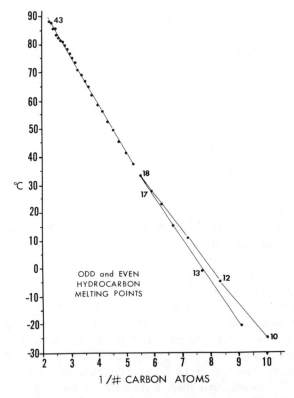

Figure 9.4 Plot of melting points of hydrocarbons vs 1/# carbon atoms. Note convergence of odd and even at 17 carbons.

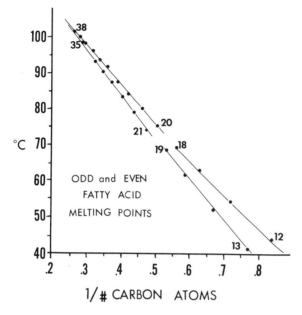

Figure 9.5   Plot of melting points of normal, unsubstituted fatty acids vs 1/# carbon atoms.

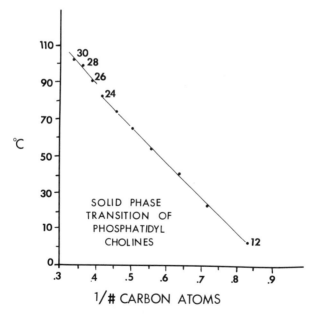

Figure 9.6   Plot of the melting points (solid-state transitions) of hydrated, disaturated phosphatidyl cholines vs 1/# carbon atoms. Values were available for $12^0 12^0$, $14^0 14^0$, $16^0 16^0$, $18^0 18^0$, and $22^0 22^0$. The other values were calculated by the fatty acid melting-point method.

normal fatty acids and phosphatidyl cholines are shown. Similar plots are obtained for alcohols, ketones, and methyl esters of fatty acids. The data for iso fatty acids gave a line without slope change from 12-29 carbons. Members of an homologous series fall on the same line because they are similar in conformation. The similarities and differences correlate well with the natural distribution of acyl chains. The fatty acid plots show conformational similarity between 12 and 18 and 20 to 38 carbons, and it is apparent the replacement of the terminal methyl by a carboxyl group causes a significant conformational change. Plants that have high levels of polar lipids with 20-28 carbon atoms combine two longer chain (20-28) acids in the same molecule, rather than mixed with the 12-18 carbon group of acids which have conformational differences. Glycerol-phospholipids of this type have very high phase transition temperatures. The significance of this is discussed later in this chapter. It is apparent that both groups of acids can be matched with spingosine in sphingomyelin that has a trans double bond. The situation with odd vs even numbers of carbons is also made clear by the plots. The odd carbon acids have lower melting points than predicted from the plot of even carbon acids up to 35 carbons where the lines merge (Figure 9.8). The odd carbon acids occur in large amounts in some bacteria. The situation appears to be like that for the different groups of even carbon acids in that odd carbon acids are placed together rather than mixed in one molecule with even carbon acids, or occur in sphinogomyclin.

Iso and anteiso fatty acids occur in themophilic and thermotolerant bacteria. The isoacids have a methyl group on the next to last carbon ($i18^0$ is 16-methyl-17^0) and anteisoacids have a methyl group on the second to last carbon ($a18^0$ is 15-methyl-17^0). The positional distribution data for thermophilic bacteria and growth data for nonthermophilic organisms such as A. *laidlawii* make it clear that both types of methyl-branched acids can be mixed with even carbon-saturated acids in the same molecule. This is not difficult to understand for the isoacids since they have melting points that are very close to the unsubstituted saturated acid with the same number of carbons (18^0=69.6°C, $i18^0$=69.5°C; 16^0= 62.9°C, $i16^0$=62.4°C), and the plots of melting points are thus closely similar. The plot for anteisoacids shows acids with 12 to 29 carbons to be similar in conformation. It is apparent that, although the anteisoacids are not similar in conformation to the normal saturated fatty acids, their conformations become compatible when incorporated into phospholipids as long as the straight-chain portion of the anteisoacids has an even number of carbon atoms, whereas isoacids are compatible when the straight-chain portion has an odd number of carbons.

The fatty acid composition of the polar lipids of many plants is much more variable than that of animals. Although some plants use 20^4, this acid is generally absent, as are 22^5 and 22^6. Plants in general contain saturated acids with 12,14,16 or 18 carbons as well as oleic, linoleic and linolenic acids ($18^1,18^2,18^3$). The relative amounts of the unsaturated fatty acids is widely variable and extensive replacements between 18^1, 18^2 and 18^3 are apparent and follow changes in environmental temperature. Some plants also have large amounts of $16^2,16^3,16^4$, and 18^4 in their polar lipids. All of these variations point to the general absence of a protein-specified, acyl chain code. Some bacteria and fungi also appear to be largely, if not entirely, without acyl chain codes. The absence of acyl chain codes makes possible extensive shifting of acyl chain composition as an adjustment to prevent too much lipid being present in the solid state at various growth temperatures.

THE POSITION AND PHYSICAL STATE OF CHOLESTEROL IN MEMBRANES

As noted in the previous section, lipid composition data show cholesterol to pack in a separate space in membranes rather than to mix with phospholipids. Each animal cell membrane has a characteristic and reproducible amount of cholesterol that is usually different from the amounts in other membranes of the same cell. There appears to be no alternative to a separate cholesterol space to explain why cholesterol is generally high in plasma membranes and low in mitochondrial membranes. If cholesterol packed with phospholipids, a packing principle based on acyl chain composition and molecular conformation should be apparent, but an extensive search for such a set of principles disclosed in fact that no such principles are shown by the data. *In vitro* data show that cholesterol preferentially interacts with unsaturated rather than saturated molecular species of phosphatidyl choline.[33] The data thus suggest that cholesterol should be higher in mitochondrial lipids since they are generally more unsaturated than those of plasma membranes, but this is not the case.

In addition to the general failure of membrane data to disclose any relationship between cholesterol and polar lipids, there is direct evidence from red blood cell studies that shows cholesterol and phospholipid to occupy different spaces that cannot be occupied by lipids of the opposite type. A portion of the phosphatidyl choline and sphingomyelin of human and dog red blood cells[34] as well as cholesterol[35] exchanges with the corresponding lipids in plasma. Also, about 40% of the red cell cholesterol can be removed by incubation in plasma that has a low free-cholesterol to cholesterol-ester ratio produced by allowing plasma to stand before use. Since phospholipid is available in plasma and some of it exchanges with other phospholipid molecules in the membrane, an increase in the phospholipid content of the membrane can be expected if phospholipid and cholesterol can occupy the same space. No such increase is observed, however. That the cholesterol space is still available is shown by the observation that cholesterol-depleted cells regain their normal cholesterol values when incubated in fresh plasma. Thus, the exchangable cholesterol of the human red blood cell clearly occupies a space that is separate from that of phospholipids and available only to cholesterol molecules. In agreement with this conclusion is the finding that, *in vivo*, bovine red cells show free exchange of labeled cholesterol, but no exchange of phospholipids.[36]

When lipids are heated to the point where transformation from the solid to the soft solid state begins, there is a volume increase as expected for organic compounds in general. This volume increase was shown for dipalmitoyl phosphatidyl choline.[37] When this phospholipid is mixed with cholesterol, monolayer studies show that the area per molecule decreases, *i.e.*, there is a "condensing effect."[38-42] This is indicative of the phospholipid being in the solid state when mixed with cholesterol. In agreement with this conclusion, data obtained with various physical methods have led authors to state that a mixture of phospholipid and cholesterol is more highly ordered than the phospholipid alone (see *e.g.,* reference 43). When order is increased, transition to the solid state occurs at a higher temperature. The use of the spin label Tempo to disclose the phase transitions of phosphatidyl choline-cholesterol mixtures did show,[44] as expected, that the first appearance of the solid phase of a mixture of cholesterol and dimyristoyl or dipalmitoyl phosphatidyl choline was always at a higher temperature than with phospholipid alone, and that the second irregularity in the plots indicative of complete transition to the solid state was at or above the solid-phase transition of the phospholipid alone. In another study[45] chlorophyll-*a* fluorescence was used as a probe. Fluoresence is not observed when chlorophyll molecules aggregate. Since the probe gave a plot very similar to that obtained with Tempo for phospholipid alone, it is apparent that it mixes with the phospholipid. Since the fluorescent intensity was reduced as cholesterol was added and became zero at about 50 mol %, it is apparent that cholesterol and phospholipid molecules mix, and that chlorophyll-*a* is excluded from regions composed of cholesterol alone or cholesterol mixed with phospholipid. It is important to note that both studies show that cholesterol and phosphatidyl choline molecules mix, since it was concluded from vapor pressure studies over monolayers that they will not mix,[46] at least under some conditions. Since the chlorophyll probe monitors only the regions consisting of phospholipid molecules not packed next to those of cholesterol, it does show that a 1/1 molar ratio is the limit for mixing of cholesterol with phospholipids in agreement with the findings by differential scanning calorimetry.[47] Both Tempo and chlorophyll studies are in agreement in that the first appearance of the solid state of phospholipid-cholesterol mixtures is above the solid-state transition of the pure phospholipid alone when the proportion of cholesterol exceeds about 20 mol %. The attempt in the chlorophyll probe studies to arrive at a lower transition temperature is not justified in view of the fact that the data were plotted arithmetically, smooth curves were obtained, and no transition other than that of phospholipid alone can be detected.

Discussions of complex formation between cholesterol and phospholipid molecules appears to be premature. Complex formation implies that molecular association is increased, and this can in general be expected to raise the phase transition temperature since additional energy is required to dissociate a complex held together by favorable conformations. A statement that appears to have caused confusion in the literature is that mixture of cholesterol with phospholipid lowers the phase transition temperature.[23] The calorimetric data presented actually show however that, as the amount of cholesterol added to dipalmitoyl phosphatidyl choline is increased, the amplitude of the phase transition of the pure phospholipid is decreased until it is no longer apparent at about 50 mol %. Thus, differential scanning calorimetry fails to disclose any transitions between about 0°C and 80°C. The failure to detect a phase transition in the mixtures is associated with an increase in nonfreezable water,[23] and thus the failure to detect a transition can be attributed to cancellation by change in polar group hydration as noted in the first section of this chapter.

The conclusions supported by the data are that cholesterol occupies a space different from that of phospholipids, and that cholesterol exists in animal cell membranes in the solid state.

THE PHYSICAL STATES
OF POLAR LIPIDS IN MEMBRANES

It has generally been assumed, without direct evidence, that lipids in membranes do not occur in the solid state. A very clear demonstration that lipids can occur in the solid state in membranes of *Acholeplasma laidlawii* has, however, been presented.[47] This model of careful and systematic investigation included determination of the minimal, optimal and maximum growth temperatures as well as phase transition temperatures of intact cells of *A. laidlawii* and lipid extracted from the cells by differential scanning calorimetry. Growth of this mutant with various fatty acid supplements established that the growth rate was not changed when up to 50% of the lipid could be shown to be in the solid state. Above 50% the rate declined, and growth stopped when over 90% of the lipid was in the solid state. It is thus apparent that solid lipids can enter membranes, and that some organisms can tolerate large amounts of solid lipids. There is however no requirement for solid lipid, since with some supplements, lipids were entirely in the soft-solid or viscous-liquid states at growth temperature.

It appears that cholesterol is the chief lipid that occurs in the solid state in animal cell membranes (see previous section). Phospholipid in the solid state appears to be somewhat less common. One well known case is dipalmitoyl phosphatidyl choline in lung. This particular species with a SS→S transition of 41°C is the predominant form of phosphatidyl choline in lung. A few analyses show phosphatidyl inositol to be composed mostly of stearic acid with some palmitic acid in contrast to the common species $18^0 20^4$ (stearoyl, arachidonyl). Distearoyl phosphatidyl inositol is estimated to begin transition to the solid at 54°C (as discussed later in this chapter). The phase transitions noted for brain cerebroside also place this lipid in the solid state, and some species of sphingomyelin also appear to exist as solids.

Many plants have highly unsaturated molecular species and probably lack solid lipids. It is not unusual however for plants to superimpose upon the unsaturated pattern in which 18^2 and 18^3 predominate (along with some 16^0 and 18^1), a pattern of long-chain saturated fatty acids (20-28 carbons). An example is the sugar beet.[48] The composition of different parts of this plant are different, and show a rather wide range of variation of the types and amounts of long-chain fatty acids in each lipid class. A common upper limit is about 35% 20-carbon and over, but phosphatidyl choline of seedling stalks was reported to have 55% 26^0-cyclopropyl. The presence of long-chain fatty acids is correlated[49] with drought resistance and growth of plants in early spring (where moisture content of the air may be low). In another study,[50] a close inverse correlation was found for chloride ion permeability and the percentage of longer-chain fatty acids in the polar lipids of grape stock roots. The data indicate that plants utilize longer-chain acids in polar lipids to give molecular species that are in the solid state and form part of a water loss barrier. Water loss is also decreased by secretion of longer-chain hydrocarbons in particular to form a nonpolar cover. It is of interest that the correlations in plants are in keeping with the presence of dipalmitoyl phosphatidyl choline in lung in which saturated lipids may also add structural rigidity.

The data available for bacteria and fungi do not indicate the presence of longer-chain acids, and thus a function for solid lipids is not apparent, except perhaps for dipalmitoyl phospholipids and glycolipids.

ESTABLISHMENT OF CHAIN LENGTH EQUIVALENTS FOR UNSATURATED FATTY ACIDS AND THE CONFORMATIONS OF ACYL CHAINS AT DIFFERENT TEMPERATURES

The normal (unsubstituted), saturated fatty acids form a series in which chain length increases by well-defined increments. It is apparent that unsaturated fatty acids have a compatible conformation with saturated acids since together they form most of the molecular species found in membranes of animals in particular. Molecular conformational analysis requires that chain length equivalents (CLEs) of the unsaturated acids relative to the saturated acids be established. Such equivalents can be determined by the nature of the replacements of the unsaturated acids observed when diet is varied. The major findings on a fat-free and fat-free plus 18^3 diets were noted in a previous section. The data plus plant lipid fatty acid replacement show:

$$
\begin{aligned}
\text{CLEs} \quad 18^0 &= 18^1 = 18^2 = 20^3 = 20^4 = 20^5 \\
16^0 &= 16^1 = 16^2 = 18^3 = 18^4 \\
14^0 &= 14^1 = 14^2 = 16^3 = 16^4 \\
12^0 &= 12^1 = 12^2 \\
20^0 &= 20^1 = 20^2 = 22^3 = 22^4 = 22^5 = 22^6
\end{aligned}
$$

The CLEs established in this way are fully checked and confirmed by other forms of data analysis.

Animal diet data provide lengths when chains are in the viscous liquid conformation, as do most plant data. It is also necessary to know CLEs in the soft solid and solid states. The approach to this problem is to examine the melting-point behavior of binary mixtures of fatty acids with different chain lengths. The data required were in fact found in the literature since binary mixtures were studied extensively as an aid in establishing purity of long-chain fatty acids. The general nature of the findings is shown by data in reference 51 in which melting point values for the mixtures palmitic-stearic ($16^0 + 18^0$), palmitic-margaric ($16^0 + 17^0$) and margaric-stearic ($17^0 + 18^0$) were presented. The mixtures gave the three types of melting-point plots reported in the literature. The plots are for values between the melting points of the two fatty acids and show: (1) little or no lowering of the melting point below that of the lowest melting acid ($17^0 + 18^0$); (2) a distinct lowering of the melting point below that of the lowest melting acid with a single minimum (eutectic) at about 1/1 molar ratio (16^0+17^0); 3) a distinct lowering of the melting point below that of the lowest melting acid with two minima (eutectics) at about 1/1 and 3/1 (lowest/highest melting) shown by 16^0+18^0. These are general findings, and the general explanation of chain conformations follows some simple general rules. The data are explained by each carbon chain being able to adopt three conformations that give rise to chain-length equivalents that may be designated as, *e.g.,* with stearic acid:

$18^0 = 18^0$ solid state (shortest length)

$18^0 = 19^0$ viscous liquid state (medium length)

$18^0 = 20^0$ the forced and most extended conformation (longest length)

When examined between the melting points of the two fatty acids, the acid with the higher melting point will be in the solid-state conformation (*e.g.,* $18^0=18^0$), and the lower melting acid will be in the viscous liquid conformation (*e.g.,* $16^0=17^0$). With the mixture 16^0+18^0, two minima are observed as noted above. The packing arrangements are thus:

$18^0 = 18^0$ $18^0 = 18^0$ $16^0 = 17^0$ $18^0 = 19^0$

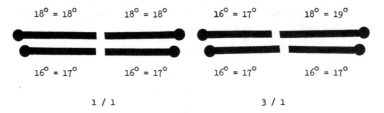

$16^0 = 17^0$ $16^0 = 17^0$ $16^0 = 17^0$ $16^0 = 17^0$

1 / 1   3 / 1

Diagram 2

In both cases, packing is such that each pair of molecules in the bilayer is flanked by an adjacent pair from which it differs in length by two carbon atoms (one on each side of the bilayer). These mismatches cause packing to be less ordered, and thus cause a lowering of the melting point by 4.0 to 6.5°C. The mismatch at 3/1 $(16^0/18^0)$ gives a slightly greater melting-point lowering effect because there is only one possible arrangement of the molecules, whereas at 1/1 some packing can be $18^0 18^0$ next to $18^0 18^0$ and $17^0 17^0$ next to $17^0 17^0$ that will not show the lowering effect. If this explanation is correct, a mixture of 17^0 and 18^0 in which 18^0 is the higher melting (62.8°C and 61.2°C in the data from reference 51) should not show any appreciable melting-point lowering since $17^0=18^0$ and $18^0=18^0$ and there is no chain-length mismatch. This is indeed the case. A small lowering of the melting point (about 0.3°C) is not surprising in view of the fact that the conformation of odd and even carbon acids is not exactly the same as noted earlier. As expected from the above explanation, the mixture 16^0+17^0 should show the chain-mismatch effect because the melting points are $16^0=62.7^\circ$ and $17^0=6l.2^\circ C$. Thus, $16^0=16^0$ and $17^0=18^0$ gives the 2-carbon mismatch. This mixture shows melting-point depression below that of the lowest melting acid from 8-10% up to 98% 17^0 since the melting points of the two acids are close together. There is, however, only one minimum at about 58% 17^0. The second minimum, at about 3/1 $(17^0/16^0)$, is abolished. This is attributable to the molecules adopting, in part, the conformations $17^0=17^0$ and $16^0=17^0$ that abolishes the eutectic. Previously, eutectics were explained as due to clustering or compound formation. This is clearly incorrect since, when the conformations are favorable and molecular interaction is increased (clustering), the effect will be to raise the melting point since more energy is required to separate molecules undergoing the transition from the solid state.

It is to be emphasized that, although each acyl chain has a preferred conformation at any given temperature, chains may be forced to adopt other conformations. Acyl chains must pack one carbon forward or backward as depicted above. Thus, a mixture of 15^0 and 18^0 can utilize the favored conformations. However, in the mixture 14^0+18^0, 14^0 is forced to adopt the fully extended and less favored 16^0 conformation. This forcing is possible only when the ratio of 18^0 to 14^0 is high. As it drops below 5/1 (16.7% 14^0), 14^0 reverts to its favored conformation $(14^0=15^0)$ and a separate phase of 14^0 is formed.

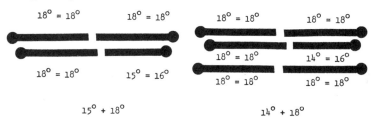

Diagram 3

It is apparent that molecules of 13^0 and 18^0 will not pack side by side at any molar ratio. Such mixtures do however show a eutectic. In such cases, bilayers of the shorter acid are dispersed between bilayers of the longer acid, and eutectics are produced from size differences between pairs of bilayers.

Chain-length equivalents for acids with trans double bonds and methyl branches can be established from mixed melting-point data. Thus, mixtures of stearic acid and elaidic acid ($\Delta^9 18^1$ trans) do not show depressions below the lower melting (elaidic) acid. Mixtures of elaidic acid and palmitic acid show melting-point depression with one minimum at about 73% elaidic acid.[52]   The data establish:

elaidic acid = 18^{1t} = 17^0 (solid) = 18^0 (viscous liquid) = 19^0 fully extended

$\qquad\qquad 18^{1t}$ + 18^0 is (17^0 = 18^0) + (18^0 = 18^0) (no melting-point lowering)

$\qquad\qquad 18^{1t}$ + 16^0 is (17^0 = 18^0) + (16^0 = 16^0) (typical lowering)

In a similar manner, the data[53] show that $i18^0$ (16 methylheptadecanoic acid) has the chain-length equivalent $i18^0=18^0$ solid and 19^0 viscous liquid, since the mixture $i18^0+16^0$ shows melting-point lowering ($i18^0=18^0$ and $16^0=17^0$) whereas $i18^0+17^0$ does not. This type of equivalence appears to extend to other methyl-branch positions since $i19^0$ with the methyl group at the 2 or 4 positions shows melting-point depression when mixed with 17^0 ($i19^0=19^0$ solid with $17^0=18^0$ viscous liquid).

The mixed melting-point data[54] for cis unsaturated fatty acids cannot be used to define their behavior unambiguously because the melting points of the pure acids used do not correspond to those presently accepted. It appears, however, that mixtures of cis unsaturated fatty acids show little or no melting-point lowering (no eutectics) because there is no chain-length difference (e.g., 18^1+18^2) and changes in conformation occur (e.g., 18^3+18^2).

Mixed melting-point data are available for a number of phospholipid molecular species.[55,56]   When incorporated into a double-chain phospholipid molecule, an additional variable is introduced since molecules can adopt conformations that differ with respect to the alignment of the two chains. Thus, conformational analysis of polar lipid molecules consists of defining the degree of mismatch between the position 1 and 2 chains, i.e., the extent to which they differ from the matched position in which both ester groups are directly across from each other, the polar groups extend forward, and are parallel to the long axis of the molecule. As the positions of the chains are shifted, the polar group orientation changes to an angle to the long axis of the molecule. Binding of water molecules is maximal in the matched (M) conformation and decreases as the polar group moves to more acute angles.

When two molecular species of the same lipid class with similar conformations are mixed, the melting-point plots can be expected to be similar to those of fatty acids. The data for saturated molecular species of phosphatidyl cholines show this to be the case.[55]   The spin label Tempo was used to determine the temperature at which transition to the solid state was first detectable, and when the transition to the solid state was complete. The data were presented as phase diagrams at different molar ratios. The diagrams for $18^0 18^0$ PC plus $16^0 16^0$ PC and $16^0 16^0$ PC + $14^0 14^0$ PC were similar and consisted of two smooth curves, separated by up to 5-6°C. The upper line in all cases was very close to the mean value of the SS→S transitions of the two species at each molar ratio. Lowering of the transition temperature below that of the lowest melting component did not occur. As expected from fatty acid data showing 18^0 plus 14^0 to form separate phases at some ratios, $18^0 18^0$ PC mixed with $14^0 14^0$ PC shows two phases when the ratio $18^0 18^0/14^0 14^0$ is less than 3/1.

Data for equimolar mixtures of dioleoyl PC ($18^1 18^1$) and $22^0 22^0$, $18^0 18^0$, $16^0 16^0$ and $14^0 14^0$ PC were obtained by differential scanning calorimetry.[56] The data show clearly that $18^1 18^1$ PC is different in conformation from the saturated species. All mixtures gave similar scans in that the peak of the saturated species disappeared and a new peak a few degrees lower appeared in its place. Thus, some $18^1 18^1$ molecules mixed with all of the molecules of the saturated species, but there was also a separate phase of $18^1 18^1$ because the typical peak at -20°C was apparent. The data are typical for forced acyl chain and molecular conformations discussed below in detail.

Phase-transition temperatures are available for a number of molecular species of several lipid classes.[18,55-57] The data show that species of different lipid classes with the same fatty acids may have the same or different transition temperatures. Thus, when the fatty acid composition is the same, PC, PG, PS and DPG give the same transition temperatures. However, the transitions for PE, PA and diglyceride are similar and differ from those of the PC group. There are thus three conformational groups, the PC type, the PE type and the Sph type. It is apparent that transitions are determined by the combination of fatty acid and molecular conformation and not by the polar group except indirectly by an influence on conformation. Good illustrations are provided by the $18^0 18^1$ combination. $18^0 18^1$ PE and $18^0 18^1$ diglyceride have the same transition temperature (about 35°C) whereas $18^0 18^1$ PC is different in conformation with a transition at about 11°C.[57]

When molecular conformations are the same, i.e., when chains are matched or mismatched to the same degree, the transitions should depend entirely upon the transitions of the acyl chains and thus be directly related to the melting points of the fatty acids. This is indeed the case.

The SS→S transition of one saturated fatty acid species of PC can be calculated from that of other species, and the difference between the melting points of the fatty acids multiplied by 2. Thus, since the melting points of stearic and palmitic acids are 69.6°C and 62.9°C respectively:

$$18^0 18^0 PC = 16^0 16^0 + 2(69.6\text{-}62.9)$$
$$= 41.0 \quad + 13.4 = 54.4°C$$
$$vs = 54°C \text{ reported}$$

When molecular conformations are different, the calculated and observed values will differ. Thus, the difference of 22°C between transition values for $16^0 16^0$PE (63°C) and $16^0 16^0$PC (41°C) represents two different conformations. A similar difference of about 22°C was reported for $18^0 18^1$PE and $18^0 18^1$PC.[57] Conformational differences (polymorphism) are also apparent within a lipid class. Thus in one study, [58] $18^1 18^0$PC was found to have a transition at about 11°C whereas in another it was found to have a transition at 22°C.[59] The difference of 11°C between the values represents a conformational difference that is half that of the PC-PE differences.

The SS→S transition of $18^1 18^1$PC (dioleoyl) begins at -20°C. The value calculated for $18^0 18^1$PC is thus

$$18^0 18^1 PC = 18^1 18^1 PC + (69.6 - 16.3)$$
$$= -20° + 53.3° = +33.3°C$$

The value reported is 11°C[58] that is 22°C lower than the calculated value. Thus, the conformations of these two species is different and shows the 22°C difference noted above for PC vs PE $16^0 16^0$.

The value calculated for the SS→S of $16^0 16^1$PC from $18^0 18^1$PC is

$$16^0 16^1 = 18^0 18^1 - (69.6 - 62.9) - (16.3 - 0.0)$$
$$= 11.0° - 23.0° = -12°C$$

whereas the value reported[60] is about 32°C or 44°C (2 x 22) higher. When $16^0 16^1$PC is calculated from $16^0 16^0$PC the value obtained is SS→S of

$$16^0 16^1 = 16^0 16^0 - (62.9 - 0.0)$$
$$= 41.0 - 62.9 = -21.9°C$$

that is 22 + 32 = 54°C higher (or about 5 x 11 = 55°C). The numerous calculations of this type that are possible invariably show a multiple of 11°C that can be taken as the value for a mismatch of chains by one carbon atom.

The absolute conformation can be assigned from X-ray diffraction data that demonstrated $12^0 12^0$PE to have the acyl chain in position one extending beyond the position two chain by four carbon atoms.[89] Conformations can be designated as M (Matched) or 1F,2F,3F, and 4F when the position one chain extends beyond the position two chain and as 1B,2B,3B and 4B when the chain in the two position extends beyond the position one chain. With PE $16^0 16^0$ as 2F (derived from the comparison of $12^0 12^0$ and $16^0 16^0$PE SS→S transition temperatures), the 22°C difference between PC and PE $16^0 16^0$ places PC $16^0 16^0$ as matched (M). Since the calculations show that $14^0 14^0$, $16^0 16^0$ and $18^0 18^0$PC are similar in conformation, all are matched. The value for $18^1 18^1$PC SS→S becomes

$$18^1 18^1 PC = 18^0 18^0 PC - 2(69.6 - 16.3)$$
$$= 54.0 - 2(53.3) = -52.6°C$$

The value reported is $-20°C$ or $32.6 = 33°C$ (3 x 11) higher. Thus, $18^1 18^1 PC$ is assigned as M + 3 = 3F. This new conformation then determines the SS→VL transition. The difference between the SS→S and VL→SS values for $18^1 18^1 PC$ is $49°C$ ($-20°$ and $+ 29°C$). This is very close to (4 x 11) + 5.5 = $49.5°C$. The $5.5°C$ (11 ÷ 2) effect is assignable to the chain in position one going from the $18^1 = 18^0$ to the $18^1 = 19^0$ conformation and the conformation change is to 4F as transition to the VL state begins. It is apparent that the $11°C$ effect is caused by a $5.5°C$ change at the ester group end plus a $5.5°C$ effect at the methyl end. The second peak shown for $18^0 18^0 PC$ by calorimetry is at $59.5°C$ in some cases. This is also a $5.5°C$ effect in the M conformation explainable by the chain in position one retaining the $18^0 = 19^0$ length and the chain in position two adopting the $18^0 = 18^0$ conformation. This explanation also provides a reason for the conformational differences observed for $18^0 18^0 PC$ that in some cases has a SS→S of $59.5°C$ rather than $54°C$. In this polymorphic form, the conformation is 1F with the chains in both positions in the $18^0 = 18^0$ conformation.

That $5.5°C$ must be subtracted for each carbon atom shortening of the chain in position one when conformations are the same is shown by the calculations for $16^0 18^1 PC$ from $18^1 18^1 PC$ or $16^0 16^0 PC$ and fatty acid melting points, or as the mean of $16^0 16^0 PC$ and $18^1 18^1 PC$. In each case, the calculations give a value of $27°C$, that is $11°C$ higher than the observed value of about $16.0°C$. This is not due to a difference in molecular conformation because the data considered in the following section show that $16^0 18^1$ can pack next to $18^1 18^1$. The $11°C$ difference is caused by the chain in position one being two carbons shorter.

ESTABLISHMENT OF PHASE-TRANSITION TEMPERATURES, MOLECULAR CONFORMATIONS, AND MIXED-SPECIES PACKING PRINCIPLES FOR POLAR LIPIDS

Molecular conformational analysis was described earlier and examples were provided to show the approach used to assign the transition temperatures and conformations given in Tables 9.1-9.3. Each combination of fatty acids gives rise to two different conformational groups of glycerolphospholipids. One group consists of PC, PG, PS, PI and DPG. The other group is PE and PA (that are like diglycerides). Thus, the designations in the tables indicate the groups as PC or PE types. All 18^1 species listed are for the Δ^9 isomer (oleic acid) from which the values for the Δ^{11} isomer (cis vaccenic acid) can be calculated by subtraction of $1.8°C$ for each 18^1 chain.

It is important to note that one species may adopt more than one conformation. Thus, different polymorphic forms of pure lipids may be obtained by

Table 9.1   Transition Temperatures and Conformations for Saturated Species of Phospholipids

LC[a] Type	MS[b]	SS→S °C	MC$_s$	MC$_{ss}$	CC$_{ss}$
PC	26°26°*	91.0	3B	M	27°26°
	25°25°*	81.8	3B	M	26°25°
	24°24°*	83.2	3B	M	25°24°
	23°23°*	73.0	3B	M	24°23°
	22°22°	74.0	3B	M	23°22°
	20°20°*	65.6	3B	M	21°20°
	18°18°	54.0	3B	M	19°18°
	16°16°	41.0	3B	M	17°16°
	14°14°	23.0	3B	M	15°14°
	12°12°	3.2	3B	M	13°12°
	17°17°	37.4		M	18°17°
	15°15°	19.4		M	16°15°
	a17°a17°	16.7		2F	19°18°
	i18°i18°	98.0		4F	19°18°
PE	18°18°	87.0	4F	3F	19°18°
	16°16°	63.0	3F	3F	17°16°
	14°14°	45.0	4F	2F	15°14°
	12°12°	30.7	4F	3F	13°13°
Sph[c]	14°24°	42.1		4F	15°25°
	14°22°	35.5		3F	15°23°
	14°20°	23.3		2F	15°21°
	14°18°	27.5		1F	15°19°
	14°16°	21.0		M	15°17°

[a]Abbreviations: LC type = lipid class type as PC (=PG, PS, PI, DPG), PE (=PA) or Sph; MS = molecular species with the position one acid given first; SS→S = temperature at which the transition from the soft solid to solid state begins. MC$_s$ = molecular conformation in the solid state (the position of the fatty acid in position one relative to that in position two). MC$_{ss}$ = molecular conformation in the soft solid state. M refers to the matched conformation in which the ester groups are directly across from each other and the polar group is parallel to the long axis of the molecules, and 1F, 2F, 3F, 4F refer to the position one chain extending beyond the position two chain by 1, 2, 3 or 4 carbon atoms. CC$_{ss}$ is the carbon chain conformation of position one and two fatty acids in the soft solid state. In all the saturated species, the position two acid retains the conformation characteristic of the solid state of a fatty acid, and the position one acid adopts the conformation of the viscous liquid (VL) state. The designations a and i before the carbon chain number refer to anteiso and iso fatty acids.

[b]SS→S values marked * were calculated by the fatty acid melting-point method described in the text. The SS→VL transition of the PC-type species begin immediately after the SS→S transition and are spread over a 5.5°C range by DSC. The VL→SS transitions of the PE species will begin 33.0° higher than the value given for the SS→S transition. Sph appears to exist in the S and SS states only in the physiological range.

[c]Sph species with monoenoic acids are most probably all below 0°C since the melting points of these acids are far below those of the corresponding saturated acids.

Table 9.2 Transition Temperatures and Conformations for Unsaturated Species of Phospholipids[a]

PC Type				PE Type			
MS	SS→S	MC_{VL}	CC_{VL}	MS	SS→S	MC_{VL}	CC_{VL}
$16^0 18^1$	15.6	4F	$18^0 18^0$	$16^0 18^1$	4.6	3F	$18^0 18^0$
$18^1 18^1$	-20.0	4F	$20^0 18^0$	$18^1 18^1$	-31.0	3F	$20^0 18^0$
$18^0 18^1$	11.3	3F	$20^0 18^0$	$18^0 18^1$	0.3	2F	$20^0 18^0$
$18^0 18^2$	-10.0	3F	$20^0 18^0$	$18^0 18^2$	-21.0	2F	$20^0 18^0$
$16^0 18^2$	-5.7	4F	$20^0 18^0$	$16^0 18^2$	-15.7	3F	$18^0 18^0$
$18^2 18^2$	-62.5	4F	$20^0 18^0$	$18^2 18^2$	-73.6	3F	$20^0 18^0$
$16^0 18^3$	-23.2	2F	$18^0 16^0$	$16^0 18^3$	-34.2	1F	$18^0 16^0$
$18^3 18^3$	-97.6	2F	$18^0 16^0$	$18^3 18^3$	-108.6	1F	$18^0 16^0$
$16^0 20^4$	-50.2	4F	$18^0 18^0$	$16^0 20^4$	-61.2	3F	$18^0 18^0$
$18^0 20^4$	-43.5	4F	$20^0 18^0$	$18^0 20^4$	-54.5	3F	$20^0 18^0$
$16^0 20^5$	-55.1	4F	$18^0 18^0$	$16^0 20^5$	-66.1	3F	$18^0 18^0$
$18^0 20^5$	-48.1	4F	$20^0 18^0$	$18^0 20^5$	-59.4	3F	$20^0 18^0$
$16^0 22^6$	-45.2	4F	$18^0 20^0$	$16^0 22^6$	-45.2	3F	$18^0 20^0$
$18^0 22^6$	-38.5	4F	$20^0 20^0$	$18^0 22^6$	-49.5	3F	$20^0 20^0$
$16^0 16^1$	-6.2	3F	$17^0 16^0$ [b]	$16^0 16^1$	-11.7	2F	$18^0 16^0$ *
$16^1 16^1$	-74.2	2F	$18^0 16^0$	$16^1 16^1$	-85.6	1F	$18^0 16^0$
$16^0 18^{\equiv}$	26.1	M	$18^0 16^0$				

[a]Abbreviations as for Table 9.1 and $18^{\equiv}$ is the Δ^9 triple bond of stearolyic acid. The transition temperatures and conformations were derived as described in the text.

[b]Can occur in membranes as $18^0 16^0$.

Table 9.3 Transition Temperatures for Equimolar Mixtures of Phospholipid Species[a]

PC Type		PE Type	
MS	SS→S	MS	SS→S
$18^1 18^1$ $16^0 18^1$	-2.2	$18^1 18^1$ $16^0 18^1$	13.2
$18^2 18^2$ $16^0 18^2$	-28.5	$18^2 18^2$ $16^0 18^2$	-29.0
$16^0 18^2$ $14^0 18^2$	-29.0	$16^0 18^2$ $14^0 18^2$	-11.9
$18^0 18^1$ $18^0 18^2$	1.3	$18^0 18^1$ $18^0 18^2$	-4.8

[a]Abbreviations as for Table 9.1. Other species that are conformationally similar can also pack together. This includes various species of 20^4, 20^5, and 22^6 (Table 9.2) with species that have higher transition temperatures to cause them to be lowered as in animals prepared for hibernation. This type of mixed packing is not shown because in principle it can vary over a wide range.

evaporation from different solvents. In membranes, the space to be filled may determine (force) a conformation. An example is provided by the Na^+K^+ATPase that was delipidated and then reconstituted with different species of PG.[18] The pure PG species showed transitions like those of PC, but different values arising from different conformations were obtained with the reconstituted enzyme. Thus, $16^0 16^0$ PG gave a peak at about 41°C whereas the enzyme showed a transition at about 30°C. This is the value expected for a shift from the M to the 1B conformation.

Conformational changes cause molecular length to vary. Thus, each one-carbon shift of chain alignment produces a two-carbon length change since one carbon is lost from the chains and another from the new angle forced upon the polar group. Elaidic acid with a $\Delta^9 18^1$ trans double bond shows a wide range of conformations, and its species are discussed here rather than presented in the tables.

The SS→S values calculated for $18^{1t} 18^{1t}$ (from $18^1 18^1$), $16^0 18^{1t}$ (from $16^0 18^1$), $14^0 18^{1t}$ (from $16^0 18^{1t}$), and side by side packing as the mean of the two separate values are:

$$18^{1t}18^{1t}(4F) = \; = \; -20 + 2(43.7\text{-}16.3)$$

	= -20 + 54.8		= 34.8°C
(3F)	= 34.8 - 11.0		= 23.8°C
$16^0 18^{1t}$ (4F)	= 16.0 + (43.7-16.3) + 11.0		= 54.4°C
(3F)	= 54.4 - 11.0		= 43.4°C
$14^0 18^{1t}$(4F)	= 54.4 - (54.4 - 44.2) - 11.0		= 33.2°C
(3F)	= 33.2 - 11.0		= 22.2°C
$18^{1t}18^{1t}$ next to $16^0 18^{1t}$(4F)			
	= 34.8 + 54.4 + 2		= 44.6°C
(3F)	= 44.6 - 11.0		= 33.6°C
$16^0 18^{1t}$ next to $14^0 18^{1t}$(4F)			
	= 54.4 + 33.2 + 2		= 43.8°C
(3F)	= 43.8 - 11.0		= 32.8°C

In three separate studies of *E. coli* mutants grown with an elaidic acid supplement,[7,10,11] transition temperatures were reported for PE monolayers and total lipids extracted from membranes as well as whole cell values for growth rate, growth temperature, respiration, transport, spin label motion and X-ray diffraction spacing. The values reported were: 44°, 43°, 38.7°, 38.0°, 37.7°, 32.4°, 31.0°, 30.7° and 28.0°C. The values are assignable as SS→S transitions of:

43 - 44°C	= $18^{1t}18^{1t}$ next to $16^0 18^{1t}$(4F)		= 44.6°C
	and $16^0 18^{1t}$(3F)		= 43.4°C

$37.7 - 38.7°C$ = mixture of peaks at   = $38.0°C$
$33.2°, 33.6°, 34.8°, 43.4°$
and $44.6°C$ equally weighted
$30.7 - 32.4°C = 16^0 18^{1t}(3F)$ = $32.8°C$
$28.0°C$ = mixture of peaks at $22.2°, 23.8°$,
$33.2°, 33.6°, 34.8°$ equally weighted   = $29.5°C$

The major problem in the studies was the relatively small number of widely spaced values that prevented recognition of all transitions.

The data for mycoplasma strain Y indicate an even wider range of conformations of 18^{1t} species. This organism will incorporate 18^{1t} essentially as its only fatty acid (about 97%), or about equal amounts of even carbon acids with 10 to 20 carbons and 18^{1t}. At first glance, it might appear that such a wide range of chain lengths would cause molecular length to vary, but this is not the case since

$$18^{1t}12^0(M) \ = \ 17^0 13^0 \qquad\qquad = \ 30 \text{ carbons}$$
$$18^{1t}14^0(1B) = \ 17^0 15^0 \text{ - 2 carbons} = \ 30 \text{ carbons}$$
$$18^{1t}16^0(2B) = \ 17^0 17^0 \text{ - 4 carbons} = \ 30 \text{ carbons}$$
$$18^{1t}18^{1t}(2B) = \ 17^0 17^0 \text{ - 4 carbons} = \ 30 \text{ carbons}$$
$$18^0 18^{1t}(3B) = \ 19^0 17^0 \text{ - 6 carbons} = \ 30 \text{ carbons}$$
$$20^0 18^{1t}(4B) = \ 21^0 17^0 \text{ - 8 carbons} = \ 30 \text{ carbons}$$

Growth on 10^0 requires that it be in the extended conformation.

$$18^{1t}10^0 \qquad = \ 18^0 12^0 \qquad\qquad = \ 30 \text{ carbons}$$

Although increase in chain length increases the volume of the hydrocarbon portion of the molecule, the change in conformation causes less water to be bound to the polar groups, and closely similar molecular volumes are maintained.

Even though transition temperatures were not reported for species of 22^4, 22^5, or 22^6, their conformations can be determined from dietary-induced replacements, and the transitions calculated by the melting-point method.

The major questions about the packing principles of lipids are: 1) Do molecules of different lipid classes pack next to each other? 2) Which molecular species of each lipid class pack next to each other? The high degree of reproducibility of quantitative lipid class data for animal cell membranes and some organs indicates compartments (unit) that hold in general only one lipid class. The data indicate, as noted above, a protein conformational code that specifies particular lipid classes. Even in plants where a lipid class code appears to be absent, the strong preference for the most compact and stable arrangement (achieved by packing molecules with the same polar group next to each other) probably causes molecules of the same lipid class to pack next to each other in membranes. *In vitro* studies of lipid class mixtures are of limited value because the restrictions imposed by membranes are removed, and molecules are forced by use of higher temperatures and physical means (sonication, shaking with glass beads) to adopt less favorable conformations.

The types of molecular species that pack next to each other are shown rather clearly by data for membrane composition and *in vitro* mixing of different species. Even *in vitro* under forcing conditions, $18^1 18^1$ PC has little tendency to mix with saturated species of PC,[56] and membrane composition and phase transition data do not indicate side by side packing of such species. The incompatibility of these species is expected from the large conformational differences between the disaturated and diunsaturated species (Tables 9.1 and 9.2). Membrane composition data do not indicate disaturated species to pack next to monounsaturated species. This is to be expected from the conformational differences disclosed by the analysis of phase transition temperatures.

Data for *E. coli* and *A. laidlawii* show very clearly that the disunsaturated species ($18^1 18^1$, $18^2 18^2$) preferentially pack next to a monounsaturated species two carbons shorter ($16^0 18^1$, $16^0 18^2$, $16^0 18^3$). A good example is provided by *A. laidlawii* cells grown with an 18^1 (oleic acid) supplement.[3] The membrane lipid fatty acid composition was 12^0 (2.2%), 14^0 (6.6%), 16^0 (22.1%), 18^0 (4.5%), and 18^1 (64.4%). Although $18^1 18^1$ and $16^0 18^1$ are clearly major species, the differential scanning calorimetry data showed that there were no transitions at -20°C ($18^1 18^1$ SS→S) or +16°C ($16^0 18^1$ SS→S). Rather, there was a transition that fused with the ice peak at about -4°C, but was clearly a little higher. This is in keeping with the mean value of the SS→S transitions of $18^1 18^1$ and $16^0 18^1 = -20° + [(20+16)/2] = -2°C$. Thus, equal molar amounts of the two species would require that the 18^1 value ÷ 3 equal 16^0 value (with all 18^1 and 16^0 as $18^1 18^1$ and $16^0 18^1$). This is indeed the case since 18^1 ÷ 3 = 64.4 ÷ 3 = 21.5% vs 22.1% reported. The data also show clearly disaturated species packing next to each other.

Monolayer studies show that pure species of disaturates have smaller limiting cross-sectional areas than species with one unsaturated fatty acid, which in turn have smaller areas than $18^2 18^1$ and $18^3 18^3$,[57,62] although $18^1 18^1$ gives about the same area as $18^1 18^0$.[63] Despite these differences, monolayer studies of the mixed molecular species of PE derived from *E. coli* grown on various fatty acid supplements showed in all cases a limiting area of 50 Å^2.[7] It thus appears that mixing of the diunsaturates $18^2 18^2$ and $18^3 18^3$ with $16^0 18^2$ and $16^0 18^3$ causes a reduction of the molecular cross-sectional area. This provides a reason for the packing preference $18^2 18^2$ with $16^0 18^2$, and $18^3 18^3$ with $16^0 18^3$ disclosed by the *E. coli* and *A. laidlawii* data in particular. The exceptional volume relationship of $18^1 18^1$ is in keeping with its packing alone or with $16^0 18^1$ as shown by the membrane composition data.

The packing principles of molecular species in animal cell membranes is shown by the data[64] for rat liver PC (Table 9.4). In the control

Table 9.4 Molecular Species of Rat Liver PC on Corn Oil and Fat-Deficient Diets

	$16^0 20^4$	$18^0 20^4$	$18^1 20^4$	$16^0 20^3$	$18^0 20^3$	$18^1 20^3$	$16^0 16^0$	$18^0 16^0$
Corn Oil 360 hr	5.2	22.4	40.6	6.1	none			none
		69.1%						
FDD	5.2	7.5		14.2	28.4	5.4	2.5	3.0
		12.7%			48.0%		5.5%	

	$16^0 18^2$	$18^0 18^2$	$18^1 18^2$	$16^0 18^1$	$18^0 18^1$	$16^1 18^1$	$18^1 18^1$	Recovery
Corn Oil 360 hr	13.7	10.2	3.1	4.3	1.4	none		101.8%
		27.0%			5.7%			
FDD	1.6	2.2		10.2	6.5	2.3	7.6	96.6%
		3.8%			26.6%			

	$20^4 + 20^3$	$18^2 + 18^1$	Saturated	Recovery
Corn Oil	69.1%	32.7%	none	Difference
FDD	60.7%	30.4%	5.5%	
	- 8.4%	- 2.3%	+ 5.5%	5.2%

animals (fed the deficient diet supplemented with corn oil high in linoleic acid), there are three groups of molecular species (20^4, 18^2 and 18^1). Animals on the fat-deficient diet produce additional species (20^3, $16^0 16^0$ and $18^0 16^0$) and replace 18^2 with 18^1 species. The data show that $16^0 18^1$ and $18^0 18^1$ can replace $16^0 18^2$ in the bulk phase lipid, and that 20^3 or 20^4 species can replace 18^1 and 18^2 species, although $18^1 18^1$ replaces $18^0 20^4$ to some extent. The explanation for this specificity appears to be related to the differences in conformation and cross-sectional area between the two groups. The appearance of two disaturated species on the deficient diet shows a forcing of the appearance of species that will be in the solid state at body temperature. The presence of both $16^0 16^0$ and $18^0 16^0$ suggests the molecular-length equivalent replacements:

$$16^0 16^0 (3F) \text{ or } (3B) = 16^0 20^4 (4F)$$
$$18^0 16^0 (3F) \text{ or } (3B) = 18^0 20^4 (4F)$$

Such replacements could be the result of cross-sectional area matching by the saturated species.

In general, the fatty acid composition data for animal cells indicate that the replacements and packing principles shown clearly for PC, PE and PG are followed (as expected) by other glycerolphospholipids.

Sphinogolipids present a different type of problem. The phase transitions reported for brain cerebroside[84] show this group of lipids to be in the solid state at body temperature. The data for sphingomyelin[85] show some transitions to be above body temperature also. The mismatch rule derived from glycerolphospholipid data applies to sphingolipids as well. Since the short chain of sphingosine corresponds to the fatty acid in position one of a glycerolphospholipid and sphingosine has the length equivalent to a 14-carbon acid, $5.5°C$ must be subtracted for each additional carbon atom in the fatty acid chain over 14 at each conformation (Table 9.1). The trans double bond, like that of elaidic acid allows the conformation to change as fatty acid chain length is increased so that molecules with 16-24 carbon acids can have the same bilayer length.

THE POSITIONS OF COENZYME Q
AND FAT-SOLUBLE VITAMINS
IN MEMBRANES

The roles of coenzyme Q and retinal are most clearly defined. Coenzyme Q functions in the electron transport system in mitochondria and thus appears to pack into the polar-lipid space, probably next to some particular species. The only method available to arrive at a possible packing principle is to associate the presence of a particular type of phospholipid with the presence of the coenzyme. Since the special feature of mitochondrial polar-lipid composition is the high level of diphosphatidyl glycerol, it is reasonable to suggest that coenzyme Q packs next to molecules of diphosphatidyl glycerol. In the retina, there is a high level of species of 22^6 and thus, the association of retinal with species of this acid is suggested.

It is commonly assumed that vitamin E protects membrane lipids from autoxidation. If so, vitamin E should pack with some species of polar lipid. It is apparent at once however that such packing must be a special feature that would be coded for by protein since membranes such as those of human red blood cells have most of the common species of the various phospholipid classes and vitamin E is at most a trace component (which has, however, been reported to be an essential dietary component for prevention of rat red blood cell hemolysis[65]). The data for fatty acid composition changes of the polar-lipid classes of rat brain, heart and liver mitochondria on a vitamin E-deficient diet[66] suggest that the vitamin may be related to linoleic acid and 22^6 levels because these acids either remained near control levels or decreased, whereas arachidonic acid levels remained near control levels or increased.

It is tempting to suggest that vitamin K packs with some particular molecular species of polar lipid (*e.g.,* arachidonic acid species since vitamins E and A appear to be involved with other polyunsaturated fatty acids), and that vitamin D, due to its structural similarity to cholesterol, serves some special packing function with cholesterol. In contrast to the other suggestions for which there is data, similar roles for vitamins K and D must be classed as speculative rather than interpretive since there is no direct data to support the correlations.

The alternatives to fat soluble vitamins being required for membrane lipid packing are their participation in biosynthesis, or polar-lipid transport to membranes. It is apparent that these are important areas for future research.

CORRELATION OF TUMOR CELL MEMBRANE COMPOSITION AND STRUCTURAL FEATURES WITH THE POTENTIAL FOR RAPID GROWTH

A key feature of the change of normal cells to tumor cells capable of rapid growth is a change of the cell surface that causes the cells to be unresponsive to normal growth control by hormones, and prevents them from forming strong cell-cell interactions that allows the cells to metastasize. Metabolic studies have shown various combinations of energy metabolism to be compatible with rapid growth.

One feature of tumor cell lines that has emerged as a major and common, if not invariable, change is the characteristic alteration of acyl chain composition of membrane lipids. When tumor cells are grown in an animal or a tissue culture medium containing serum, they have varying amounts of linoleic and archidonic acids. However, the tumor cells, unlike normal cells, can be grown in a medium devoid of serum or exogenous lipid. When grown in a lipid-free medium, the cells have little or no linoleic or archidonic acids.[79-83] Also, unlike the response of normal cells to a fat-free diet that causes 20^3 to appear as a replacement for arachidonic acid, the tumor cells do not in general produce 20^3. Thus, the tumor cells are strikingly similar to bacteria such as *E. coli* and *A. laidlawii* (as discussed in earlier sections) that do not have a protein conformational code for specific acyl chains. The tumor cells respond to supplements of linoleic and linolenic acid like bacteria in that both fatty acids appear in membrane lipids, but may differ[83] in that fatty acids may be chain elongated (18^2 to 20^2 and 22^2 and 18^3 to 20^3) and desaturated (18^2 to 20^4 and 18^3 to 20^4 and 22^4).

The reversion to the more primitive uncoded membrane protein can be visualized as follows for oncogenic viruses and chemical carcinogensis. Lipid-containing viruses that are not oncogenic reproduce as noted above by replacement of host cell plasma membrane protein with virus protein followed by close apposition of the viral nucleic acid core to its protein, and a budding process that results in the production of a virus particle (consisting of a central nucleic acid core covered by a lipoprotein membrane). In contrast, the oncogenic lipid-containing viruses enter the cell and the nucleic acid core becomes incorporated into the host cell genome. The viral nucleic acid directs production of its primitive type of membrane protein that replaces host cell membrane protein, but migration of the viral nucleic acid core does not take place, and budding cannot occur. In this way, the host cell becomes transformed to a cell with a primitive type of membrane protein that is uncoded for specific acyl chains, and lacks hormone receptors to the extent to which virus protein replaces normal cell membrane proteins.

Carcinogenic chemicals such as hydrocarbons enter the hydrocarbon region of cell membranes and decrease the ability of normal cells to carry out their functions. Abnormal function of the immune system is of particular importance because spontaneous mutations to a more primitive type of membrane protein have an increased chance to survive. When such mutants arise, a tumor cell population develops. The difference between viral oncogensis that results in the production of the same type of tumor cell in all cases, and the wide range of tumor cell types produced by chemical carcinogens is thus explained as the latter being dependent upon a variety of different types of spontaneous mutations.

SOME GENERAL COMPOSITIONAL
AND STRUCTURAL FEATURES OF MEMBRANES

In previous sections, the properties of lipids alone and in membranes could be considered without regard to details of membrane structure, since incorporation of lipids into membranes does not alter the bulk phase properties of the lipids. Discussion of membrane functions must, however, be based on a detailed model of membrane structure. Such a model was developed and tested as described in this and the next section.

Extensive investigations have established some general properties of membranes of all types of organisms. All membranes are composed of lipids, proteins, water, and mono- and divalent ions (Na^+, K^+, Ca^{++}, Mg^{++}). Membrane proteins are divisible into two major groups, the intrinsic and the extrinsic. The extrinsic proteins bind through ionic and

hydrogen bonds to the intrinsic proteins from which they can be disso-
ciated by solutions of high ionic strength and by pH adjustments. After
dissociation, the extrinsic proteins are typical water-soluble proteins.
In contrast, the intrinsic proteins bind to lipids. Dissociation of the
lipid-protein complex is possible with detergents that destroy membrane
integrity in contrast to stripping extrinsic protein that does not alter
the structure observed by thin-section electron microscopy by ordinary
methods. The intrinsic proteins are not water soluble, although at least
some of them (e.g., the proteolipid protein by myelin) can be obtained
in water-soluble form by dialysis against aqueous solutions.

It is now clear that the "railroad track" or dark-light-dark appearance
of membranes by thin-section electron microscopy is due to the staining
of intrinsic proteins since lipids can be extracted without appreciable alteration of the structure observed. The extrinsic proteins can be visualized
by special methods that avoid their removal during preparation for electron microscopy as a fuzzy, amorphous layer on one side of the membrane. The layer of extrinsic protein is not to be confused with the
thickening of the outer surface of plasma membranes caused by treatment
with permanganate that oxidizes the carbohydrate moieties of glycoproteins extending from the outer surface only. The asymmetric distribution
of glycoprotein carbohydrate moieties can be visualized by electron microscopy when lectins that bind to specific carbohydrate sequences are made
visible by chemical linkage to ferritin. Extrinsic proteins are localized
entirely on the inner surface whereas the carbohydrate moieties of glycoproteins and glycolipids are positioned on the outer surface to serve
cell surface functions such as cell-cell recognition.

The asymmetric distribution of the carbohydrate portions of glycoproteins and glycolipids (outer surface only) and extrinsic proteins (inner
surface only) of plasma membranes are examples of a general feature of
membrane structure (asymmetry). It has been found that enzyme activities and specific binding sites are present entirely on either the outer or
inner surface of membranes.

Intrinsic proteins are divisible into two categories, proteins that pass
through (span) the membrane, and those that occur only on the inner
or outer surface. When the molecular weights of total membrane proteins are determined by sodium dodecyl sulfate-gel electrophoresis, a
wide range with molecular weights up to 200,000 or more may be found.
In contrast, after stripping the extrinsic proteins, generally only two
molecular weight regions, i.e., about 100,000 and about 50,000 (in some
cases about 25,000) are observed. It is thus apparent that the sizes of
intrinsic proteins are restricted.

The close similarity of the molecular weights of intrinsic proteins of the $Na^+ K^+$ ATPase (from brain, kidney and the rectal salt gland of the shark), the Ca^{++} ATPase (from skeletal muscle), the human red blood cell, and liver microsomes suggests that in general, intrinsic proteins fall into two molecular-weight ranges (50,000 and 100,000) and that the 50,000 molecular-weight protein may be replaced by one of 25,000 or perhaps even 12,000-13,000 molecular weight.   The larger membrane proteins have been associated with the production of intramembraneous particles (IMPs) by freeze-fracture-etching and appear to pass through the membrane, whereas the smaller proteins appear on either the inner or outer surface only.

One of the most notable achievements of electron microscopists and protein and enzyme chemists is the demonstration of repeating units. A repeating unit can consist of a larger unit, *e.g.,* ABC, in which A,B,C,AB and BC are also repeating units. One of the most striking repeating units is the oligomycin sensitive ATPase of mitochondria (for review see reference 70). This enzyme system is seen by electron microscopy after negative staining to consist of a rounded head piece that is joined by a stalk to the membrane sector of the enzyme. The head pieces are spaced at regular intervals and the enzyme has been shown to have a quantitatively reproducible protein composition. The ATPase functions with the electron-transport system that constitutes another type of repeating unit consisting of a precisely arranged sequence of components in reproducible amounts.

Most of the endoplasmic reticulum of skeletal muscle is a Ca^{++} ATPase (pump), that is composed of two intrinsic proteins with molecular weights of about 50 and 100,000 to which are bound (one side only) several acidic, Ca^{++} binding, extrinsic proteins. Negative staining shows knobs at regular intervals. Thus, this pump has been shown by electron microscopy and protein composition to be a repeating unit. The pump was delipidated and reconstituted to full activity with dioleoyl PC.[71]

An example of a plasma membrane that is composed mostly of one enzyme is the $Na^+ K^+$ ATPase of the proximal convoluted tubule cells of the kidney. The basolateral portion of the plasma membrane is ATPase whereas the brush-border portion has a variety of transport systems. This ATPase is composed of two intrinsic proteins (about 50 and 100,000 molecular weights). These outstanding examples show that various membranes consist of repeating units.

It is now generally accepted that the intramembraneous particles (IMPs) produced by freeze-fracture etching represent proteins that pass through the membrane. IMPs appear to be composed of lipid as well as protein, since they are not formed if lipid is extracted from the membrane prior to freeze-fracture.

Lipid-protein interaction is now generally accepted to involve both the polar groups and the carbon chains of the lipid. Thus, the lipid molecules are parallel to the protein molecules rather than perpendicular as depicted in some early models. As noted in previous sections, lipid-protein interaction does not appear to alter the bulk-phase properties of the lipid. Also, the data show rather clearly that lipids are present as a bilayer.

Membrane components have been observed to be mobile by observation of the rate of mixing after cell fusion, observation of the extent of aggregation after treatment with an agent such as a multivalent antibody, and alteration of IMP distribution. Complete mixing of the originally separate halves of two fused cells was observed to require 30-40 minutes. On the other hand, treatment of lymphocytes with agents that bind to plasma membranes can cause complete aggregation of membrane surface components in about 5 mins. The movement has been referred to as "fluidity." Since membranes are hydrated solids held together by various types of noncovalent bonds, mobility appears to be a more accurate term, and the rate of movement is dependent upon the strength of the interaction between membrane components (proteins) rather than their fluidity. Movement of membrane components is temperature sensitive. The cessation of movement below a certain temperature is attributed to a membrane phase transition that increases the strength of interaction of membrane components.

A major area of confusion with regard to the arrangement of the lipoprotein complex in membranes is whether the polar groups of lipids are exposed or covered by protein. Studies of human red blood cells indicate that lipid polar groups are covered by protein, since there was no indication by cell electrophoresis of exposed groups other than the carboxyl groups of the sialic acid moieties of the glycoproteins, and chemical reagents that do not pass through the membrane do not react with the amino groups of lipids. Also, the pancreatic type of phospholipase does not degrade the lipids of intact red blood cells unless the membrane is stretched by exposure to a hypotonic solution that causes the cells to swell.

DERIVATION OF A GENERAL MODEL FOR MEMBRANE STRUCTURE FROM LIPID CLASS COMPOSITION AND OTHER DATA AND ITS USE TO PROVIDE EXPLANATIONS FOR MEMBRANE FUNCTIONS

The highly reproducible lipid class composition data of animal cell membranes is indicative of a protein conformation code that specifies particular lipid classes. Such specificity has been shown for lipid dependent enzymes. Fatty acid composition data also provides strong evidence for protein conformational codes specifying particular types of acyl chains. It is thus possible for the lipid-class data to disclose the existence of lipid compartments of particular sizes and shapes.

The repeating units in membranes will contain a reproducible number of lipid molecules. The total number of molecules can be determined by a two-step derivation. In the first step, a multiple of the total number is obtained by a ratio fit method. The ratio of each value in a phospholipid class analysis to all other values gives an overall fit to a single multiple. The multiple series found in all cases was 1.099, 0.549, 0.275, etc. The multiples correspond to 91, 182, 364, etc. molecules. In the second step, the approximate number of molecules is calculated from quantitative lipid and protein data. Since data for human red blood cells are particularly well established, they can be used with confidence. The weight ratio of lipid to intrinsic protein is 1/1, and the molar ratio of cholesterol to phospholipid is 0.85. The mean molecular weights of the proteins are 100,000 and 50,000. With two moles of the 100,000 M.W. protein associated with phospholipid and two moles associated with cholesterol, and two moles of the 50,000 M.W. protein (one on the outer and one on the inner surface of the membrane), the total is 500,000 Daltons. When converted to molecular weight units and divided by the mean molecular weight of cholesterol and phospholipid (700 + (384) x .85 ÷ 2 = 548), the values are 331 molecules total with 180 of phospholipid and 151 of cholesterol. Thus, the correct multiple appears to be 0.549 that corresponds to 182 phospholipid molecules.

It is to be noted that the molar ratios of the two intrinsic proteins are fixed by the weight percentages of the proteins. In the red cell as well as the Na^+ K^+ and Ca^{++} ATPases, and other membranes that contain cholesterol, the higher molecular weight protein (100,000) is about 80% of the total weight. It appears that human red blood cells do not differ appreciably from other membranes that contain the same amount of cholesterol.

The sizes and shapes of the units can be determined in two ways. One way is to determine all of the possible sums of one or more units that give 91 (the number of molecules in one-half of the bilayer). The other is to show that all possible sums of the phospholipid class values for all membrane analyses give certain percentages that are the same. Both methods gave the same answer, *i.e.,* that there are two units of equal size that have 28 molecules on each side of the bilayer arranged 4 by 7, and one unit that has 35 molecules on each side of the bilayer arranged 7 by 5. Thus, each of the smaller units has 56 molecules or

30.8% of the total and the larger unit contains 70 molecules or 38.5% of the total. The analysis of all possible sums of phospholipid class values disclosed that all animal cell membrane polar lipid analyses gave sums that were very near 30.8% and 69.3% (30.8 + 38.5%) or 38.5% and 61.6% (30.8 + 30.8%). Thus, the phospholipid class composition data for animal cell membranes fix the sizes and shapes of the compartments with a high degree of certainty.

The derivation used for animal cell membranes cannot be followed completely for microorganisms and plants, although the ratio fit method gave the same multiple for their membranes. The method used for the highly coded animal cell membranes to determine compartment sizes was applied to the data[90] presented as molar ratios for polar lipids of leaves of twenty plant species. The analysis indicated that the compartments in these plants are the same size as those of animals. However, more data are required for microorganisms and plants before it can be stated with certainty that they are always the same as those of animal cells.

In the derivation of compartment sizes, the sizes of the smallest units were derived as if different lipid classes and all molecular species of each lipid class packed into units together. This is not the case, however, as the considerations of packing principles show. The phospholipid class composition data indicate that at least 24 units of 182 molecules (4368 molecules total) are required, and the value is compatible with fatty acid composition data, although no conclusive way of fixing the exact number from acyl chain composition data has been found.

The size of cholesterol compartments can be closely approximated, but cannot be fixed with complete certainty. Four cholesterol molecules packing with their side chains overlapping and their hydroxyl groups engaged in hydrogen bonding provide a length about equivalent to an average phospholipid bilayer and gives two polar ends from hydroxyl groups that correspond to the polar groups of phospholipids. For the other dimensions to be similar to those for phospholipid compartments, the other dimensions would be 3 x 7 molecules to give a total number per compartment of 84 molecules.

Lipid composition data cannot be used to determine the orientation of the lipoprotein complex in membranes. Since all lipid-protein interactions appear to involve polar groups and carbon chains, the bilayer must be turned perpendicular to the plane of the membrane if polar groups are exposed, and parallel to the plane if polar groups are not exposed. Because the weight of evidence appears to favor polar groups not being exposed (see the preceding section) and there are advantages provided by this orientation (see below), the parallel orientation was chosen for the schematic model shown in Figure 9.7 that illustrates the smallest repeating unit (182 molecules). Only intrinsic proteins are shown and their carbohydrate moieties that project from one surface of the membrane are not shown.

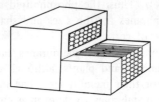

Figure 9.7 Schematic representation of the smallest repeating unit in an animal cell membrane. There are three lipid compartments. Two of these are the same size (56 molecules each arranged 4 x 7 x 2), formed by intrinsic protein that passes through the membrane. The third compartment, which contains 70 molecules (7 x 5 x 2), is formed by intrinsic protein that does not pass through the membrane. See text for discussion.

In Figure 9.7, the two compartments that contain 56 molecules each are depicted as box-like (B) units. The compartment that contains 70 molecules is shown as a sandwich-like (S) unit. Each small repeating unit is thus composed of one B unit with two compartments and one S unit. This L-shaped unit packs with a similar unit to give a larger box-like unit containing 364 molecules (Figure 9.8).

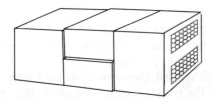

Figure 9.8 Schematic representation of the interaction of two L-shaped units shown in Figure 9.7 which contain 182 molecules to form a larger unit consisting of 364 molecules. These units pack side by side in both directions to form the membrane (see Figure 9.9).

The model shows the membrane with potential polar pores formed by the hydrated polar groups of the phospholipids. There is also a hydrocarbon space that polar molecules are not compelled to enter when passing through the membrane. The model is in keeping with the electron microscopic appearance of membranes since it will show with thin sections the "railroad track" appearance. The model also shows why extraction of lipid prior to workup does not change the appearance of the electronmicrograph appreciably, since lipid is entirely covered by protein and only protein will be stained. The B units in the model are about 75 Å in all three dimensions, and constitute the protein passing through the membrane that gives rise to IMPs. IMPs are about 85 Å square, but this includes the shadowing material required to make them visible.

One of the most important and strictest tests of a model is its ability to explain the reversible processes of stretching. This is readily explained by separation of units (Figure 9.9).   Since polar groups are exposed

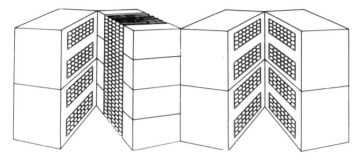

Figure 9.9   Schematic representation of a membrane that is stretched. The polar groups of the phospholipids are exposed in the stretched state, and water and external ions enter the polar pores.

when the membrane is stretched, it is apparent why a phospholipase that does not degrade phospholipids of intact human red cells in an isotonic medium can degrade the lipids of these cells when they are placed in a hypotonic medium that causes them to swell but not hemolyze.[72]   As noted in the preceding section of this chapter, protein-protein interaction involves ionic ($-NH_3+$ and $-COO^-$) and hydrogen bonds, as well as non-polar (conformational) contributions.   Alternate back and front separation is thus possible with alternation of bonding types.

Two major functions of membranes are the control of molecular movement into and out of cells and subcellular compartments, and conduction of impulses.   Conduction involves three main features.   One is generation of an impulse, another is how ion movements propagate the impulse, and the other is how impulses pass from node to node in myelinated axons in which Na^+ and K^+ movements are confined to the nodes. In the model depicted in Figure 9.10, generation of the impulse is by addition of excess positive or negative charges by a metabolic process or the presence of a transmitter.   When protons are removed from the amino groups of lipids and proteins, units that are held together by $-NH_3+$ and $-COO^-$ interaction separate.   The separation that is caused by charge repulsion

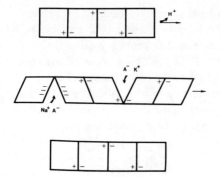

Figure 9.10 Schematic representation of the events in impulse conduction discussed in detail in the text.

is transmitted mechanically to adjacent units that also separate (Figure 9.10). The excess negative charge causes Na^+ (and water) to move into the phospholipid polar group region, but the negative charge of the units prevents entry of external anions. When charge repulsion is neutralized by Na^+, the units return to their normal position with Na^+ ions trapped in the polar region. Na^+ can move through the uncharged inner membrane surface. As it does so, the negative charge is restored to the phospholipid polar groups and it is passed on to other units in the direction of impulse transmission. The present model has a special feature for ion movements. The long continuous rows of lipid polar groups allow charge transfer to take place rapidly without actual movement of the ion initiating the imbalance. This provides a means for passage of an impulse from node to node in myelinated axons. This type of charge transfer is analogous to the rapid movement of protons in ice.[73] Movement of K^+ is passive and is caused by the mechanical opening of the pore barrier to its movement into the membrane pore.

The ion exchange reactions in impulse transmission are:

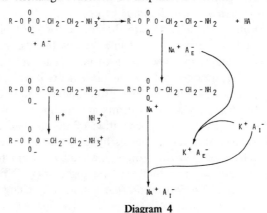

Diagram 4

Impulse propagation is by movement of protons in the polar group region of the membrane, and ionic balance on both sides of the membrane is maintained by Na^+ and K^+ interaction with internal (A_I^-) and external (A_E^-) anions.

The mechanism of action of general anesthetics is readily visualized with the present model. Small polar molecules such as those of diethyl ether can enter the polar-group region of membranes and interrupt the continuous ion path responsible for impulse propagation. Foreign molecules of this type cannot only insert themselves between the charged groups that disrupt the continuous path, but cause some separation of units that allows external ions to enter and cause charge dissipation. Interruption of the ion path is possible with inert gases that are general anesthetics. Xenon is the most potent of the inert gases. Its effectiveness is attributable to its size (2.2 Å atomic radius) that causes it to fit in a clathrate-type space between the phospholipid polar groups. This insertion blocks the continuous ion path and ion channels in keeping with data showing that xenon stops Na^+ movement.[74] Xenon has been found to associate preferentially with subcellular particulates, and to have a greater solubility in membranes than it has in aqueous or lipid environments.[75]

The action of local anesthetics with either plus or minus charges can be visualized readily since these molecules can interrupt the $-NH_3^+$ $-COO^-$ links between proteins of adjacent units and cause separation of units and charge dissipation of impulse transmission.

Anesthetics can also act by entering the hydrocarbon space of membranes. The presence of foreign molecules in this space can force lipid molecules to elongate and cause unit separation and charge dissipation of impulse transmission. At the beginning of this chapter, the lipid "free" (vibrational) space was estimated to be about 9-12% of the lipid space. The space available to small anesthetic molecules is similar to that for larger molecules. Thus, the maximum molar ratio of pentanol to phospholipid molecules was found to be 4/6.[76] The ratio of carbon atoms with the average chain length for phospholipids being 18 becomes 20 (4 x 5) and 216 (18 x 2 x 6). Thus, pentanol molecules occupy about 9% of the space filled by pentanol and phospholipid. It is to be emphasized that investigations of the mode of action of anesthetics led to the recognition of a relationship to lipid space in the later part of the nineteenth century (for review see reference 77), and various relationships to lipid-free volume have been demonstrated recently.[78]

The entrance of small anesthetic molecules alters enzyme activity and lowers the phase transition temperature of the lipid in the membrane.[91,92] Activity of the mitochondrial ATPase was reduced to about 20% of control activity,[91] and the phase transition temperature of the enzyme was reduced from 16.8°C to 12°C by diethyl ether.[92]   Since both adamantane and cholesterol lower the transition temperature by 5-6°C, it is apparent that small anesthetic molecules have about the same space available to them (as noted above), and that they reduce transition temperatures to about the same extent.

Passage of molecules across membranes can be visualized with the present model as follows. Simple diffusion is explained as more or less random separation of units to form a polar pore through which polar molecules can enter, whereas nonpolar molecules diffuse through the hydrocarbon space. Facilitated diffusion is explainable by the presence of a binding site near the potential pore. When the units separate and a pore is formed, binding affinity is decreased and the molecules enter the pore. Active transport is energy dependent and thus requires an energizing unit. There are two different types of transport systems. One arrangement is to have the specific binding site on the energizing unit (e.g., $Na^+ K^+$ and Ca^{++} ATPases). The other is when the binding site is on another protein next to or near the energizing unit. With the $Na^+ K^+$ ATPase type arrangement, hydrolysis of ATP produces an ion imbalance that causes the units to separate. When the specific binding site is not on the energizing unit that creates the ion imbalance, opening of the pore is accompanied by separation of adjacent units brought about mechanically as described above and illustrated in Figure 9.10.

The controlling effects of polypeptide hormones can be visualized as their specific binding sites being located on proteins that are associated with a particular multienzyme complex that includes adenyl cyclase. Hormone binding causes pores to open and the entrance of external ions activates adenyl cyclase that produces cyclic AMP. The prostaglandins are molecules that can be expected to enter certain specific regions of the hydrocarbon space of adenyl cyclase and cause inhibition of the enzyme. The change of ion balance produced by an increase or decrease of cyclic AMP could be transmitted to other parts of the membrane by the mechanism described above for impulse transmission. Such transmission could extend from the plasma membrane to other membranes through direct connections. Since each hormone produces specific effects that are mediated by a common messenger (cyclic AMP), communication between the plasma membrane and other cell compartments, if not through direct membrane connections, must be through organized regions of the cytoplasma whose physical state is controlled by specific regions of the membranes. If organized cytoplasmic channels are induced by interaction with membranes, altered ionic balances could cause the channel to go through reversible sol-gel transformations that would pass along the channel by the charge-transfer mechanism described above.

Attempts to explain some intracellular ion movements also make the idea of a continuous path from one membrane to another attractive. Thus, in heart muscle, Ca^{++} is released from the plasma membrane to the contractile elements, and Ca^{++} is taken up by a Ca^{++} pump in the endoplasmic reticulum. Since there are direct connections between the plasma membrane and the endoplasmic reticulum, return of Ca^{++} to the plasma membrane can involve ion movement along the inner surface of the endoplasmic reticulum. The latter membrane could be covered with a continuous coat of Ca^{++} ions and entry of additional Ca^{++} would force Ca^{++} to pass along the membrane to open sites. This mechanism provides a rapid and specific means of ion movement.

The transmission of signals from the plasma membrane to other parts of a cell along specific paths is related to the mobility of membrane components. Movement of membrane units is easily visualized with the model presented here because units are free to slide in either direction in the plane of the membrane. The rate of slide would depend upon the strength of protein-protein interactions holding the units together. The strength of plasma membrane protein-protein interactions can be compared by treatment of a cell with an agent such as a multivalent antibody that tends to aggregate and thus cause membrane units to aggregate. This type of comparison has shown that lymphocytes have units held together by relatively weak bonds that allow complete aggregation within five minutes whereas aggregation is not apparent with fibroblasts. It is apparent that cells with freely mobile units will not be able to maintain a number of specific cytoplasmic-plasma membrane connections.

ESTABLISHMENT OF LINEAR RELATIONSHIPS FOR PHYSICAL PROPERTIES AS A FUNCTION OF TEMPERATURE, AND CHANGES WITH TIME IN BIOLOGICAL SYSTEMS

The basis for relationships to temperature and time are in general incompletely understood. As a result of efforts to establish relationships of membrane lipid phase changes to temperature, and changes of membrane lipids with age, a method of graphic analysis was developed that can be used to establish functions in general. The findings by graphic analysis are then correlated with other data, and incorporated into a general interpretive framework.

The graphic method for function analysis consists of plotting data for a relationship in all possible ways, except that, since log A vs B and log 1/A vs B in general give equivalent lines, only log A is plotted since it is easier to use. The routine plots are thus A vs B, A vs 1/B, 1/A vs B, 1/A vs 1/B, log A vs B, log A vs 1/B, A vs log B, 1/A vs log B, and log A vs log B. When the relationship is to time or temperature, log time and log temperature are not plotted since these are arithmetic rather than exponential. The plot giving a linear relationship with the smallest number of slope changes, and with values close to the line (no scatter), is selected as the correct function. Each function shows characteristic distortions when values are plotted incorrectly, and these features become a part of the proof of function. The typical distortions were established with model plots of lines with different slopes and intercepts. One of the most dramatic and easily recognized features is the large degree of scatter with breakup into two or more lines when the function 1/A vs 1/B is plotted log A vs 1/B.

The simplest case is when only one plot shows one or more straight lines without a slope change and values fall close to the line. Some relationships give straight lines without a slope change in more than one way. This can be the case when the range is small. When the function is A vs B and lines pass through the origin, lines passing through the origin are obtained on a 1/A vs 1/B plot, and lines at a 45° angle are obtained when log A vs log B is plotted on log-log paper. When two sets of values (A_1 and A_2) are available, and the function is A_1 vs 1/B and A_2 vs 1/B, the proper plot is A_1 vs A_2. However, $1/A_1$ vs $1/A_2$ and log A_1 vs log A_2, also give good lines without point scatter. This characteristic distinguishes the A vs 1/B function, and thus provides good proof of the function. In all cases with an adequate number of values the function 1/A vs 1/B will give a straight line when plotted A vs B, but scatter is introduced. However, scatter may not be detected when a small number of values are available, and the two plots may appear to be equivalent. In this case, plotting log A vs B and A vs log B will give a slope change in both cases, and scatter will generally be apparent on one of the plots.

When all functions are tested and the relationship is found to show at least one slope change, the plot giving the smallest number of slope changes is selected. It is generally recognized that plots of spin label motion in a lipid vesicle or membrane show slope changes at characteristic temperatures. The slope change arises from a lipid phase transition. Plots of other relationships also show slope changes attributable to structural changes.

Physical properties depend upon precise structural principles that give rise to linear relationships that may be arithmetic or exponential. It is common in homologous series, such as fatty acids, for the effect of adding one or two carbon atoms to decrease as chain length increases. This is the case for melting points. In this case, the relationship is an inverse reciprocal one. Plots of melting point and log melting point (Figures 9.4-9.6) against the reciprocal of the number of carbon atoms shows that the correct function is:

melting point ($^{\circ}$C or $^{\circ}$K)

vs

1/# of carbon atoms

Although plots of melting points of hydrocarbons, fatty acids, and similar homologous series commonly show slope changes indicative of conformational differences, the plot for melting points of iso fatty acids gives a linear relationship without slope change, and values very close to the line, from 12 to 29 carbon atoms. Convergence of odd and even fatty acid lines also show that conformational changes occur as chain length is increased. Graphic analysis shows that other physical properties such as density, refractive index, heats of crystallization, heats of the α to β form transition of saturated fatty acids, and boiling points follow the A vs 1/# carbon atoms function. The melting points of the saturated dicarboxylic acids with even numbers of carbon atoms decrease as chain length is increased. Since the effect of adding two carbon atoms decreases as chain length increases, the relationship is still to 1/# carbons. However, since the melting point goes down as chain length is increased, the functions expected are:

1/melting point ($^{\circ}$C or $^{\circ}$K) or log melting point

vs   1/# carbon atoms

Graphic analysis shows the function to be exponential.

The precision of the structural features determining the boiling points of organic compounds is widely recognized, and formulas for calculation of boiling points with the necessary constants are given in handbooks of chemistry. Graphic analysis can be used to show conformational changes in homologous series that cause the observed and calculated values to differ.

Graphic analysis is also useful for the estimation of values for missing members of an homologous series, and selection of the most accurate values when reported values for one member are different. An example is the plot for melting points of hydrocarbons vs 1/# carbon atoms. The plot shows convergence of odd with even at 17 carbons and linear periods from 12-18, 22-43, 44-60 and above 60 carbons. Although the values for members up to 43 carbons are generally very close to the line and values are available for all members of the series, there are missing members above 44 carbons, and reported values vary in some cases. The plot of the data makes it rather clear which values are the most accurate, and good estimates of values for missing members can be obtained from the plot.

Mixed melting point data for members of an homologous series provide valuable information on molecular conformations. When the melting points of mixtures of two fatty acids differing by two carbon atoms are determined at different molar ratios, presentation of the data has been as:

$$\text{mol \% vs melting point (}^{\circ}\text{C)}$$

Although this is the correct function and eutectics are clearly visible on such plots, slope changes indicative of conformational changes can not be determined accurately from the plots. It is to be expected that all ratios of the acids will show the melting point lowering effect that reaches its maximum at about a 3/1 ratio. That this is the case is shown by the plot of mol % versus the difference between the calculated melting point for mixtures if there were no effect on conformation, and the observed value. This plot shows linear periods with abrupt slope changes, and can be used to fix ratios at which conformational changes occur.

That some functions are exponential has been widely recognized. Examples are log retention time vs # carbon atoms used in gas-liquid chromatography, log # atoms decaying vs time for radioactive isotopes, and log activity vs $1/^{\circ}\text{K}$ for catalytic activity including that of enzymes. Graphic analysis discloses other exponential functions that provide a broader base for an interpretive framework. A log function is followed when there is a constant characteristic of the system such as constant half life for radioactive decay, and constant doubling time for bacterial growth as a function of time. The constant feature in physical properties appears to be a conformational factor that increases in magnitude with chain length and causes an exponential change in physical properties. Thus, retention time at constant temperature becomes an exponential function of the number of carbon atoms, and catalytic activity changes exponentially as a function of temperature. Graphic analysis confirms that the activity of enzymes follows the log vs $1/^{\circ}\text{K}$ function. The relationship to temperature appears thus to be caused by the conformational factor increasing as temperature is reduced. When temperature is held constant, the properties of a series of related substances will reflect the exponential structural component. An example is determination of the molecular weights of proteins by Sephadex column chromatography in which elution volume is a function of log molecular weight of the protein.

Graphic analysis of physical properties such as density as a function of temperature frequently presents the problem of many slope changes such as those noted above for the density of water. Some regions of the relationship appear, however, to make the function clear because the slope of the line is correct to show a slope change when plotted incorrectly. This is the case for the density of water between -3.0 and 0°C and 7-11°C in particular. In the case of water, the plot of log vapor pressure vs 1/°K is easily established as correct since a linear relationship is obtained without slope change over a wide range, and all other plots are curves or a series of straight lines with different slopes. This appears to be the case for the vapor pressure of many organic and inorganic compounds since the log-reciprocal relationship is widely recognized and tables of constants for use in log-reciprocal relationships are given in chemistry handbooks. Since it is difficult to see how interdependent physical properties could follow different functions, it can be expected from the vapor pressure data that other physical properties will follow the log-reciprocal relationship, and this expectation is confirmed by graphic analysis.

Plots of 1/density vs °C for oleic acid indicate this to be the correct function. Rather striking confirmation of the log-reciprocal function was obtained with viscosity data for a variety of organic and inorganic substances. If, as expected from the results for vapor pressure, the log-reciprocal relationship is correct for organic and inorganic compounds in general, a selection of diverse compounds and elements should prove the point. Plots of log viscosity vs 1/K for toluene and sodium nitrate did in fact show the relationship to be log (Figures 9.11 and 9.12). A linear relationship without slope change and values falling very close to the line was obtained for toluene between 0 and 110°C, for sodium nitrate between 308 and 408°C and for mercury between 40 and 197°C. The plot of the viscosity of air (Figure 9.13) was linear from 0 to 400°C. In each case, all other plots

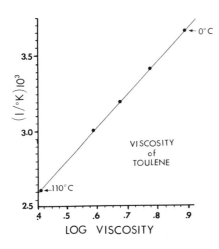

Figure 9.11 Plot of **log** viscosity of toluene vs 1/°K to show the linear relationship up to the boiling point (110.6°C).

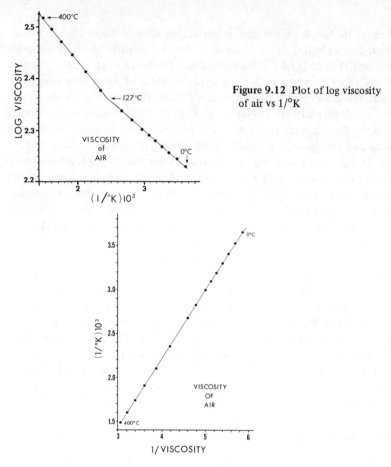

Figure 9.12 Plot of log viscosity of air vs 1/°K

Figure 9.13 Plot of log viscosity of sodium nitrate vs 1/°K to show that inorganic compounds follow the same function as organic compounds from its melting point (308°C) to the temperature at which it decomposes.

gave curves or a series of lines with slope changes. The data are particularly good for establishing function since the range is broad for the regions that do not show slope changes. It thus appears that, in general, density, viscosity and related properties will be found to follow various related functions.

It is to be stressed that physical properties that are not dependent upon conformational changes do not change exponentially. One of the most important exponential functions for membrane research is spin label motion in lipid bilayer vesicles and membranes discussed earlier.

Enzyme reactions are treated in general as following a nonexponential course, even though the relationship of substrate (S) to velocity (V) determined by plotting 1/S vs 1/V gives a curve rather than a straight line in some cases. Since enzyme activity follows the log vs 1/ K function, it can be expected that conformational factors may cause exponential kinetics in some cases. That this is indeed the case was shown by replotting data presented in the literature as arithmetic plots giving curves. Glutamine synthetase of *R. capsulata*[93] is an example of the function

$$\log 1/S \text{ vs } \log 1/V.$$

That an inhibitor can change kinetics from arithmetic to exponential is shown by the data for the effect of dATP on the activity of ribonucleotide (cytidine-5'-phosphate) reductase of *A. quadruplicatum*. In the absence of an inhibitor, the enzyme was shown to follow arithmetic kinetics[94] When dATP is added, reaction rate measured as product formation is shown by graphic analysis to follow the function

$$\log \text{ dCDP concentration}$$
$$\text{vs}$$
$$\text{dATP concentration.}$$

The activation of methanol dehydrogenase by ammonium chloride[95] is shown clearly by graphic analysis to follow the function

$$\% \text{ activity vs } \log NH_4 \text{ Cl concentration.}$$

These clearcut examples show that enzyme kinetics is exponential in some cases.

Growth of some microorganisms is known to follow a log vs time relationship, although this relationship is not apparent in the early phases of growth or as the organisms go into the stationary phase. The log growth phase is the result of a constant doubling time and is followed by *E. coli*. Some variations in medium composition cause the slope of the log vs time line of *E. coli* to change.[96] As *E. coli* goes into the stationary phase, its lipid composition changes and graphic analysis of the changes reported[97] for fatty acids shows that these follow the function: log vs 1/time. The reciprocal relationship arises from a steady decline in biosynthetic rates as the organisms approach the stationary.

An important feature of growth in general is that the enzymes producing DNA, RNA, lipids and other cell components are controlled by activators and inhibitors. This gives rise to four different relationships for both arithmetic and exponential changes. Since the determinant regulator may increase or decrease with time, the relationship becomes 1/time when the regulator decreases with time. When the component being regulated changes in the same direction as the regulator, the relationship is either component vs time or 1/time depending upon the direction of change of the regulator. When the change in the component measured is in the reverse direction to that of the regulator, the relationships can be either 1/component vs time or 1/time.

When growth of microorganisms does not follow the log vs time relationship, values are presented in the literature as plots of cell number, or lipid composition changes against time. The plots are either a series of straight lines or curves. Graphic analysis of the data presented in this way disclosed other functions. The changes in fatty acid composition of *C. lipolytica* with time after a shift down in growth temperature[98] follow the function mol % fatty acid vs 1/time. Outgrowth of germinated spores of *B. subtilis*[99] measured as DNA (mg/ml) followed the function log DNA vs 1/time. The plot showed slope changes at 85 and 105 minutes that correlated reasonably well with the times observed microscopically for the first and second synchronous nuclear division times of 90 and 110 minutes. Subsequent cell division occurred without a change of slope. The growth of *M. xanthus* measured as incorporation of labeled thymidine and valine (100) followed the function

1/thymidine and 1/valine incorporation

vs

1/time

The values gave a linear relationship without slope changes as did the plot

1/thymidine incorporation

vs

1/valine incorporation

The growth function can be changed by temperature as shown by the data for a thermophilic bacterium (101) grown at different temperatures. At 52°C the function was log uridine incorporation vs time. Whereas at 65°C the function was log uridine incorporation vs 1/time. This response is in contrast to the response of *E. coli* to changes in the medium that causes slope changes[96] rather than changes of function. These examples show that bacterial growth functions can vary over the full range of possibilities.

Some changes in composition of animal cells and organs with time occur over a short time span in response to food intake and other variables. Other changes occur gradually over the entire life span or a major portion of it. Graphic analysis of the data obtained in the author's laboratory for changes with age of human and mouse brain water, lipid composition, and mouse organ weights showed several relationships. Human brain lipid composition followed the function log lipid value vs 1/age. Most lipid values gave one line from fetal life to 98 years of age. Some plots showed one slope change. When a slope change was noted, it was found that specific lipid value sums gave lines without a slope change. The slope changes could thus be shown to arise from replacement of one lipid by another. The relationships of lipid values to each other followed the function log lipid A vs log lipid B. The data for mouse brain lipid was found to follow the function 1/lipid value vs 1/age, and lipid values plotted against each other followed the function 1/lipid A values vs 1/lipid B value. Lipid values were found to increase throughout life. Thus, it appears that regulatory factors decrease with time making the relationship vs 1/time, and lipid values going up when regulators go down makes the function 1/lipid value when it is arithmetic as it is for mouse brain. When the relationship is exponential, log lipid and log 1/lipid both give lines without slope changes so that log lipid can be used.

Water content of mouse brain followed the function

$$1/\text{water content (\% fresh weight)}$$

vs

$$1/\text{age}$$

In this case, the regulatory factors decrease with age to make the function 1/age. Since water content decreases with age and total, nonlipid solid increase with age, the function for nonlipid solid becomes reciprocal, and since water content has a direct inverse relationship to solids, the function for water is also reciprocal. The water content of human brain followed the log-reciprocal relationship.

The weights of mouse organs were found to follow the function log weight vs 1/age. Since organ weights increase with age, it appears that regulatory factors decrease with time. Data from the literature for lipid, DNA and RNA values were used to establish functions for other organs. Total phospholipids of mouse liver[102] clearly followed the function 1/total phospholipid vs 1/age and increased throughout life as noted for brain. Liver DNA also followed the double reciprocal function. Since DNA content decreases with age, it appears that it has a direct inverse relationship to another component that increases with age. Since membrane mass increases with age, DNA levels may be inversely related to membrane mass and hence to total lipid. RNA values also appear to follow the double reciprocal function. The double reciprocal function is thus the most common relationship for animal organ composition. This function is particularly easy to prove because there is a striking introduction of scatter when the values are plotted log vs 1/age, and plots of, for example, lipid A vs lipid B give lines without slope change, but scatter is introduced. It is important to note that expression of lipid values as a percent of the total lipid introduces scatter. It is thus necessary to plot absolute (millimolar) amounts to establish the relationships among the lipid classes and fatty acids.

Analysis of animal organ data is complicated by a range of variability not found in the other functions discussed above. Distribution within the normal range is clearly not random about an overall mean value. Rather, values commonly form parallel lines that indicate distinct subgroups. This is understandable for lipids since they occur in compartments of reproducible size, and replacement of one lipid by another is incremental. Subgroups for the other components appear to be determined by regulatory factors that are produced in incremental amounts.

Analysis of data in general by the graphic method appears to be basic to the definition of proper functions, analysis of molecular conformations, and the study of metabolic regulatory mechanisms. Since each function has distinctive features, the proper function can be defined unambiguously when an adequate number of data points is available.

Functions for physical properties depend upon the type of molecular interaction. Thus, the functions for the viscosity and density of air are arithmetic, whereas the function for the vapor pressure of mercury is exponential. Air molecules do not associate (cluster) whereas mercury molecules do and there is a constant structural feature. The exponential function is thus attributable to molecular association. The plot log vapor pressure of mercury vs $1/^{\circ}K$ is linear without a slope change from $28^{\circ}C$ to $1300^{\circ}C$ and changes from 0.002359 mm to 835.9 atmospheres with a halving (doubling) interval of $10^{\circ}C$. That the function for the vapor pressure of many substances is exponential has been widely recognized because most molecules cluster and the structural effect is constant over a wide temperature range.

In the liquid state, three types of molecular interactions are possible. One is uniform molecular interaction (no clusters) that gives rise to the viscous nature of substances such as oleic acid, and an arithmetic function for density at different temperatures. Another is when molecules cluster, and the intra- and intercluster interaction effects go in the same direction. The function in this case is exponential. The third possibility is clustering with the intra- and intercluster effects going in opposite directions. When two log functions determine a property and go in opposite directions, the function becomes arithmetic.

The effects of structure on function are illustrated by the functions for fatty acid melting points, molecular volumes, density and retention times in gas chromatography. The functions are arithmetic for melting point, density and molecular volume. As noted above, melting point vs $1/\#$ carbon atoms is the proper function since the melting point increases with a decreasing increment as chain length is increased. Molecular volume increases at a constant increment per carbon atom that is characteristic of the A vs B function, and the proper linear plot is volume vs # carbon atoms. Since density and volume are inversely related, the function is density vs $1/$# carbon atoms. The functions are arithmetic because the twisted conformation prevents the effect of chain elongation from being constant. Above their boiling points, the hydrocarbon chains are fully extended, and the effect of chain elongation follows a constant structural feature that gives rise to the log retention time vs # carbon atoms function that is well known in gas chromatography. The increment per carbon atom increases and there is a characteristic doubling length. Interaction between the hydrocarbon chains and the stationary phase is analogous to clustering of molecules of the same type.

The exponential function for catalytic reactions is attributable to a change in the binding of substrate going in the same direction as that of the product, whereas the function is arithmetic when the changes are in opposite directions. The effects of regulatory factors on bacterial growth and changes with age in animals are thus attributable to the effects on substrate and product binding of rate-limiting reactions.

SUMMARY

1. The data showing that the physical (bulk phase) properties of lipids are not altered appreciably by incorporation into membranes is reviewed. The data show that the physical properties (phase transitions as temperature is lowered) of membranes are largely determined by lipid.

2. It is noted that there is a "free" (vibrational) space in the bulk-phase lipid in membranes, and that foreign molecules can enter this space and alter membrane structure and function. The size of this free space can be as high as 9-12% of the total lipid space. It is noted that, despite the broad implications of the existence of this membrane space, its existence has gone unrecognized except by those who have studied the mode of action of anesthetic molecules (covered in a later section).

3. The three physical states of lipids are defined as viscous liquid (VL), soft solid (SS), and solid (S). The transitions from one state to another are designated as VL→SS and SS→S. It is emphasized that phase transition temperatures can be defined accurately only by the correct plots, and that failure to use the proper function will give misleading results. It is emphasized that phase transitions disclosed by plots may cause only a slight, temporary change of slope, and that it is necessary to have values at 1°C intervals. The nature of such transitions is explained as one structural modification producing a compensatory structural change. It is noted that major changes in the slope of the line on an appropriate plot arise when there is no compensation. Arrhenius type

plots of the vapor pressure of water are presented. The vapor-pressure plot is essentially one long line with only very small, temporary shifts typical of the compensated type of plot. Thus, the constant activation energy for dissociation of water molecules from liquid clusters arises from counter-balancing changes in cluster size and structure. The density plot of water shows a number of phase changes which for water are definable as variations in cluster size. It is further shown that caution must be used when plots are prepared using the ratio of spin label motion in the hydrocarbon phase to that in the polar phase since transitions of water may modify the slope of the line.

4. Qualitative and quantitative variations of membrane lipids are examined and it is noted first that, in general, all organisms use the same polar groups because packing into membranes is under strict space and conformational limitations. Also, the highly reproducible values for membrane lipid class composition, and the nature of the acyl chain replacements on fat-free diets are shown to be indicative of protein conformational codes in animal cell membranes that specify particular polar groups and acyl chains. These codes are absent in plants that readily adapt for growth over a wide range of environmental temperatures. It is shown that plots of the melting point in $^\circ$K against $1/\#$ carbon atoms discloses for hydrocarbons, alcohols, ketones, fatty acids, methyl and ethyl esters of fatty acids, and phopholipids a series of straight lines with abrupt changes in slope at specific chain lengths. The chain lengths that fall on the same line have conformational similarity. It is further shown that the conformational similarity of chains disclosed by such plots correlate with their natural occurrence in membrane lipids.

5. Cholesterol is shown to occupy a separate space from polar lipids in membranes. Both *in vivo* and *in vitro* data show clearly that phospholipids and cholesterol molecules do not pack next to each other in membranes, and that cholesterol occurs in membranes in the solid state.

6. The data that show some bacterial cell membranes to be highly tolerant of the presence of lipid in the solid state in their membranes, and the use of polar lipids in the solid state by plants as a part of a defense against water loss are considered, and the existence of solid lipid in animal cell membranes is noted.

7. The first steps in the conformational analysis of polar lipid molecules are presented. The chain lengths of unsaturated fatty acids relative to those of saturated fatty acids are established by analysis of the replacements observed for animal cell membranes on a fat-free diet, and temperature-induced replacements in other organisms. Mixed melting-point data for fatty acids of different chain lengths are then shown to

disclose three acyl chain conformations for each acid, and phospholipids
are shown to have the same characteristics. It is shown that the lowering of the melting point below that of the lowest melting component of
a binary mixture (a eutectic) is caused by a chain-length mismatch, *i.e.*,
the packing side by side of two chains that differ in length by one carbon atom. It is further shown that a **eutectic** is not observed if the
ratio of the acyl chains in a mixture favors conformations that cause
molecules to have the same length. It is pointed out that the explanation previously offered for the eutectic, clustering or compound formation, is incorrect since increased molecular interaction makes dissociation
take place at a higher temperature. It is stressed that, although there
are favored chain conformations at different temperatures, conformations
may be forced to change when the proper ratios of components of a
binary mixture are used.

8. The way that phase transition temperatures and molecular conformations (the relative positions of the two acyl chains) are established
from the data for molecular species of polar lipids obtained by chemical
synthesis, and bacterial and fungal mutants grown on different fatty acid
supplements is described. It is shown that the transition temperatures of
molecular species with conformational similarity can be calculated with
a simple formula that relates the melting-point differences between the
fatty acids of the species to its transition when incorporated into a polar
lipid molecule. When the calculated value differs from the measured
value, the difference can be used to show the conformational difference
between the species. It is also shown that the membrane acyl chain
composition data show a strong preference for packing of mixed molecular species such as $18^1 18^1$ next to $16^0 18^1$.

9. A brief consideration of the possibilities for packing coenzyme Q
and the fat-soluble vitamins with certain molecular species of polar lipids is
presented. The principles suggested are derived from the association of
special lipid composition features.

10. It is pointed out that studies of the fatty acid composition of
lipids of tumor cells derived from animal cells show that the tumor cells
have reverted to the more primitive type of membrane protein that does
not have a code specifying specific acyl chains. This change is disclosed
only when the tumor cells are grown in appropriate media.

11. Some general features of membrane structure disclosed by extensive investigations of all types of organisms are described.

12. The way in which a detailed model of membrane structure was
derived from lipid class composition data and the considerations in the

previous section are described. The ways that the model depicts membrane stretching, impulse transmission, transport, and the action of anesthetics and polypeptide hormones is described.

13. A method of graphic analysis that can be used to determine the linear relationships of physical properties to temperature, and changes with age in biological systems is described. The method disclosed that the proper plot for melting points of lipids as a function of chain length is melting point vs $1/\#$ carbon atoms. Other related properties such as heats of crystallization, the heat of the α to β transition of fatty acids, and boiling points were shown to follow the same relationship. The value for density, vapor pressure, and viscosity at different temperatures was shown to follow the log vs $1/^\circ K$ function in some cases.

Graphic analysis disclosed that the rates of enzyme reactions can be exponential since when the plot of substrate (S) concentration and velocity (V) as $1/S$ vs $1/V$ is a curve, log $1/S$ vs log $1/V$ is linear. The relationship of an inhibitor to activity can follow the function log produce formation vs concentration of inhibitor, and enzyme activation can follow the function % activity vs log concentration of activator.

Analysis of bacterial growth data that does not follow the well known log vs time relationship disclosed various functions depending upon the organism and growth conditions. Examples of the functions A vs 1/time, log A vs 1/time, and 1/A vs 1/time are presented.

Changes with age of lipids, water, DNA, and RNA and organ weights of animals were shown to follow the functions log lipid vs 1/age in human brain, 1/lipid vs 1/age in mouse brain and other organs, 1/water content vs 1/age, 1/DNA and 1/RNA content vs 1/age. The relationship of these functions to changes in regulatory factor levels is discussed.

ACKNOWLEDGMENTS

The membrane structure model presented in this chapter was first presented by the author at the Intra Science Research Foundation Symposium on Membranes held in December 1974. The model and its derivation were also presented before the staff of the division of Neurosciences at the City of Hope National Medical Center in a series of lectures, and at the University of California at Riverside, California in 1975.

REFERENCES

1. Steim, J. M., Tourtellote, J. C. Reinert, R. J. McElhaney and R. L. Rader. *Proc. Nat. Acad. Sci. U. S.* 63:104 (1969).
2. McElhany, R. N., J. DeGier and E. C. M. VanDerNeut-Kuk. *Biochem. Biophys. Acta.* 298:500-512 (1973).

3. McElhaney, R. N. *J. Mol. Biol.* 145-157 (1974).
4. Hsung, J. C., L. Huang, D. J. Hoy and A. Haug. *Can. J. Biochem.* 52:974-980 (1974).
5. James, R. and D. Branton. *Biochem. Biophys. Acta.* 323:378-390 (1973).
6. DeKuryff, P. W. M., VanDuck, R. W. Goldbach and L. L. M. Van Deenen. *Biochem. Biophys. Acta.* 330:269-282 (1973).
7. Overath, P., H. W. Schairer and W. Stoffel. *Proc. Nat. Acad. Sci. U. S.* 67:606-612 (1970).
8. Overath, P. and H. Traube. *Biochemistry.* 12:2625-2634 (1973).
9. Nascimento, G., Z. E. Zehner and S. J. Wahil. *J. Supramol. Str.* 2:646-660, (1974).
10. Schechter, E., L. Letellier and T. Gulik-Krzywicki. *Eur. J. Biochemistry.* 49:61-76 (1974).
11. Linden, C. D., A. D. Keith and C. F. Fox. *J. Supramol. Str.* 1: 523-534 (1973).
12. Henry, S. A. and A. D. Keith. *Chem. Phys. Lipids.* 7:245-265 (1971).
13. Eletr, S., M. A. Williams, T. Watkins and A. D. Keith. *Biochem. Biophys. Acta.* 339:190-201 (1974).
14. Wunderlick, A. Ronai, V. Speth, J. Seelig and A. Blume. *Biochemistry.* 14:3730-3735 (1975).
15. Ashe, G. B. and J. M. Steim. *Biochem. Biophys. Acta.* 233:810-814 (1971).
16. Raison, J. K. "Rate Control of Biological Processes," *Soc. Exp. Biol.* XXVII (1973).
17. Blazyk, J. and J. M. Steim. *Biochem. Biophys. Acta.* 266:737-741 (1972).
18. Kimelberg, H. and D. Papahadjopoulos. *J. Biol. Chem.* 249:1071-1080 (1974).
19. Lee, A. G., N. J. M. Birdsell, J. C. Metcalf, P. A. Toon and G. B. Warren. *Biochemistry.* 13:3699-3765 (1974).
20. Wisnieski, B. J., Y. O. Huang and C. F. Fox. *J. Supramol. Str.* 2:593-608 (1974).
21. Wisnieski, B. J., J. G. Parker, Y. O. Huang and C. F. Fox. *Proc. Nat. Acad. Sci. U. S.* 71:4381-4385 (1974).
22. Ladbrooke, B. D., T. J. Jenkinson, V. B. Kamat and O. Chapman. *Biochem. Biophys. Acta.* 161:101-109 (1965).
23. Ladbrooks, B. D., R. M. Williams and D. Chapman. *Biochem. Biophys. Acta.* 150:333-340 (1968).
24. Azuma, K. and T. Yoshizawa. *Biochem. Biophys. Acta.* 249:135-143 (1971).
25. Snipes, W., S. Person, A. Keith and J. Cupp. *Science.* 187:64-66 (1975).
26. Nicoloides, N. and F. Laves. *J. Amer. Oil Chemists Soc.* 40:400-413 (1963).
27. Vandenheuvel, F. A. *Chem. Phys. Lipids.* 2:372-395 (1968).
28. Suzuki, K. in *Inborn Errors of Sphingolipid Metabolism.* S. M. Aronson and B. W. Volk, Eds. (New York: Pergamon Press, 1967), pp.215-230.

29. Rouser, G., G. Kritchersky, A. Yamamoto and C. F. Baxter. in *Advances in Lipid Research Vol. 10.* D. Chapman, Ed. (New York: Academic Press, 1972), pp.262-360.
30. Rouser, G., G. J. Nelson, S. Fleischer and G. Simon. in *Biological Membranes.* D. Chapman, Ed. (New York: Academic Press, 1968), pp.5-70.
31. Kuiper, P. J. C. *Plant Physiol.* 45:684-686 (1970).
32. Yamamoto, A., M. Isozaki, K. Hirayama and Y. Saki. *J. Lipid Res.* 6:295-300 (1965).
33. DeKruyff, B., R. A. Demal, A. J. Stutboom, L. L. M. VanDeenen and A. F. Rosenthal. *Biochem. Biophys. Acta.* 307:1-19 (1973).
34. Reed, C. F. *J. Chem. Invert.* 47:749 (1968).
35. Murphy, J. R. *J. Lab and Chem. Med.* 65:756 (1965).
36. Winterborn, C. C. and R. D. Batt. *Biochem. Biophys. Acta.* 152:412 (1968).
37. Trairble, H. and D. H. Haynes. *Chem. Phys. Lipids.* 7:324-335 (1971).
38. Leathes, J. B. *Lancet.* 268:853 (1925).
39. Adam, N. R. and G. Jesson. *Proc. Roy. Soc. Sci. A.* 120:473 (1928).
40. de Bernard, L. *Bul. Soc. Chem. Biol.* 40:161 (1958).
41. Van Deenen, L. L. M., W. M. T. Houtsmuller, G. H. De Hass and E. Mulder. *J. Pharm. Pharmacol.* 14:429 (1962).
42. Shak, D. O. and J. H. Schulman. *J. Lipid Res.* 8:215 (1967).
43. Cogan. U., M. Shinitzky, G. Weber and T. Nishida. *Biochemistry.* 12:521-528 (1973).
44. Shimshick, E. G. and H. M. McConnell. *Biochem. Biophys. Res. Commun.* 53:446-451 (1973).
45. Lee, A. G. *FEBS Letters.* 62:359-363 (1976).
46. Gershfeld, N. L. and R. E. Pagano. *J. Phys. Chem.* 76:1244-1249 (1972).
47. McElhaney. *J. Mol. Biol.* 84:145-157 (1974).
48. Kylin, A., J. C. Kuiper and G. Nanson. *Physiol. Plant.* 26:271-278 (1972).
49. Kuiper, P. J. C. and R. Stuiver. *Plant Physiol.* 49:307-309 (1972).
50. Kuiper, P. J. C. *Plant Physiol.* 43:1367-1371 (1968).
51. Smith, J. C. *J. Chem. Soc.* 625-627 (1936).
52. Smith, J. C. *J. Chem. Soc.* 974-980 (1939).
53. Cason, J. and W. R. Winans. *J. Org. Chem.* 15:148-158 (1950).
54. Stewart, H. W. and D. H. Wheeler. *Oil and Soap.* 18:69-71 (1941).
55. Shimshick, E. J. and H. M. McConnell. *Biochemistry.* 12:2351-2360 (1973).
56. Phillips, M. C., B. D. Ladbrooke and D. Chapman. *Biochem. Biophys. Acta.* 196:35-44 (1970).
57. Stoffel, W. and H. D. Pruss. *Hoppe Seyleis Z. Physiol. Chem.* 350:1385-1393 (1969).
58. Phillips, M. C., H. Hauser and F. Paltauf. *Chem Phys. Lipids.* 8:127-133 (1972).
59. DeKruff, B., R. A. Demel and L. L. M. Van Deenen. *Biochem. Biophys. Acta.* 255:331-347 (1972.

60. Soutat, A. K., H. J. Pownall, A. S. Hu and L. C. Smith. *Biochemistry*. 13:2828-2836 (1974).
61. Rodwell, A. *Science*. 160:1350-1352 (1968).
62. Demel, R. A., W. S. M. Geurts Van Kessel and L. L. M. Van Deenen. *Biochem. Biophys. Acta*. 266:26-40 (1972).
63. Demel, R. A., L. L. M. Van Deenen and B. A. Pethica. *Biochem. Biophys. Acta*. 135:11 (1967).
64. VanGolde, L. M. G., W. A. Pieterson and L. L. M. Van Deenen. *Biochem. Biophys. Acta*. 152:84-95 (1968).
65. Jager, F. C. and U. M. T. Houtsmuller. *Nutr. Metabol.* 12:3-12 (1970).
66. Fujta, T., M. Yasuda, Y. Kitamura and S. Shimamura. *J. Pharm. Soc. Jap.* 92:670-676 (1972).
67. *Handbook of Chemistry*. N. A. Lange, Ed. (New York: McGraw-Hill Book Co., 1969), pp.1199-1166 and 1470-1473.
68. Drost-Hansen, W. *Ann. New York Acad. Sci.* 204:100-112 (1973).
69. Dreyer, G., E. Kahrig, D. Kirstein, J. Erpenbeck and F. Lange. *Naturwiss.* 56:558-559 (1969).
70. Senior, A. E. *Biochem. Biophys. Acta*. 301:249-277 (1973).
71. Warren, G. B., P. A. Toon, N. J. M. Birdsall, A. G. Lee and J. C. Metcalf. *Proc. Natl. Acad. Sci.* 71:622-626 (1974).
72. Lankisch, P. G. and W. Vogt. *Biochem. Biophys. Acta*. 270:241-247 (1972).
73. Eigen, M. and L. DeMaeyer. *Proc. Royal Soc. London Ser A.* 247:505-533 (1958).
74. Mullens, L. J. *Leck Proc.* 27:898-901 (1968).
75. Kwan, E. and A. Trevoe. *Proc. Western Pharmacol. Soc.* 12:29-82 (1969).
76. Seaman, P., S. Roth, H. Schneider. *Biochem. Biophys. Acta*. 225:29-82 (1969).
77. Henderson, V. E. *Physiol. Rev.* 10:171 (1930).
78. Stern, S. A. and H. L. Frisch. *J. Applied Physiol.* 34:366-373 (1973).
79. Geyer, R. P., A. Bennett and A. Rohr. *J. Lipid Res.* 3:80 (1962).
80. Lengle, E. and R. P. Geyer. *Biochem. Biophys. Acta*. 260:608 (1972).
81. Kagarva, Y., T. Takaoka and H. Katsuta. *J. Biochem.* 68:133-136 (1970).
82. Bailey, J. M., B. V. Howard, L. M. Dunbar and S. F. Tillman. *Lipids*. 7:125-134 (1972).
83. Cowen, W. F. and F. P. Heydrick. *Exptl. Cell Res.* 72:354-360 (1972).
84. Clowes, A. W., R. J. Cherry and D. Chapman. *Biochem. Biophys. Acta*. 249:301-317 (1971).
85. Shipley, G. G., L. S. Avecilla and D. M. Small. *J. Lipid Res.* 15:124-131 (1974).
86. Ubbelhode, A. R. *Melting and Crystal Structure*. (Oxford: Clarendon Press, 1965).
87. Hildebrand, J. H. and R. L. Scott. *Regular Solutions*. (New Jersey: Prentice Hall, Inc., 1962).

88. Hildebrand, J. H. and R. L. Scott. *The Solubility of Nonelectrolytes.* 3rd ed. (New York: Dover Publications, Inc., 1964).
89. Hitchcock, P. B., R. Mason, K. M. Thomas and G. G. Shipley. *Proc. Natl. Acad. Sci.* 71:3036-3040 (1974).
90. Roughan and R. D. Batt. *Phytochem.* 8:363-369 (1969).
91. Curatola, G., L. Mazzanti, A. Bigi, M. Familiari and G. Lenaz. *Bull. Soc. Itl. Biol. Sper.* 50:1305-1310 (1974).
92. Parenti-Castelli, G., A. M. Sechi and G. Lenaz. *Bull. Soc. Itl. Biol. Sper.* 50:1705-1710 (1974).
93. Johansson, B. C. and H. Guest. *J. Bacteriol.* 128:683-688 (1976).
94. Gleason, F. K. and J. M. Wood. *J. Bacteriol.* 128:673-676 (1976).
95. Patel, R. N. and A. Felix. *J. Bacteriol.* 128: 413-424 (1976).
96. Sloan, J. B. and J. E. Urban. *J. Bacteriol.* 128:302-308 (1976).
97. Cronan, J. E., Jr. *J. Bacteriol.* 95:2054-2061 (1976).
98. Kates, M. and M. Paradis. *Can. J. Biochem.* 51:184-197 (1973).
99. Keynan, A., A. A. Berns, G. Dunn, M. Young and J. Mandelstram. *J. Bacteriol.* 128:8-14 (1976).
100. Kimachi, A. and E. Rosenberg. *J. Bacteriol.* 128:69-79 (1976).
101. Souza, K. A., L. C. Kostin and B. J. Tyson. *Arch. Microbiol.* 97:89-102 (1974).
102. Hrachovec, J. P. and M. Rockstein. *Gerontologia.* 3:305-326 (1959).

CHAPTER 10

EFFECTS OF ENVIRONMENTAL AGENTS
ON MEMBRANE DYNAMICS

John R. Rowlands, Ph.D. , Catherine J. Allen-Rowlands
and Emily M. Gause

Southwest Foundation for Research & Education
P.O. Box 28147
8848 West Commerce St.
San Antonio, Texas 78284

INTRODUCTION

Membranes are responsible for a whole variety of biological phonomena. They provide a barrier towards diffusion of small and large molecules into the cell, are involved in concentrating metabolites and metal ions, and are intimately associated with processes that are responsible for energy transduction, information transfer and recognition.

A number of concepts of the structure of biological membranes have been proposed over the years as additional compositional and physical data on membranes have become available. One feature which many of the proposed models have in common, and one for which the experimental evidence is in most cases incontrovertible, is a lipid bilayer structure. In this lipid bilayer, the polar groups of the phospholipids are oriented at the (extracellular) aqueous interface and the hydrocarbon chains of the fatty acid esters are perpendicular to this interface; another layer of similar structure in a "mirror image" orientation provides the inner half of the bilayer structure oriented toward the intracellular aqueous interface. The current "working model" of membrane structure incorporating the findings of many investigators has been formalized by Singer and Nicolson[1] as the Fluid Mosaic Model of membrane structure, and basically pictures proteins as floating in a fluid bilayer matrix. The fluidity of this bilayer can be affected greatly by temperature and/or by exogenous agents. It has been shown by several investigators that many membrane functions are affected by changes in lipid fatty acid composition and that these changes in function can be directly correlated with changes in the physical properties of the membrane lipids.

One of the major advances in cellular level studies in the past few years has been the realization that membranes are extremely dynamic structures. This realization has been gained largely by the application of physical techniques such as nuclear magnetic resonance, fluorescence spectroscopy, and electron spin resonance spin labels to the study of membranes.

As a result of these studies, it has become increasingly clear that there is a crucial interdependence of the three major membrane components (*i.e.*, lipid, protein and water) in the determination of membrane function. The importance of water in the lipid bilayer of the membrane has been recently demonstrated by both nuclear magnetic resonance and electron spin resonance techniques. For example, Jost *et al.*[2] have shown by spin label studies that water penetrates into the lipid bilayer of membranes and that it plays an important role in determining the electrical properties, as well as the fluidity and ordering of the membrane system.

Since the plasma membrane is what separates the cell from its environment, it is logical to suppose that it is the first site of attack of pathologic agents whether physical, chemical or biological. Environmental contaminants are capable of reacting or interacting with membrane components in several ways. For example, lipophilic compounds can intercalate into the phospholipid bilayers and cause changes in lipid fluidity. Polyvalent metal ions can bind to specific sites in the phospholipid head groups, causing either an expansion or contraction of the membrane surface. Certain metal ions, *e.g.*, Cd^{2+}, Hg^{2+}, are also able to bind to specific sites in membrane proteins, *e.g.*, -SH groups.

Thus, by their ability to bind to specific sites on membrane-bound proteins or phospholipid head groups, or to intercalate into phospholipid bilayers, these agents are potentially capable of modifying important membrane functions. For example, changes in activity of membrane-bound enzymes can be visualized to take place either by direct reaction of the contaminant with the enzyme, or through an indirect mechanism whereby reaction of the agent with lipid components causes fluidity changes which, in turn, modify the amplitude and/or the periodicity of the low frequency oscillations which are associated with protein conformational changes occurring during catalysis by a given enzyme.

In this chapter, we shall confine ourselves to a discussion of the application of the electron spin resonance spin label technique to studies of membrane dynamics with particular reference to the perturbing effects of environmental agents.

THE ELECTRON SPIN RESONANCE SPIN LABEL TECHNIQUE.

Electron spin resonance (ESR) spectroscopy has been used extensively for many years in biological and biophysical research. However, the technique can only be applied to systems that contain some paramagnetic component since the presence of unpaired electrons is required. Except for free radical intermediates in certain redox reactions and certain metalloproteins, biological systems are diamagnetic and hence not amenable to study by the ESR technique. Recently, a new approach has been developed for introducing paramagnetic species into normally diamagnetic biological systems through the use of relatively stable nitroxide free radicals. By incorporating these nitroxide spin labels into different molecules, the free radical probe molecules can then be introduced into the biological system either by covalent binding to specific sites in membrane protein molecules, or by noncovalent intercalation into membrane lipids. In either case, the specific type of spin resonance signal that is observed from the nitroxide spin label is dictated by its immediate environment.

Three classes of useful parameters are present in nitroxide spin label spectra—the g tensor, the nitrogen hyperfine coupling tensor, and the widths of the individual ESR lines. From their combinations, information can be obtained about the orientation and mobility of the nitroxide.

The first two parameters may be described by the spin Hamiltonian (omitting the nuclear Zeeman term) where g and A are the g and hyperfine coupling tensors,

$$H = \beta H \cdot g \cdot S + hS \cdot A \cdot I$$

respectively. The conventional axis system for nitroxides is defined below. The unpaired electron is considered to occupy a molecular orbital composed of the $p\pi$ orbitals of nitrogen and oxygen. The observed values for the components of the hyperfine tensor indicate that a substantial fraction of the unpaired electron is localized on the nitrogen atom and, therefore, suggest that the NO three-electron π-bond has polar character, as represented here:

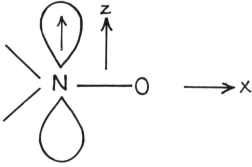

Because the molecular orbital containing the unpaired electron is made up in part of a degenerate oxygen pπ orbital, the g tensor for the nitroxide moiety is expected to be anisotropic ($g_{xx} \neq g_{yy} \neq g_{zz}$). The hyperfine coupling tensor is also anisotropic and is most often nearly axially symmetric ($T_{zz} \neq T_{xx} \approx T_{yy}$) because of the occupation by the unpaired electron of a molecular orbital of π-symmetry. Thus, the magnetic field value at which the ESR spectrum of a nitroxide occurs and the separations between the hyperfine lines will depend very much on the orientation of the free radical with respect to the applied magnetic field.

Because of the ionic character of the nitroxide bond, the values of the g- and hyperfine-tensor components of a given spin label will vary with the polarity of the environment. In general, the isotropic hyperfine splitting constant will increase and the isotropic g factor will decrease as the polarity of the solvent increases.

A spin label ESR spectrum is extremely sensitive to the nature and rate of the motions the label undergoes. If a nitroxide rotates symmetrically at a rate greater than the frequency corresponding to the largest differences between the principal components of the hyperfine coupling tensor ($\gg g_{xx} - g_{zz}$ $\beta H h^{-1} \approx 29$ MHz for X-band spectrometers operating at fields of about 3.3kg), the isotropic parameters a_o and g_o are observed and the ESR lines are narrow and of equal width. However, when the rate of rotation about any of the axis becomes comparable to these differences, changes in individual line widths and positions occur. Thus, it is obvious that nitroxide ESR spectra are very sensitive to the rate of molecular rotation—covering a range of correlation times from 10^{-10} sec (spectrum of three narrow lines of almost equal width) to 10^{-7} sec (a strongly immobilized spin-label spectrum). This range of correlation times includes those of most biological molecules, both large and small, and herein lies the very general applicability of the technique to conformational problems in molecular biology.

Measurements of Correlation Time for Rotational Motion

For cases in which the spectra are essentially isotropic—i.e., the label is relatively free to tumble, the spectral analysis is made using the following relationship:

$$\tau_c = 6.5 \times 10^{-10} \, (W_0) \left[\left(\frac{h_0}{h_{-1}} \right)^{1/2} - \left(\frac{h_0}{h_1} \right)^{1/2} \right]$$

where W_0 is the width in gauss of the center line, h_0 is the center line amplitude, h_{-1} that of the low field line, h_{+1} the high field line, and τ_c the rotational correlation time.

Measurements of Amplitude Frequency Order Parameter

However, if a nitroxide free radical becomes bound within a molecular configuration which inhibits tumbling of the nitroxide and serves to orient the nitroxide spatially, then a very different type of ESR spectrum is obtained. When this anisotropic type of spectrum is obtained, orientations of the orbital of the unpaired electron, both parallel and perpendicular to the applied magnetic field, are observed; and, in addition, line broadening is observed.

A completely different type of spectral analysis is required for this anisotropic type of spectrum. Suitable methods of analysis have been developed by Seelig and Hasselbach,[3] and Hubbell and McConnell[4] by adaptation of single-crystal experience. Briefly, this analysis provides for calculation of what the isotropic coupling constant a' would be from measurement of the experimentally obtained tensors, $T_\parallel$ and $T_\perp$; and derivation of an order parameter S, which is expressed as:

$$S = \frac{T_\parallel' - [T_\perp' \,(\text{approx.}) + C]}{T_\parallel' + 2[T_\perp' \,(\text{approx.}) + C]} \cdot 1.66$$

$$C = 4.06 - 0.055 \,[T_\parallel' - T_\perp' \,(\text{approx.})] \text{ MHz}$$

or

$$S = \frac{1}{2} \frac{3 \,(T_\parallel' - T_\perp')}{(T_\parallel - T_\perp)} - 1$$

in which $T_\parallel$ and $T_\perp$ represent values obtained when the same nitroxide label molecule is oriented within a crystal where the precise orientations are known

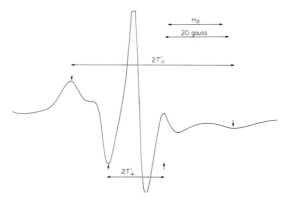

Figure 10.1 ESR spectrum of 5-doxyl stearic acid spin label diffused into intact alveolar macrophages.

ESR SPIN LABEL STUDIES OF MEMBRANES

Membrane Lipids

X-Ray diffraction studies have shown the presence of substantial regions of lipid bilayer in a number of biological membranes, including myelin,[5-7] retinal rods,[8] erythrocytes,[7] synaptosomes,[7] sarcoplasmic reticulum,[7,9] purple membrane of *Halobacterium halobium*,[10] and in lipid cytochrome C complexes.[11,12] Such studies do not allow a quantitative assessment of the bilayer content of the membrane. It has, however, been shown that a large majority of the lipid in *Acholeplasma laidlawii* is free to undergo a thermal transition from a gel to a liquid crystalline state, analogous to that in a lipid bilayer.[13]

As a working model for the membrane, the bulk of the lipid can be taken to be in a bilayer form, with a fraction of the lipid immobilized around the membrane proteins. It is further assumed that some proteins span the membrane, while others do not. These concepts follow the fluid-mosaic model of Singer and Nicolson.[1]

Studies in which spin-labeled probes are incorporated into the membrane suffer from similar problems to nuclear magnetic resonance (NMR) studies, since it is not known what proportion of the lipid environment of the membrane is being sampled by the probe. For example, it is known that in mixed lipid bilayers, spin-labeled fatty acids are excluded from any pools of lipid in the gel phase in preference for pools of lipid in the liquid crystalline phase.[14] Spin-labeled lipids and fatty acids will therefore probably only report on the properties of the more "fluid" of the lipids in the membrane. Using fatty acids spin-labeled at different positions in the chain, it has been found that the "fluidity" increases towards the center of the membrane in *Acholeplasma laidlawii*,[15] yeast,[16] viruses,[17-19] mitochondria[20] and sarcoplasmic reticulum.[3]

The results of ESR experiments involving the incorporation of spin-labeled fatty acids or lipids into lipid bilayers have been interpreted in terms of an order parameter, S_n, which is related to the average orientation of the nitroxide radical by the equation:

$$S_n = 1/2(3 \cos^2 \bar{\theta} - 1).$$

Here, n is the number of carbon atoms between the carbonyl carbon and the labeled carbon, θ_n is the angle between the nitroxide $2_p\pi$ orbital and the normal to the plane of the bilayer at some time, and the bar denotes that the time average of the angle is taken. If the C-C bonds preceding the labeled carbon are all *trans* and perpendicular to the plane of the bilayer, $S_n = 1$. If the motion of the spin label is isotropic, then $S_n = 0$.

For phospholipid spin labels incorporated into bilayers of dipalmitoyl-lecithin above the thermal transition, it has been found that log S_n shows an approximately linear decrease with increasing n = 8. Beyond n = 8, the decrease in log S_n becomes increasingly more marked.[4] These results suggest that the region of the chain up to n = 8 is effectively all *trans*, but that the probability of a non-*trans* conformation increases rapidly with increasing n beyond this point.

The rapidly increasing disorder towards the center of the bilayers creates interesting packing problems. Because of its greater disorder, the volume occupied by a $-CH_2-$ group towards the center of the bilayer will be greater than that for a $-CH_2-$ group near the glycerol backbone region. The increase in volume towards the center of the bilayer can be accommodated in two ways: (a) by a bend in the fatty acid chains, with the upper portion of the chain tilted with respect to the bilayer plane,[21] and, (b) by a decreased packing density in the glycerol backbone region, perhaps with the extra space being taken up by water.

On the basis of studies using oriented multilayers of egg lecithin containing spin-labeled phospholipids, it has been suggested that in the liquid crystalline phase, the upper portion of the labeled fatty acid chain is titled *ca.* 30° from the normal to the bilayer, whereas the lower portion is nearly perpendicular to the bilayer.[21] On the average, the bend occurs at about bond 8, and persists for a time longer than 10^{-8} sec. Such a bent chain implies the area occupied at the bilayer surface by a $-CH_2-$ group in the first half of the chain is greater than that occupied by a $-CH_2-$ group for the lower portion of the chain, but at the same time the packing of the ordered, upper portion of the chain is still relatively tight.

Spin label data can potentially provide information about water penetration into the bilayer, since spin label coupling constants are sensitive to the polarity of the environment. Studies with spin-labeled fatty acids and lipids incorporated into phospholipid bilayers have in fact been interpreted as showing that water molecules penetrate into the fatty acid chain region to at least the C-2 position.[22]

In addition to fast internal motions within lipid molecules in the liquid crystalline phase, there is ESR spin label[23] and NMR[24] evidence for a fast diffusion of the lipid molecules in the plane of an unperturbed lipid bilayer.[23-25] Diffusion has also been shown to occur in lipid systems in the gel phase, although the rates are unknown.[26]

Estimates have been made of the rate of lateral diffusion of lipid molecules in biological membranes. The rate of lateral diffusion of spin-labeled lipids incorporated by fusion into sarcoplasmic reticulum membranes was estimated by extrapolation from experiments performed at 50-70°C to be *ca.* 7 x 10^{-8} cm^2 sec^{-1} at 40°C.[27] Proton NMR experiments yield an estimated lower limit on the rate of lateral diffusion as 6 x 10^{-9} cm^2 sec^{-1} at 80°C.[24] The rates of diffusion of spin-labeled fatty acids in liver microsomal membranes was estimated to be *ca.* 11 x 10^{-8} cm^2 sec^{-1} at 30°C[28] and in *E. coli* membranes *ca.* 3 x 10^{-8} cm^2 sec^{-1} at 40°C.[29]

The average distance travelled per second x^{-2} by a molecule in a two-dimensional lipid lattice is related to the diffusion coefficient by the equation:

$$D = x^{-2}/2.$$

Thus, if the lipids in a 1-μ-long cell can be characterized by a self-diffusion coefficient of *ca.* 10^{-8} cm^2 sec^{-1}, a lipid molecule can move from one end of the cell to the other in the order of seconds.

The rate of lipid flip-flop has been measured for spin-labeled phosphatidyl-cholines incorporated into excitable membrane vesicles prepared from the electroplax of *Electrophorus electricus.*[30] The rate of transfer of the spin-labeled lipids from the inner to the outer surface of the membrane was found to be characterized by a half-time of *ca.* 5 min. at 15°C. This rate is an order of magnitude faster than the corresponding rate in pure phospholipid vesicles.[31]

Membrane Proteins

The observed translational freedom of motion for at least some of the lipids in biological membranes suggests that some membrane proteins will also be freely diffusing. Using a "free-volume" model for the diffusion, it is estimated that a cylindrical protein of molecular weight 100,000 will diffuse a factor of 100 more slowly than the lipid molecules.[29]

An accurate measurement of a protein diffusion rate in the surface of a membrane has been reported for rhodopsin in the retinal rod membrane,[32] where the diffusion coefficient was calculated to be *ca.* 4 x 10^{-9} cm^2 sec^{-1} at 20°C. E-Ray evidence indicates that the average separation between nearest-neighbor rhodopsin molecules in the disc membrane is *ca.* 70 Å.[8] The average time τ between collisions with another rhodopsin molecule can then be estimated as:

$$\tau = s^2/4D$$

where s is the distance travelled between collisions. Assuming a diameter for rhodopsin of *ca.* 45 Å, s = 25 Å, and collision frequency between rhodopsin molecules is calculated to be in the range of 10^5-10^6 collisions per second. Although it is too early to assess the full significance of such high collision frequencies, it is clearly possible that coupled enzyme systems such as that of the electron transport chain might rely upon high frequency collisions in performing their function rather than being spatially fixed with respect to each other. Thus, it has been suggested that the cytochrome b_5 and NADH-cytochrome b_5 reductase in endoplasmic reticulum are randomly distributed, rather than bound in a "complex" or fixed array. Translational diffusion of reductase and cytochrome within the membrane are then required prior to their interaction.[33]

A high rate of lateral diffusion has also been estimated for antigens on the cell surface.

Lipid-Protein Interactions

Although the molecular mechanisms that regulate the interaction of phospholipids with membrane-bound proteins are not clearly understood, the importance of lipid-protein interactions to the functional role of membranes is clear. For example, there exists a wealth of data which demonstrates that the activity and stability of membrane enzymes may be altered by the phospholipid changes.[34-36] Although it was initially thought that membrane-bound enzymes had an absolute requirement for specific phospholipids, it is now generally accepted that it is a specific physical environment that they require. The specific physical environment that is necessary for the proper function of membrane-bound enzymes is directly related to the fluidity of the membrane lipid. For example, Eletr, Zakin and Vessey[37] have shown that Arrhenius plots of the activities of the two hepatic microsomal enzymes glucose-6-phosphatase and UDP-glucuronide transferase showed discontinuation at 19°C. UDP-glucuronide transferase showed a further discontinuity at 32°C. These authors also carried out studies of the order parameter (S) as a function of temperature using lipophilic fatty acid spin labels and showed that changes in slope were obtained at 19°C and 32°C in intact neurosomes. The activity of lactate dehydrogenase in *E. coli*[38] has been shown to depend upon the degree of unsaturation of their membrane lipids, which is directly related to the fluidity of the lipid. Rowlands *et al.*[39] have recently measured sodium potassium ATPase activity in rat alveolar macrophages and shown that three discontinuities exist within the temperature range 4-40°C. Figure 10.2 shows Arrhenius plots of enzyme activity as a function of temperature (assayed in suspension); three different regions of ATPase activity energy are seen. Above 24°C, a value of 17.3 kcal/mole is obtained and below 10°C is found to be 16.8 kcal/mole. The activation energy observed for the alveolar macrophage (AM) from 24-37°C is close to the value of 14.0 kcal/mole reported by Charnock, Doty and Russell[40] for rabbit kidney ATPase. However, these results indicate that below 10°C, the AM has a lower energy of activation than the rabbit kidney enzyme or other purified enzyme preparations. In the temperature region between 10 and 24°C, the AM also manifests a third region of very low energy of activation. The value of E_a obtained from the plot in Figure 10.2 is 6.2 kcal/mole. The authors are not aware of any ATPase for which activation energies this low have been reported; and their observation of it here could reflect a unique feature of the macrophage membrane. In fact, it is between 12 and 20°C that macrophages first are able to initiate phagocytosis. At 20°C, phagocytosis is about 6% of that occurring at 37°C; from 20-37°C the rate increases markedly, going from 6 → 100%. Again, at 37°C there is a change of slope such that the value at 43.5°C is 112% of that at 37°C. It can be seen from Figure 10.2 that there is a change energy of activation between 37 and 42°C. Phagocytosis is an energy-dependent process and plasma membrane ATPase has been suggested to act as a "mechano-enzyme," making phagocytosis possible through the conversion of chemical energy in the form of ATP to the mechanical energy required for attachment and ingestion.[41]

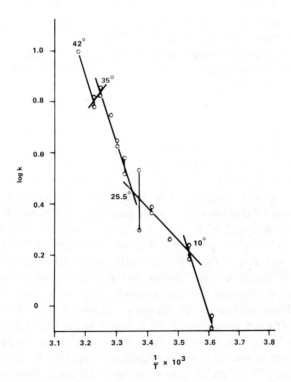

Figure 10.2. Arrhenius plot of alveolar macrophage ATPase activity.

Changes in fluidity of membrane lipids were examined by labeling intact AMs with the nitroxide spin label 5-doxyl stearic acid and monitoring changes in spectral parameters as a function of temperature. Arrhenius plots of variation of order parameters S for AMs labeled with 5-doxyl stearic acid are shown in Figure 10.3. It can be seen that multiple slope

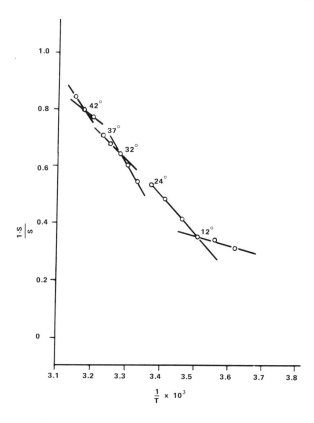

Figure 10.3 Arrhenius plot of alveolar macrophage lipid fluidity as monitored by stearic acid spin label 12, 3.

deflection points are indicated, some more pronounced than others. There is some variation between individual animals as to the exact temperature for each inflection; however, it is felt that all these transition points are real and that they all represent physical changes in membrane structure. Wisnieski et al.[42] have also reported multiple phase transitions and have attempted to correlate the transition temperatures with physiological events which occur at the cell surface (antigen diffusion or Con A binding) or require participation of protein structures which span the entire membrane ($Na^+K^+Mg^{++}$ - ATPase, aminoisobutyric acid transport, or adenylate cyclase). These workers concluded that of the five characteristic membrane-transition temperatures observed, the transitions at $22°C$ and $38°C$ represented phase transitions of the outer monolayer. When lipids were extracted from these cells, only two transitions were obtained: one at $34-35°C$ and one at $14-17°C$. Their suggestion is in accord with the reported sidedness, or asymmetry, of cell membranes with respect to phospholipid composition.[43,44] Measurements by the authors were conducted on intact cells, whereas Wisnieski et al.[42] employed isolated membranes which might contain inside-out vesicles as well as outside-out vesicles.

Though there appears to be a correlation between enzyme activity and bulk membrane fluidity established in these studies, the fluidity properties of membrane lipids is by no means homogenous. Aside from the question of pools of different lipids in heterogeneous chemical distributions, there is strong evidence for a shell of "immobilized" lipid surrounding membrane-bound proteins. The properties of the bound lipid rather than that of the free lipid would be expected to ultimately control enzyme activity. Spin label experiments of membrane fluidity do not reflect these lipid responses of the membrane. Evidence for an immobilized lipid shell comes from studies of the binding of Tempo to the sarcoplasmic reticulum membrane. The amount of Tempo bound is ca. 80% of the amount by the equivalent amount of extracted lipid.[45] Since the lipid: protein molar ratio in sarcoplasmic reticulum is 90:1, there is enough lipid to form approximately three lipid shells around each molecule, of which only one is immobilized. Similarly, for the cytochrome oxidase-lipid complex, there is evidence from studies with spin-labeled fatty acids for a single bilayer shell of immobilized lipid surrounding the protein, the remainder of the lipid forming a normally fluid bilayer.[2,46]

A similar kind of mosaic structure has been suggested for the cytochrome P_{450}-cytochrome P_{450} reductase system of liver microsomes. Spin-labeled fatty acids incorporated into the membrane showed a rapid rate of diffusion at $30°C$ which is evidenced by their diffusion to and subsequent reduction by membrane enzymes. The activation energy for the reduction of the nitroxide-labeled fatty acids by the reductase was found to decrease abruptly above $32°C$, suggesting that either the enzyme system was enclosed by an immobilized phospholipid shell below $32°C$, which undergoes a transition to a fluid state at $32°C$ or that a thermally-induced conformational change took place at this temperature.[28] The possibility that a thermally-induced protein conformational change caused the observed change in activation energy was ruled out by showing that no change in activation energy was observed in the reduction of the water-soluble spin label Tempo phosphate by the reduction enzyme.

The version of the spin-label technique adopted in this work provides a powerful tool for the investigation of lipoprotein complexes within membranes. There have been numerous reports in the last several years of the reduction of lipophilic nitroxide labels when bound to intact cells.[47] It is thus possible to utilize this nitroxide reduction to study lateral diffusion in intact cells.

The nitroxide reduction technique has been used to examine the effect of environmental agents upon alveolar macrophages and for preliminary studies of the mechanism of action of the peptide hormone ACTH upon Y-1 tumor adrenal cells.[48] In both studies, the lipophilic spin label 5-doxyl stearic acid was used. In these studies it was observed that as long as care was taken to preserve the viability of the cells during the labeling process, the free radical decayed rapidly. The same spin label is known to be stable for periods of a day or more when diffused into phospholipid liposomes or into cells which have lost their viability. From measurements of the kinetics of the decay of the spin label in adrenal cells and in alveolar macrophage cells, the characteristics of the decay suggest that the decay process is enzymatic in nature. The possibility that the decay process consisted of ascorbic acid into the lipid bilayer, was excluded by measurements of the effect of $10^{-4} M$ ascorbic acid upon the decay kinetics. Trypsinization of cells prior to labeling is known from measurements of the order parameter to cause the cell membrane to become more fluid. Trypsinization of adrenal tumor cells prior to label-ing caused the radical to decay far more rapidly, suggesting that the fluidity of the membrane plays an important role in the decay kinetics. Figure 10.4 illustrates the decay characteristics of adrenal tumor cells measured in several different experiments, as explained in the legend. In each case, although the total kinetics is complex, there is a portion of each decay curve in which the decay is exponential and appears to fit first order kinetics. To determine the effect of temperatures on the process, the rate constant for this pseudo first order region in AMs was plotted against the reciprocal of the temperature (Figure 10.5). It can be seen from the figure that there is a definite change in slope occurring at approximately 20°C. Figure 10.6 illustrates a plot of $2T_{\parallel}$ versus T (°C) measured for macrophages obtained from the same group of animals from which the kinetic data were obtained. Here again the measured $2T_{\parallel}$ which is linearly related to the order parameter (S) shows a change of slope at the same temperature (20°C), indicating that a lipid phase trans-ition occurs at this temperature. Evidently, the decay of the spin probe is related to the membrane fluidity of the viable cells.

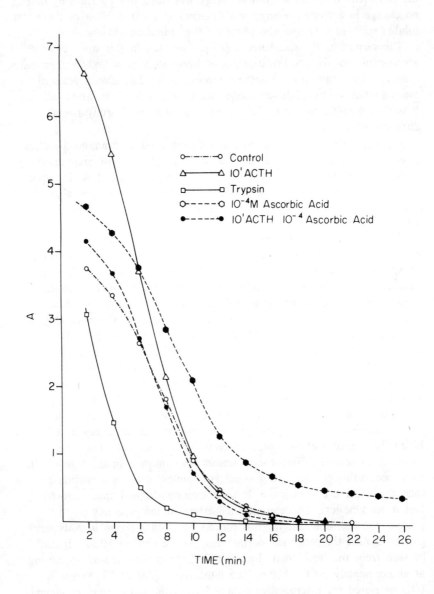

Figure 10.4. Amplitude of signal versus time (minutes). Y^1 adrenal tumor cells.

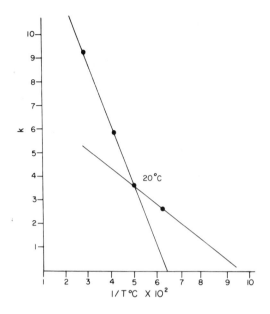

Figure 10.5. Rate constant for decay of spin label (pseudo first-order region) versus $1/T°C$ for alveolar macrophages.

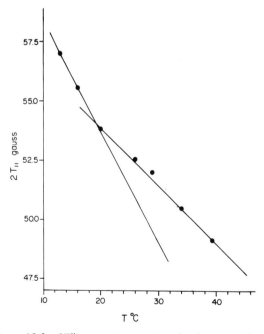

Figure 10.6. 2T|| versus temperature alveolar macrophages.

EFFECTS OF EXTERNAL PERTURBATION ON MEMBRANE DYNAMICS

If we accept the premise that the dynamic properties of membranes which have been described are a necessary and important factor to the functional efficiency of the cell, then any external agent which modifies these dynamic properties is potentially capable of exerting a toxic effect. While the physiochemical nature of the interaction of a given agent with different cell types might be the same, *i.e.*, covalent binding to membrane proteins or intercalation in membrane lipids, etc.; the affinity of the agent might differ markedly between cell types due their wide differences in membrane composition and functional characteristics. Thus, it is extremely difficult to predict *a priori* the biological effect which might be most significant for any pollutant. An understanding of the biochemical and biophysical mechanisms by which environmental agents interact with different cell types, when correlated with the corresponding physiological response of these cell types, would, however, greatly enhance our ability to predict the *in vivo* pharmacology of environmental agents. In order to illustrate the type of information that is available from biophysical studies of the effects of environmental agents on membrane dynamics, we shall discuss results obtained in our laboratories utilizing two cell types— the rat alveolar macrophage and the murine-derived Y-1 adrenal tumor cell.

Alveolar Macrophage

Alveolar macrophages, located on the air side of the pulmonary alveoli, are important cells in defense of the lung against inhaled particulate matter, including potentially infectious agents and particles to which may be adsorbed potentially hazardous chemicals. Macrophages are also important in cooperative interactions with other cells, particularly lymphocytes, in mediation of immune responses, both locally, as in the lung, and systemically.

Y-1 Adrenal Tumor Cell

The Y-1 adrenal tumor cell is representative of cell types that are responsive to peptide hormones. Little, if any, attention has been placed to date on the effects of environmental agents on neuroendocrine mechanism, which are known to modulate metabolic, behavioral and immune processes. Hormones are intimately interdependent in their physiologic effects throughout the body. In general, hormones are aligned in patterns of antagonistic and synergistic relationships with each other. Thus, the overall activity of any given physiologic process would depend on the critical relative balance among the interdependent hormones which influence the process, rather than on the absolute level of any single hormone.

Environmental agents which can interact with membrane components of the neuroendocrine system (*i.e.,* adrenal, pituitary, CNS) have potential to alter neurohormonal mechanisms controlling and/or modulating the dynamics of the endocrine systems. It has been documented that many disease states in man and animals are associated with decreased or increased hormonal sensitivity. Since hormone-receptor interaction is the first step in the action of the hormone, the disruption of either CNS or target organ cellular membranes by environmental agents could significantly disrupt the normal hormonal cascade of the endocrine axis.

Before we discuss the effect of environmental agents upon these systems, we shall briefly review the status of research on peptide hormone plasma membrane receptor interactions with reference to the effect of peptide hormones on membrane dynamics. The relevence of studies of the effect of peptide hormones on membrane dynamics to environmental problems is that they provide an excellent model to demonstrate the profound effect that can be exerted on cellular properties by the binding of picomole to nanomole concentrations of a molecule to cellular receptors.

PEPTIDE HORMONE-MEMBRANE RECEPTOR INTERACTIONS

The classical model for membrane hormone-receptor interactions suggests that there are two protein or lipoprotein membrane-bound components: (a) the hormone receptor, which is generally thought to be exposed to the outer surface of the membrane, and (b) the adenyl cyclase system, which catalyzes the production of the nucleotide adenosine $3':5'$-cyclic monophosphate (cAMP) and is considered to protrude from the inner surface of the plasma membrane. The biologic role of cAMP has been defined in terms of a second messenger concept. In general, hormones such as ACTH are thought to act upon the target cell (adrenal) membrane receptors in a highly specific manner to activate the adenyl cyclase system. The subsequent production of cyclic nucleotides (and possibly other processes) act as the second or intracellular messenger to trigger the "physiologic" response of the target cell--the production of hormones.[49] This conventional model for membrane hormone-receptor interaction is based on the general assumption of a highly static arrangement of the receptor-adenyl cyclase system and that their properties, and hence interactions, change in a specific manner by external perturbations, *i.e.,*hormone interaction. In this conventional model, little importance is placed upon the dynamic properties of membranes.

Hormone-receptor phenomena have previously been studied, for the most part, utilizing a highly specific, isotopically-labeled hormone, a suitable receptor preparation, and an appropriate means for separating hormone-receptor complex from the hormone. The physiochemical characteristics of "pure" receptor structures derived from these types of studies are as follows: (1) the receptor sites specifically bind the corresponding hormone with a high degree of affinity; (2) the receptor sites are finite in number; (3) they are exposed to the external plasma membrane interface; (4) hormone binding is rapid and reversible and can be correlated directly or indirectly to biological processes of the cell.[50-53]

These receptor proteins are intimately associated with and influenced by the lipids of the plasma membrane.[52] The extracellular site of the hormone receptor has been demonstrated by covalently linking peptide hormones, such as ACTH[54] and insulin,[55] to inert polymers while maintaining the hormones biologically active. These receptor proteins of target-tissue plasma membranes are generally specific for its trophic hormone. For example, adrenal cell preparations that bound ^{125}I-ACTH did not bind other iodohormones.[56-58] Furthermore, cell extracts prepared from tissues other than adrenal did not bind ^{125}I-ACTH. The presence of an ACTH-sensitive adenyl cyclase system in adrenal cell extracts was also shown to be correlated with ACTH receptor content[56-58] of the plasma membrane. The close physical relationship within the plasma membrane of the hormone receptors to the adenylate cyclase has been demonstrated by solubilization of the hormone receptors with the enzyme as a single functional unit.[59,60]

Hormone-induced conformational changes of membrane-bound proteins (*i.e.,* receptors and/or enzymes) have been examined by various technical procedures. Using phase contrast microscopy, a morphological activation of the plasma membrane has been demonstrated in the cultured mouse adrenal tumor cell whereby the presence of ACTH in the incubation produced rounding up of the cells.[61] Bovine growth hormone produced conformational changes in the proteins of rat liver[62] and human erythrocyte[63,64] plasma membranes, as determined by the physical measurements utilizing circular dichroism and spectrofluorescence techniques. The direct correlation of the growth hormone-induced phospholipid distribution and conformational changes in membrane proteins, using specific fluorescence probes, with membrane enzyme activity in isolated liver membranes has been demonstrated by Ruben *et al.*[65] The liver membrane response to growth hormone was destroyed by sonication and enzyme treatment suggesting the need for some biological organization on hormone-induced activation of membrane-bound enzymes.

At present, the translation of hormone-receptor interaction into the biological action of the target cell has not been elucidated. To our knowledge, most studies presented in the literature have not been designed to consider both the role of membrane structural and/or fluidity changes upon the physiologic responses of the cell to include the response of target cells to trophic hormone. The characteristic fluidity of the plasma membrane phospholipid matrix provides the framework for another model to describe the mechanism of hormone-receptor interactions which might explain activation of the same enzyme system by multiple hormones.[52,66] This model assumes that biological membranes are in a relatively fluid state, and that direct stoichiometric interaction of receptor and adenyl cyclase components is not required. Interaction of the hormone with the receptor (H·R) imparts to that receptor increased affinity and specificity for the adenylate cyclase (AC). Formation of the hormone-receptor adenylate cyclase complex (H·R-AC) would be the second independent step whose rate would be dependent both upon the H·R and AC, and the rate of lateral diffusion of these protein or lipoprotein components. Lateral diffusion would be affected by temperature, cations, lipid components, etc., all of which modify the fluidity of the membrane. An alteration in the receptor protein conformation, as a result of hormone-receptor interaction, might induce an alteration in the structure of the lipid matrix of the membrane. Activation of the adenyl cyclase system could occur as a result of a change in its lipid environment, *i.e.,* a receptor-induced "field effect." This model system affords an explanation for: (a) basal activity of cells as a result of the constrained state of the active form of the adenyl cyclase system existing in the absence of trophic hormones; (b) negative feedback or desensitization to hormone as a result of altered lipid matric fluidity functional membrane protein changes; and (c) the spectrum of hormones that activate the same adenylate cyclase in cell systems such as the isolated fat cells.[67,68] If the hormone-receptor interaction induces membrane changes, the plasma membrane would act as the transducer in peptide hormone action to induce conformation changes in other plasma membrane proteins, and thus modulate the biological responses of the cell. For instance, if the rates of formation of H·R-AC complex are sufficiently slow, even at concentrations of H which saturate all R, "lag" periods in the expression of the biological response may be explained by the fluid state of the membrane.

Schriere-Muccillo *et al.*[69] and Oliveira *et al.*[70] have recently reported their results of a spin label study of the binding of Angiotensin II to smooth muscle plasma membranes. Using a nitroxide spin label which is known to bind to -SH sites on membrane proteins, they report that increases in the ratio of strongly immobilized to weakly immobilized spin label were induced by binding of the peptide hormone Angiotensin II. They point out that such a change is consistent with hormone-induced membrane protein conformation changes. In studies in which they used the lipophilic spin label, 5-doxyl stearic acid, they report that the probe molecule experiences two environments—one of a high degree of mobility, and another in which motion was hindered (*i.e.*, membrane-bound). They report that the ratio of the highly mobile to membrane-bound components decreased in the presence of hormone and the effect was dose dependent. These authors made no attempt to measure possible changes in order parameter which might indicate hormone-induced fluidity changes. They also found that in order to see any spin label differences between control and hormone-bound membrane systems, peptide hormone levels of 10^{-5}-10^{-3}M, were necessary. Although the authors recognized the fact that their experiments were conducted at unrealistically high hormone concentrations, such that nonspecific binding was being monitored, they claimed that they were able to detect hormone-receptor interaction.

During the past year, we have conducted preliminary experiments in which we have used the spin label technique in conjunction with measurements of cyclic AMP and steroids in attempts to define the membrane events that take place in the ACTH-induced stimulation of Y-1 adrenal tumor cells.

Spin label experiments conducted to date include: (a) the use of the protein specific spin labels 4-isothiocyanato-2, 2, 6, 6, -tetramethyl piperidinoxyl $I_{(103)}$ and ACTH-induced membrane conformational changes; (b) the use of the lipophilic spin labels 5-doxyl stearic acid $I_{(12,3)}$ and 16-doxyl stearic acid $I_{(1,14)}$ to study the effect of ACTH on bulk membrane fluidity; (c) the use of both $I_{(12,3)}$ and $I_{(103)}$ for measurements of the effect of ACTH on the nitroxide reduction kinetics. The possibility that ACTH binding to the Y-1 tumor cell plasma membrane induced conformational changes in membrane protein was initially investigated. In these initial experiments, the spin label $I_{(103)}$ was covalently bound to the adrenal cell membranes during an overnight incubation at 4°C. As illustrated in the figure (Figure 10.7), changes in the correlation time (τ_c) were observed for all ACTH-bound cells when compared to the corresponding control. The observed changes in correlation time of the spin-labeled membrane protein of the ACTH-treated cells is in all cases consistent with ACTH-induced protein conformational changes. The maximum change in τ_c was observed at an incubation time at which cAMP and steroid production were both approaching their maximum rate (Figures 10.8 and 10.9). The possibility that membrane fluidity changes could also be observed as a function of ACTH incubation time was investigated. In these preliminary experiments, order parameter (S) measurements were made at only three incubation times: 0, 30, 120 minutes, using the two stearic acid derivatives $I_{(12,3)}$ and $I_{(1,14)}$. In these experiments, spin labeling was accomplished by incubating the cells at 4°C for periods of 4 hours with the appropriate label. A decrease in fluidity, *i.e.*, an increase in S, was consistently found for the 30 min.

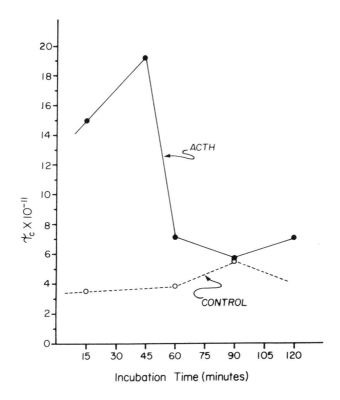

Figure 10.7. Changes in correlation (T_C) as a function of incubation times with ACTH compared to controls.

incubation experiments, both at the surface of the membrane $I_{(1\,2\,,3)}$ and at the center of the bilayer $I_{(1\,,1\,4)}$. The fluidity profiles for the 0 and 120 min. incubation periods were found to be, within experimental error, identical. Using labeling procedures which retained the viability of the cells, it was consistently observed that the nitroxide labels were rapidly reduced and that just as previously observed in studies of the alveolar macrophage, the label reduction was enzymatic. A comparison of the effects of ACTH upon order parameter and upon the kinetics of reduction of a lipophilic spin label when compared with the kinetics of reduction of an aqueous soluble spin label allows one to investigate the effect of ACTH binding upon bulk fluidity of membrane lipids, activation energy of membrane-bound enzymes, and the physical properties of the phospholipid halo surrounding membrane-bound enzymes. Figure 10.10 illustrates the

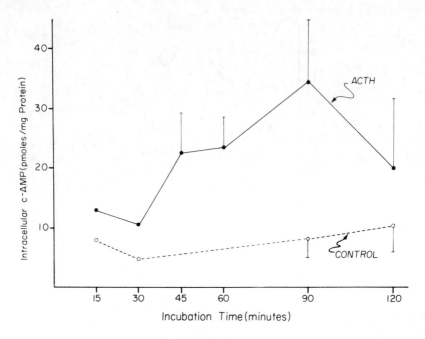

Figure 10.8. Changes in intracellular c-AMP as a function of incubation times with ACTH compared to controls.

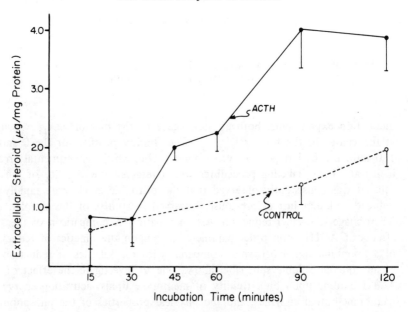

Figure 10.9. Changes in extracellular steroid as a function times with ACTH compared to controls.

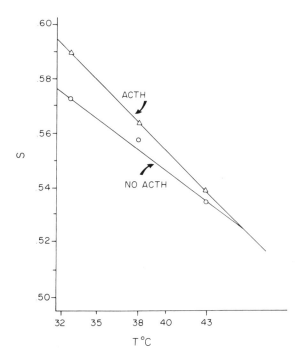

Figure 10.10. Order parameter (S) as a function of temperature in Y-1 adrenal tumor cells.

order parameter versus temperature observed for the spin label $I_{(12,3)}$ for 10-min. incubations in the presence or absence of ACTH. The order parameter in the presence of ACTH is observed to be consistently higher than observed in its absence throughout the temperature range investigated. Furthermore, both order parameter versus temperature plots fall on straight lines throughout the temperature range, so that we can infer that no phase transitions in bulk phospholipids occurred in this temperature range. Measurements of the kinetics of the reduction of the protein label $I_{(103)}$ in the presence and absence of ACTH (incubation time, 10 min.) are illustrated in Figure 10.11. The rate constants were calculated from the slope of a plot of the logarithm of the amplitude of the signal versus time. It can be seen from the figure that the activation energy for the nitroxide reduction drops from 11.25 kcal/mole to 6.00 kcal/mole in the presence of ACTH. This drop in activation energy by a factor of two is fully consistent with an ACTH-induced conformational change of the "nitroxide reductase" enzyme. Finally, the kinetics of reduction of the

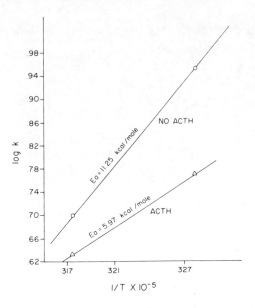

Figure 10.11. Arrhenius plot of Y-1 adrenal tumor cell reduction of protein spin label $I_{(103)}$.

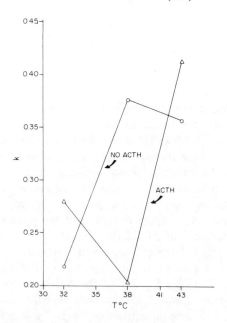

Figure 10.12. Rate constant (k) for Y-1 adrenal tumor cell reduction of lipophilic spin label $I_{12,3}$ as a function of temperature.

lipophilic label 5-doxyl stearic acid is illustrated in Figure 10.12; the variation of k with temperature is complex. In the absence of ACTH, the rate constant initially rises between 32° and 38°C and then remains approximately constant in the temperature range 38° to 42°C. In the presence of ACTH, however, a significant drop in the rate constant between 32° to 38°C, followed by a sharp rise in the rate constant between 38° and 42°C was observed.

The rate reduction of the lipophilic spin label depends upon several factors, in particular the collision frequency and the activation energy for the enzymatic reduction. Since the spin label molecules can be assumed to be initially relatively homogenously distributed in the bulk membrane lipid, the collision frequency is determined by the rate at which the spin label molecules can diffuse to the enzymatic sites. This is determined both by the lateral diffusion coefficient in bulk lipid and the lateral diffusion coefficient in the phospholipid "halo" surrounding the membrane-bound enzyme. Since the fluidity of the "halo" is known to be less than that of bulk lipid, the rate determining step therefore will be governed by the lateral diffusion rate through this important region. The observed changes in order parameter versus temperature, which were obtained on the same sample as the kinetic data, show that no discontinuities occur either in the ACTH-bound or control cells. The rate of reduction of the water soluble label $I_{(103)}$ does not depend upon diffusion through the phospholipid matrix, but depends solely upon enzyme activation energy, which as previously mentioned, decreases in the presence of ACTH. Since no discontinuities in bulk lipid were observed in the order parameter versus temperature experiments, one would expect that if there were no difference in the physical properties of the phospholipid "halo" between control and ACTH-treated cells, then the kinetics of reduction of 5-doxyl stearic acid would follow qualitatively the same pattern with respect to temperature, both in the presence or absence of ACTH. However, the gross dissimilarities observed necessarily imply that significant changes in the physical properties (e.g., fluidity, dimensions) of the phospholipid "halo" have occurred as a result of the ACTH-induced membrane-bound enzyme conformational change. It is evident that similar studies could be conducted to investigate the effect of environmental contaminants upon the fluidity of membranes and the kinetics of reduction of lipophilic and hydrophilic spin labels. Such experiments, when correlated with characteristic physiological response of the cell line under study, would lead to significant advances in our understanding of the molecular biology and pharmacology of environmental agents.

EFFECTS OF FLUOROCARBONS ON
MODEL MEMBRANES AND INTACT CELLS

Certain volatile fluorocarbon compounds are frequently and routinely inhaled by large numbers of people due to use of these compounds as aerosol propellants. When inhaled in aerosol or gaseous form, the propellants are capable of penetrating far enough into the respiratory tract to come into direct contact with alveolar macrophages. Alveolar macrophages represent an important primary host defense mechanism and in this capacity these cells depend heavily upon plasma membrane activity for migration, activation, phagocytosis and attachment to substrate tissue.

Other fluorocarbon products are routinely used as inhalation anesthetics. Anesthesiologists have been reported to have, as a group, a higher than expected suicide rate.[71] Whether this fact is due in part to their occupational exposure to waste anesthetics is at this time a matter of conjecture. Acute exposure of human volunteers to subanesthetic levels of methoxyflurane, enflurane or isoflurane was shown to give rise to impairment of memory functions.[72] Ultrastructural changes in the rat central nervous have been detected after exposure for eight weeks to 10 ppm halothane[73] and differentiation in cultured mouse neuroblastoma cells exposed for 72 hrs. to 0.3 to 2.1% halothane was impaired.[74]

In all of these examples, it is highly suggestive that fluorocarbon alterations in membrane structure and function play an important role.

Trudell et al.[75] have reported an ESR spin label study of the effect of halothane and methoxyflurane on phospholipid model membranes, using spin-labeled phosphatidylocholines and measuring the effect of anesthetics on the amplitude frequency order parameter S. Their results show that anesthetics produce disorder in phospholipid bilayers (decrease in S) and that the disorder has a linear dose-response relationship and occurs in a range of lipid anesthetic concentrations used to produce clinical anesthesia. They suggest that the mode of action of inhalation anesthetics is to produce disorder in the lipid region of a nerve membrane. They point out that the anesthetic might indirectly affect membrane protein. Membrane proteins of highly hydrophobic nature are solvated by the hydrocarbon chains of the lipid bilayer. This area of solute-solvent interaction has been termed the phospholipid "halo". The authors point out that anesthetics which produce perturbations in the hydrocarbon chains of the bilayer which solvates the membrane protein may alter the tertiary structures of hydrophobic proteins essential to nerve impulse transmission in a manner analogous to the allosteric inhibition of enzymes. Gause and Rowlands[76] have reported the results of a spin label study of the effects of several fluorocarbon inhalants upon intact alveolar macrophages. They found that when washed alveolar macrophages suspended in a balanced salt solution (Hanks') or saline were exposed to fluorocarbon-21 (dichlorofluoromethane) in the concentration range of $10^{-5} M$ up to $10^{-2} M$, a progressive increase in membrane fluidity (S decrease) was observed. Prior trypsinization of the cells did not significantly affect this membrane response. They also found that if alveolar macrophages are suspended in isotonic saline (or BSS), the membrane response to fluorocarbon-21 is much more marked than it is for macrophages suspended in isotonic sucrose. Sucrose appears to inhibit the response of the macrophage membrane to fluorocarbon-21 to the extent that the $\triangle$S observed is barely out of control range.

Fluorocarbon-11 (trichlorofluoromethane) was also found to affect this macrophage hydrophobic membrane site in a similar manner. Again, a pronounced disordering of the membrane is induced by this agent when cells are suspended in saline, but the effect appears to be negligible when cells are suspended in sucrose.

These authors also observed that if the macrophage pellet were contaminated with serum proteins, a quite different effect of fluorocarbon-21 exposure was observed. In this case, an apparent increase in S was observed, which corresponds to an increase in order or a decrease in membrane fluidity.

Fluorocarbons-12 (dichlorodifluoromethane) and -23 (trifluoromethane) were observed to have no effect upon the macrophage membrane when employed in analogous exposure experiments. In fact, exposure doses of fluorocarbon-12, corresponding to 5 x 10^{-2} up to 2.0 M produced no effect at all upon the cell membrane, whereas fluorocarbons-21 and -11 show a progressive effect from $10^{-5} M$ upward. The comparatively high dosages of fluorocarbon-12 used assured that even if some slight loss of exposing agent did occur due to volatilization, the cells would still be exposed to an appreciable quantity of the fluorocarbon.

Since exposure to fluorocarbons-21 and -11 caused such a marked alteration in membrane-surface fluidity for the alveolar macrophage as measured by the spin label technique, it was anticipated that this molecular scale disordering might be reflected in the nature of substrate attachment and cell to cell attachment. Scanning electron microscopy (SEM) was employed to investigate this possibility.

The authors found that while most treated cells remained intact and retained a rounded appearance, there was a great deal more spreading of membrane along the surface and a pronounced change in membrane ruffling activity. The overall appearance is as if the cells had undergone melting or dissolution of their plasma membrane.

In addition to the pronounced membrane fluidization produced by fluorocarbons-21 and -11 at concentrations from $10^{-5} M$ upward, the spin label studies also indicate participation of the medium (and optional participation of adsorbed proteins) in events occurring at the membrane surface. The membrane response to the 2-fluorocarbons was much more marked in the presence of a balanced salt solution or saline than in the presence of isotonic sucrose for the case of the alveolar macrophage.

When autologous serum was added to macrophages, a pronounced ordering effect upon the membrane surface was observed. (This effect could not be reversed by repeated washing, but could be reversed by trypsinization of the cells.) When fluorocarbon-21 was then added, another increase in ordering was observed which quickly leveled off, as if a certain number of membrane sites had become saturated.

The observed results are consistent with a fluorocarbon-induced unfolding of adsorbed proteins on the surface of the macrophage which serves to shield membrane hydrophobic regions to some degree from the fluidizing effects of fluorocarbon. When not protected by adsorbed serum protein, the macrophage membrane exhibits a pronounced dose-dependent disordering in an ionic medium (BSS or saline) and a much smaller effect in sucrose.

Fluorocarbons have been observed to "break" or perturb hydrogen bonds[77] in direct correlation with their anesthetic potency. Isotonic sucrose is considered to be a strongly H-bonding solvent and, as such, may form H-bonds with cell membrane components and compete with membrane components with respect to H-bond perturbation by fluorocarbons. It is known that the spin label employed in these studies is localized in the polar headgroup region of lipid bilayers, but is also subject to the influence of H_2O which penetrates the bilayer to at least a depth of 3-4 carbon atoms.[22]

The macrophage membrane disordering induced by fluorocarbons-21 and -11 and the accompanying cell-to-cell and cell-to-substrate attachment interactions observed could be indicative of possible enhancement by these fluorocarbons of granuloma formation and giant cell formation *in vivo*.

HYDROSTATIC PRESSURE EFFECTS ON MEMBRANES

The realization that biological organisms can survive and adapt to the extreme hydrostatic pressures encountered in the depths of the oceans has prompted a great deal of research into the biological effects of pressure and the mechanisms responsible for these effects. The effects of pressure upon bacteria, protozoa, marine eggs, marine invertebrates and fishes, and upon certain basic processes, such as cell division, have been studied.[78,79] Pressure effects upon a number of enzymes and other macromolecules also have been observed by these authors. As a rule, enzymes appear to be at least partially inactivated by high pressures, but a multiplicity of pressure effects upon intact organisms has been observed. This multiplicity of effects is not unexpected upon consideration of pressure as a parameter in the kinetics of numerous biochemical reactions which are quite different in nature. For example, if a reaction pathway contains an activated complex which represents a volume increase, then pressure would be expected to retard the rate of reaction; while if the reaction proceeds through a step involving a volume decrease, pressure will no doubt increase the reaction rate.

Many of the studies reported to date have been concerned with the effects of pressure upon cellular proteins with little consideration given to effects upon cellular lipids. In view of the importance of the physical and chemical properties of lipids to the structure and permeability properties of membranes, the effects of pressure in combination with reduced temperatures appear particularly significant. In a study of the effects of water temperature and depth on the fatty acid composition of marine ectotherms, Lewis emphasized that it is not only necessary to keep an organism's lipids liquid at low temperatures, but the lipid viscosity must be regulated because "long before a particular fat has reached its setting point, it will have passed through stages of viscosity inimical to many life processes."[80] Hydrostatic pressures have been shown to reverse anesthesia. When newts or tadpoles are placed in a chamber of water containing an anesthetic, they cease swimming but resume activity when the hydrostatic pressure in the chamber is increased to 150 atmospheres. Luminescent bacteria stop their luminescence when placed in a solution of an anesthetic. This response is restored by applying 150 atm of hydrostatic pressure to the solution. Finally, mice which have lost their righting reflex after being treated with anesthetics also regain this reflex when subjected to 150 atm of helium pressure. Trudell *et al.*,[75] in conjunction with their spin label study of anesthetic effects also investigated the effects of hydrostatic pressures as the model membranes. They were able to show that 4000 psi of helium completely reversed the disordering produced by 120 μ moles of halothane per mole of lipid. They also showed that this effect of pressure was completely reversible. The effect of hydrostatic pressure on intact alveolar macrophage cells has been reported by Gause, Mendez and Rowlands,[81] using the spin label technique. These authors observed an increase in the viscosity of membrane lipid as a function of increased hydrostatic pressure.

From a comparative study of the relative effects of decreases in temperature to increases in hydrostatic pressure, these authors were able to calculate that an increase in pressure of 1000 psi exerts an equivalent effect on membrane lipids to a reduction in temperature of 1°C.

Combining the results of these two studies we can calculate that 120 μ moles of halothane per mole of lipid exerts a disordering effect on the hydrocarbon chains equivalent to a temperature rise of 4°C.

NO$_2$ AND SO$_2$ EFFECTS ON INTACT CELLS

Nitrogen Dioxide

Specific physiological damage has been attributed to the oxidants present in the atmosphere--especially nitrogen oxides and ozone. Arioka[82] demonstrated that pulmonary damage was experimentally induced in rats by inhalation of nitrogen dioxide. He successfully demonstrated a relationship between the mortality rate and the NO$_2$ concentration, and he also showed that the blood of the exposed rats contained an elevated concentration of both metmyoglobin (4% to 6%) and potassium ions. Symon[83] has reported that elevated levels of metmyoglobin (3% to 5%) have been observed in children living in an environment containing high concentrations of oxides of nitrogen.

Studies by Thomas et al.[84] concerned with the effect of NO$_2$ on young rats have demonstrated that the inhalation of 1 ppm for one hour or 0.5 ppm for four hours leads to significant morphological changes in their lung-mast cells. The morphological changes are thought to occur both as a result of the chemical interaction of NO$_2$ with the cell membrane, and as a result of the interaction of NO$_2$ with certain specific but undefined cellular elements which lead to a loss in cell integrity.

In vitro studies aimed at elucidating products and mechanisms associated with observed *in vivo* effects have included work by Felmeister et al.[85] on surface pressure measurements of films of both saturated and unsaturated phospholipid, showed significant changes in the surface pressure surface area curves in the presence of all atmospheres studied which contain NO$_2$. They attribute their observed effects to a chemical interaction of NO$_2$ with the double bonds of lecithin.

Rowlands and Gause[86] have found that NO$_2$ reacts *in vitro* with lecithin and phosphatidyl ethanolamine to produce three different nitrogen-containing free radical species. These three radicals were quite stable in that they persisted in solution for periods of several hours to several days. In addition, a fourth free radical (single line, g = 2.0069) was observed in the reaction of phosphatidyl ethanolamine with NO$_2$. These reactions assume particular biological significance due to the function of these two phospholipids as surfactants of the alveolar lining.

These authors confirmed that the same three free radicals were produced upon exposure to NO$_2$ of any lipid compound containing a double bond.

The reaction of NO_2 with olefins at the unsaturated linkage has been recognized and has been the subject of many previous investigations by organic chemists over a period of many years. However, the results of these studies have been conflicting and confusing, and a multitude of reaction products have been reported, including dinitro compounds, nitronitrites, nitronitrates, nitronitroso derivatives, nitrosonitrites, nitrosonitrates, dinitrites and nitronitrates. Surprisingly enough, until these results were published, no one had reported the production of free radical species from this reaction, although Bielski and Gebicki[87] had recently reported observing similar free radicals which they attributed to the formation of NO_2-olefin π complexes when NO_2 was dissolved in unsaturated solvents.

Rowlands and Gause[86] provided evidence that π complexes are not involved in the reaction. (This has subsequently been confirmed by the work of Jonkman *et al.*[88]). The three types of stable nitrogen-containing free radicals were observed consistently in the reactions between NO_2 and a series of olefinic hydrocarbons and fatty acids.

In addition to these long-lived free radicals, they observed a fourth, very short-lived free radical when the reaction was carried out in a flow system through the sample cavity of the ESR spectrometer. The nature of this initial transient free radical was such that it was obvious they were observing the initial step in the reaction of NO_2 with a double bond, in which NO_2 breaks the double bond, and adds to one side of the bond, leaving an unpaired electron on the carbon atom on the other side.

The reactions of NO_2 with unsaturated linkages in lipids to produce the four different free radical species described took place in essentially nonaqueous systems; however, Rowlands and Gause[86] also observed a stable free radical species with a 13.4 gauss ^{14}N hyperfine coupling to be produced in aqueous solutions of tryptophan by exposure to less than 5 ppm levels of NO_2, an atmospheric concentration of NO_2 encountered in pollution episodes.

Interaction of NO_2 with a protein constituent such as tryptophan to produce a stable free radical has many implications. Not only are the tryptophan residues affected directly, but the stable free radical species produced might enter into secondary reactions with other sites on the protein or with neighboring molecules.

Rowlands and Gause[86] also found that both NO and NO_2 react with hemoglobin solutions to give rise to paramagnetic solutions characterized by a well defined triplet ESR spectrum. Kon[89] has published a detailed study of the NO-hemoglobin reaction. He was able to show that the appearance of the triplet ESR spectrum with a ^{14}N hyperfine coupling of 17 gauss coincided with a detergent-induced organic change in protein structure. Prior to the addition of the detergent, he showed from the

observed g factors that the complex was consistent with rhombic sym-
metry, with no evidence of ^{14}N hyperfine coupling.

From the point of view of air pollution research, these observations
are extremely interesting, as they parallel very closely some of the observations that have been made on the effects of NO_2 on whole blood.

Rowlands and Gause[86] have found that the reaction of NO_2 with hemoglobin solutions *in vitro* and in the blood of rats exposed *in vivo* to 1 to
3 ppm NO_2 gives rise to a broad resonance of *ca.* g = 2, with a nitrogen
hyperfine coupling of 16 gauss plainly observable on the high field side
of the signal. Evidently, NO_2 upon inhalation is capable of entering the
red blood cell to not only form the NO-hemoglobin complex, but to also
denature the globin moiety of the hemoglobin to give rise to the characteristic electron spin resonance spectrum characterized by Kon.[89] Thus,
there is ample available evidence that NO_2 can potentially react with both
lipid and protein components of cell membranes. In studies designed to
characterize the effect of NO_2 exposure upon membrane dynamics, Rowlands, Allen-Rowlands and Gause[39] have recently undertaken spin label
studies of the *in vitro* exposure of intact alveolar macrophage cells to
aqueous solutions of NO_2. In these studies, the effect of 10^{-4} molar
concentrations of NO_2 in saline upon both the amplitude frequency order
parameter S and the rate constant of the pseudo first-order nitroxide reduction kinetics were measured. Measurements were made at various
temperatures between 24°C and 40°C. The experiments were designed so
that both control and exposed macrophages were taken from the same
animal for each temperature measured. This procedure nullified any
possibility that observed differences could be due to variability between
animals, since each animal served as its own control. Figure 10.13 illustrates the order parameter and the rate constant versus temperature data
obtained by this procedure. The order parameter was found, as expected,
to increase for both control and exposed macrophages throughout the
range 40° → 24°C, consistent with a progressive loss of fluidity with decreasing temperature. Although the data for each temperature point was
obtained from alveolar macrophages isolated from different animals, the
discontinuities observed in the slopes of the order parameter versus temperature plots are believed real and indicative of lipid phase transitions
occurring at or near the temperatures at which the measurements were
made. Similar discontinuities have been observed when the order parameter
temperature dependence was obtained from macrophages obtained from a
single animal throughout the entire temperature range (Figure 10.3). As
illustrated in Figure 10.13, exposure of macrophages to 10^{-4} M NO_2
solution caused a definite increase in fluidity of the plasma membrane
throughout the entire temperature range although increases in fluidity over

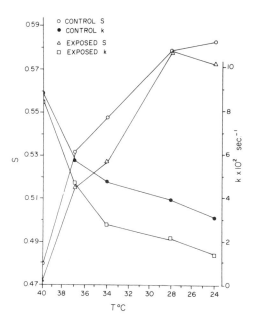

Figure 10.13. Order parameter (S) and rate constant (k) versus temperature. For control and exposed (NO_2) alveolar macrophages. For each temperature control and exposed macrophages were obtained from same animal.

control appears to be greater between 37°C and 34°C. The temperature dependence of the rate constants for nitroxide reduction of both control and exposed macrophages shows a progressive decrease with decreases in temperature. Discontinuities are observed in the kinetic data at the same temperatures at which the order parameter data indicate the existence of lipid phase transition. The existence of the discontinuities in the measured rate constants at these temperatures is not surprising since one of the factors that determines the rate of reduction of the nitroxide label is its lateral diffusion through the plasma membrane to encounter the reductase enzyme. However, since the order parameter data indicates that the bulk fluidity of the membrane has been increased by exposure to NO_2, one would expect the rate of lateral diffusion of the spin labels to be greater for the exposed alveolar macrophages. In the absence of exposure-induced conformational changes of the reductase enzyme, the rate constant for the enzymatic reduction should be greater, the more fluid the membrane. The overall temperature dependence of the rate constants for both exposed and control membranes follows this trend. However, the rate constant for the nitroxide reduction is consistently lower for the exposed cells throughout the temperature range. Hence, it may be inferred from this data that exposure of the alveolar macrophage to the NO_2 solution causes conformational changes to membrane-bound enzymes. Figure 10.14 illustrates an Arrhenius plot of the rate constant data with calculated energies of activation for the enzymatic reduction indicated.

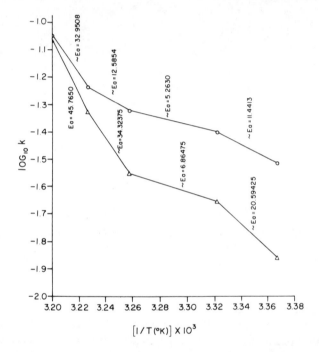

Figure 10.14. Arrhenius plot of nitroxide reduction kinetics for control and NO_2 exposed macrophages. Activation energies in kilocalories per mole.

SO₂ Effects on Intact Cells

The electron acceptor properties of SO_2 and its affinity for molecules with electron donor characteristics such as tryptophan residues of proteins has been discussed at length in a separate paper in this publication.[90] The fact that *in vivo* inhalants can affect plasma membrane activity was demonstrated in studies of the effect of SO_2 on plasma membrane-bound Na^+-K^+ ATPase activity of the rat alveolar macrophage. Physical studies of the effect of SO_2 on membrane dynamics and cell function have been reported in at least three important cell types. Gause and Rowlands,[91] have reported on the effects of *in vitro* exposure of human lymphocytes to SO_2 and bisulphite solutions, using the protein specific spin label, $I_{(103)}$, to study exposure-induced plasma membrane-bound glycoprotein alternations. Since lymphocyte plasma membranes are mechanistically involved in many immunological processes, both humoral and cellular, any alternation in the responsiveness of this membrane may prove to be of far-reaching consequence to the host. A pollutant-induced perturbation of lymphocyte membranes *in vivo* could result in a loss of immunological specificity wherein lymphocytes would not be able to (a) recognize and bind antigen (therefore, could not elaborate antibodies or participate in helper cell interactions), or (b) recognize and respond to aberrant or effete cells, thereby diminishing the host's capacity for immune surveillance.

It has been pointed out by several investigators that the long circulatory residence time of SO_2 presents ample opportunity for interaction with immunological mechanism.[92] Indeed, several studies have indicated that inhaled SO_2 results in reduced immunological function, particularly with respect to clearance of microorganisms and decrease in production of antibodies and agglutinins. Schneider and Calkins[93] have presented evidence that SO_2-induced multiple cellular aberrations in primary cultures of human peripheral lymphocytes, and concluded that exposure to moderate concentrations of sulfur dioxide could impair normal immunological functions as a result of damage to peripheral blood lymphocytes.

Gause and Rowlands[91] found that upon exposure of lymphocytes labeled with $I_{(103)}$ to SO_2, by suspension in solutions of SO_2 or HSO_3^-, the spin label spectra reflected a progressive increase in the degree of line broadening leading to the appearance of a broad single-line spectral feature. These observations indicate formation of micropatches or microaggregates of membrane protein structures at the lower concentration levels leading to the appearance and growth of the broad single-line species as the size and extent of aggregate formation proceeds with increasing SO_2 concentration. The appearance of the single-line feature occurs as a consequence of increasingly high, localized concentrations of spin-label molecules.[94]

The initiation of the process of aggregate formation by SO_2 or HSO_3^- in the medium could be detected at concentrations in the $10^{-4}M$ range, and it is probable that the sensitivity of detection could be increased by another order of magnitude by painstaking and rigorous control of experimental conditions. The cells appear to retain essentially complete viability at concentrations up to $10^{-2}M$; however, the degree of aggregation continued to increase with concentrations up to 1 M. Therefore, the aggregation observed is apparently not an active process requiring cell functions; however, the internalization of the aggregated protein probably is an active process, *i.e.*, a mechanism by which the lymphocyte is attempting to clear the membrane of denatured or nonfunctional proteins.

Chronic exposure to low levels of SO_2, thus, could induce unnaturally high rates of turnover of lymphocyte membrane proteins which, in turn, would demand increased rates of protein synthesis. The extent to which a cell can cope with these environmentally triggered demands, and still be able to maintain its membrane function, would probably reflect its capacity for increasing synthesis of messenger RNA and/or ribosomal RNA. The implications of the ability of inhaled SO_2 (or of sulfite-bisulfite employed as antioxidant and administered by injection or ingestion) to significantly and nonspecifically alter lymphocyte membrane protein are extensive, as B-lymphocyte membrane proteins are thought to serve as antigen recognition sites and to function in the internalization of specific antigens to control cellular antibody synthesis. Although the T-lymphocyte membrane structures for recognition of T-specific antigens (which may include aberrant and tumor cells, some microorganisms, fungi, etc.) are not as well understood as in the case of B-cells, the recognition mechanisms undoubtedly include membrane-bound proteins which would be susceptible to the effects of SO_2, or HSO_3^-.

The effect of *in vitro* exposure to 1.4×10^{-4} M $NaHSO_3$ solutions on both bulk fluidity and kinetics of nitroxide reduction have been measured for intact alveolar macrophages obtained from Fisher rats.[95] For measurements of bulk fluidity, order parameters versus temperature measurements were made throughout the temperature range of 4°C through 45°C. Figure 10.15 illustrates the results obtained in these studies. Bulk fluidity of the macrophage membrane appears to be increased by SO_2

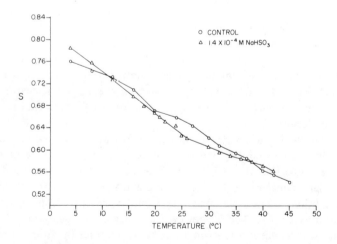

Figure 10.15 Order parameter versus temperature for control and HSO_3^--exposed macrophages. For each temperature, control and exposed macrophages were obtained from the same animal.

exposure throughout most of the temperature ranges studied. At both the lower and upper ends of the temperature range studied, an inversion in the measured order parameters occurs. The origin of the inversions appears to be related to the absence in the exposed macrophages of the discontinuities (phase transitions) that are observed in the order parameter versus temperature plot for the control macrophages.

Preliminary measurements throughout the temperature of the kinetics range $24°C$ to $16°C$ indicate that exposure to $10^{-4}M$ solutions of SO_2 facilitates the enzymatic reduction of the nitroxide label. However, a complete temperature dependence study throughout the range of temperatures reported for the effect on bulk fluidity has not been completed. The Y-1 adrenal tumor cell, as we have previously discussed, produces cAMP and steriod in response to ACTH, the peptide hormone, binding to specific receptor sites on the surface of the plasma membrane. The spin label studies that have been described indicate that ACTH binding induces a conformational change in the receptor membrane-bound protein or glycoprotein molecules. In view of the apparent affinity of SO_2 to protein molecules, it is possible that these peptide hormone-responsive cells might be particularly sensitive to exposure to environmental agents such as SO_2. In order to investigate this possibility, Rowlands et. al.[48] in a dose-response study, investigated the effect of SO_2 upon the ability of Y-1 adrenal tumor cells to produce cAMP and steroid both in the presence and the absence of ACTH.

Y-1 adrenal tumor cells were incubated in the presence of varying concentrations of $NaHSO_3$, pH6.9 both in the presence or absence of 60mU ACTH. It can be seen in Figure 10.16 that 90 min. incubations without ACTH, but in the presence of 10^{-3}-$10^{-9}M$ $NaHSO_3$, induced an increase in the mean extracellular accumulation of both steroids and cAMP. This nonspecific induction of the adenyl cyclase system with subsequent steroidogenisis was not related to sodium ions as incubation without ACTH, but in the presence of 10^{-3}-$10^{-9}M$ $NaHSO_4$, was without any effect. These findings appear to be related to the specificity of bi-sulphite/SO_2 for membrane-bound proteins. In order to examine the effect of $NaHSO_3$ on ACTH-induced cAMP and steroid production, the Y-1 adrenal tumor cells were incubated with varying concentrations of $NaHSO_3$ in the presence of ACTH. In Figures 10.16 and 10.17, the extracellular accumulation of both steroid and cAMP show a progressive increase with increasing $NaHSO_3$ concentrations from 10^{-5} - $10^{-8}M$. This potentiation of the ACTH response was observed following both 90- and 120-min incubations. Intracellular steroid production was also shown to give rise to a dose-response increase compared to control flasks, however no apparent dose response in intracellular cAMP in response to $NaHSO_3$ in the presence of ACTH was observed.

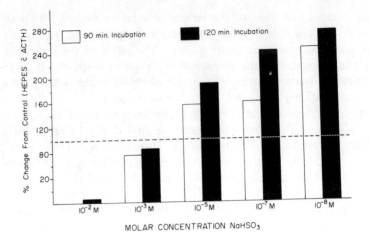

Figure 10.16. Effect of NaHSO₃ on the ACTH-induced mean extracellular accumulation of steroid compared to control (HEPES with ACTH, pH 6.9).

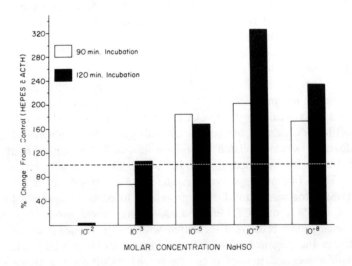

Figure 10.17. Effect of NaHSO₃ on the ACTH-induced mean extracellular accumulation of cAMP compared to control (HEPES with ACTH, pH 6.9).

Its ability to induce conformational changes in membrane-bound proteins which activate the adenyl cyclase system with concommitant steroid production. The potentiation of the ACTH response that was observed is in all probability related to the affinity of SO_2 for membrane protein. However, the elucidation of the process mechanism by which the potentiation takes place must await further studies in which both the SO_2 and the ACTH concentrations are varied in a very systematic manner. A similar and so far unexplained potentiation of the ACTH-induced production of steroid has been observed for cholera enterotoxin Y-1 adrenal cell interaction.[96]

Physical studies of the effect of SO_2/HSO_3^- on the dynamics of the plasma membrane of Y-1 adrenal tumor cells have so far been limited to comparative studies of the effect of ACTH and $10^{-7}M$ $NaHSO_3$ solutions on the kinetics of the enzymatic reduction of 5-doxyl stearic acid spin labels. Extracellular steroid levels obtained from 90-min incubations of Y-1 adrenal tumor cells with 60 mU ACTH per flask were found to be 260% of control values. Similarly, 90-min incubations with $10^{-7}M$ $NaHSO_3$ solutions in the absence of ACTH were found to stimulate steroid production of 160% of control values. Rate constants for the pseudofirst order reduction of 5-doxyl stearic acid spin label were found to be within experimenttal error identical for the ACTH and $10^{-7}M$ $NaHSO_3$ stimulated adrenal cells and to be 212% of the rate constant measured for the reduction of control cells. Whether the apparent correlation observed between ACTH and bisulphite stimulation of steroid and nitroxide reduction kinetics observed at these concentrations is fortuitous must await further kinetic measurements in the presence of varying concentrations.

METAL ION EFFECTS

The environmentally important metal ions La^{3+}, Hg^{2+} and Cd^{2+} all show a strong affinity for ligands such as phosphates and cysteinyl and histidyl side chains of proteins. All three elements inhibit a large number of enzymes having functional sulfhydryl groups, all bind to and affect the conformation of nucleic acids and all disrupt pathways of oxidative phosphopylation. The trivalent lanthanum ion, La^{3+}, by virtue of an ionic radius similar to Ca^{2+} is known to be a specific antagonist of Ca^{2+} in biological systems. Haksar et al.[97] have shown that $10^{-6}M$ concentrations of La^{3+} inhibited the calcium dependent ACTH-induced production of cAMP and corticosterone in isolated rat adrenal cortex cells. These authors showed by electron microscopic examination that the La^{3+} did not appear to penetrate beyond the plasma membrane of the adrenal cells.

Uyesaka et al.[98] have recently published the results of a study of the effects of La^{3+}, Cd^{2+} and Hg^{2+} on fluidity properties of synaptosomal membranes using the electron spin resonance spin label technique. They found that all three metal ions gave rise to an increase in the measured order parameter consistent with metal-ion-induced decrease in the fluidity of the membrane. At a metal-ion concentration of 3×10^{-3} M the three metals gave rise to a 12% (La^{3+}), 4% (Cd^{2+}) and 2% (Hg^{2+}) increase in measured-order parameter. For the case of La^{3+} these workers found that the order parameter increased hyperbolically as the concentration of La^{3+} increased and appeared to level off at a La^{3+} concentration of 4×10^{-4} M. Rowlands and Allen-Rowlands[99] have made preliminary measurements on the effect of 10^{-6} M solutions of $CdCl_2$ and $LaCl_3$ on the kinetics of the reduction of the lipophilic spin label 5-doxyl stearic acid in intact Y-1 adrenal tumor cells, both in the absence and the presence of ACTH. Their measurements indicate that in the absence of ACTH, 10^{-6} M solutions of both Cd^{2+} and La^{3+} stimulate the enzymatic reduction of the nitroxide label. For Cd^{2+}, the measured rate constant was 112% and for La^{3+}, 228% of the rate constant measured for control cells. In the presence of ACTH, 10^{-6} M Cd^{2+} was found to significantly inhibit the enzymatic reduction (28% of ACTH control), while 10^{-6} M La^{3+} solutions still appeared to be slightly stimulatory (106% of ACTH control). Thus, the effect of these ions appears to depend quite markedly upon the functional state of the cell.

SUMMARY

In this review special attention has been given to the role that the electron spin resonance spin label technique has played in determining our current awareness of the importance of the dynamic properties of membranes to cellular function. In addition, we have tried to indicate the effects that environmental agents might have on membrane dynamics by describing spin label studies of the effects of different types of environmental agents such as lipophilic agents, hydrostatic pressure, oxidizing and reducing air pollutants and metal ions, on membrane properties. Physical techniques such as electron spin resonance, nuclear magnetic resonance and fluorescence spectroscopy have proven their worth in studies of basic membrane biophysics and pharmacology of drug-membrane interactions. It is to be hoped that this review will stimulate the use of these extremely powerful techniques for environmental health research.

ACKNOWLEDGMENT

This work was supported in part by National Institute of Health Grant No. NIH1-RO1-ES01161-01 and in part by the Southwest Foundation for Research and Education, San Antonio, Texas.

REFERENCES

1. Singer, S. J. and G. L. Nicolson. *Science* 175:720 (1972).
2. Jost, P. C., O. H. Griffith, R. A. Capaldi and G. Vanderkool. *Proc. Natl. Acad. Sci., U.S.* 79:480 (1973a).
3. Seelig, J. and W. Hasselbach. *Eur. J. Biochem.* 21:17 (1971).
4. Hubbell, W. L. and H. M. McConnel. *J. Am. Chem. Soc.* 93:314 (1971).
5. Blaurock, A. E. *J. Molec. Biol.* 56:35 (1971).
6. Caspar, D. L. D. and D. A. Kirschner. *Nature, New Biol.* 231:46 (1971).
7. Wilkins, M. H. F., A. E. Blaurock and D. M. Engelman. *Nature, New Biol.* 230:72 (1971).
8. Blaurock, A. E. and M. H. F. Wilkins. *Nature* 236:313 (1972).
9. Dupont, Y., A. Gabriel, M. Chabre, T. Gulik-Krzywicki and E. Schechter. *Nature.* 238:331 (1972).
10. Blaurock, A. E. and W. Stoeckenius. *Nature, New Biol.* 233:152 (1971).
11. Blaurock, A. E. *Chem. Phys. Lipids* 8:285 (1972).
12. Blaurock, A. E. *Biophys. J.* 13:90 (1973).
13. Engelman, D. M. *J. Molec. Biol.* 58:153 (1971).
14. Oldfield, E., K. M. Keough and D. Chapman. *FEBS Lett.* 20:344 (1972).
15. Rottem, S., W. L. Hubbell, L. Hayflick and H. M. McConnell. *Biochim. Biophys. Acta.* 219:104 (1970).
16. Eletr, S. and A. D. Keith. *Proc. Natl. Acad. Sci., U.S.* 69:1353 (1972).
17. Landsberger, F. R., J. Lenard, J. Paxton and R. W. Compans. *Proc. Nalt. Acad. Sci., U.S.* 68:2579 (1971).
18. Landsberger, F. R., R. W. Compans, J. Paxton and J. Lenard. *J. Supramol. Stract.* 1:50 (1972).
19. Landsberger, F. R., R. W. Compans, P. W. Choppin and J. Lenard. *Biochem.* 12:4498 (1973).
20. Williams, M. A., R. C. Stancliff, L. Packer and A. D. Keith. *Biochim. Biophys. Acta.* 267:444 (1972).
21. McFarland, B. G. and H. M. McConnell. *Proc. Natl. Acad. Sci., U.S.* 68:1274 (1971).
22. Griffith, O. H., P. J. Dehlinger and S. P. Van. *J. Membrane Biol.* 15:159 (1974).
23. Trauble, H. and E. Sackmann. *J. Am. Chem. Soc.* 94:4499 (1972).
24. Lee, A. G., N. J. M. Birdsall and J. C. Metcalfe. *Biochem.* 12:1650 (1973).

25. Devaux, P. and H. M. McConnell. *J. Am. Chem. Soc.* 94:4475 (1972).
26. Cohn, G. E., A. D. Keith and W. Snipes. *Biophys. J.* 14:178 (1974).
27. Scandella, C. J., P. Devaux and H. M. McConnell. *Proc. Nalt. Acad. Sci.,* U.S. 69:2056 (1972).
28. Stier, A. and E. Sackmann. *Biochem. Biophys. Acta.* 311:400 (1973).
29. Sackmann, E., H. Trauble, H. Galla and P. Overath. *Biochem.* 12: 5360 (1973).
30. McNamee, M. G. and H. M. McConnell. *Biochem.* 12:2951 (1973).
31. Kornberg, R. D. and H. M. McConnell. *Biochem.* 10:1111 (1971).
32. Poo, M. M. and R. A. Cone. *Nature* 247:438 (1974).
33. Rogers, M. J. and P. Strittmatter. *J. Biol. Chem.* 249:895 (1974).
34. Martonosi, A. in *Biomembranes.* L. A. Manson, Ed. (New York: Plenum Press, 1971), p.191.
35. Vessey, D. A. and D. Zakim. *J. Biol. Chem.* 246:4649 (1971).
36. Mavis, R. D., R. M. Bell and P. R. Vagelos. *J. Biol. Chem.* 247: 2835 (1972).
37. Eletr, S., D. Zakim and D. A. Vessey. *J. Molec. Biol.* 78:351 (1973).
38. Esfachani, M. and S. J. Wakil. *Fed. Proc. Fed. Am. Soc. Exp. Biol.* 31:413 (1972).
39. Rowlands, J. R., C. Allen-Rowlands and E. M. Gause. "Effects of Pollutants on Lung Biochemistry," Submitted for publication 1976b.
40. Charnock, J. S., D. M. Doty and J. C. Russell. *Arch. Biochem. Biophys.* 142:633 (1971).
41. North, R. J. *J. Ultrastruct. Res.* 16:83 (1966).
42. Wisnieski, B. J., J. G. Parkes, Y. O. Huang and C. F. Fox. *Proc. Natl. Acad. Sci.,* U.S. 71:4381 (1974).
43. Bretscher, M. S. *Nature, New Biol.* 236:11 (1972).
44. Veriej, A. J., R. F. A. Zwaal, B. Roelofsen, P. Cumfurius, D. Kastelijn and L. L. M.van Deenen. *Biochem. Biophys. Acta.* 323: 178 (1973).
45. Robinson, J. D. N. J. M. Birdsall, A. G. Lee and J. C. Metcalfe. *Biochem.* 11:2903 (1972).
46. Jost, P. C., O. H. Griffith, R. A. Capaldi and G. Vanderkool. *Biochem. Biophys. Acta.* 311:141 (1973b).
47. Kaplan, J., P. J. Canonico and W. J. Caspary. *Proc. Natl. Acad. Sci.,* U.S. 70:66 (1973).
48. Rowlands, J. R., C. Allen-Rowlands and A. R. Parrish. "Spin Label Study of the Effects of Peptide Hormone ACTH on the Plasma Membrane of Y-1 Adrenal Tumor Cells." Submitted for publication 1976b.
49. Kahn, C. R. in *Methods in Membrane Biology.* E. D. Korn, Ed. (New York & London: Plenum Press, 1975), pp.81-146.
50. Hechter, O. and T. Braun. in *Structure-Activity Relationships of Proteins and Polypeptide Hormones.* M. Margoulies and F. C. Greenwood, Eds. (Liege: Excerpta Medica Foundation, International Congress, 1972), p. 211.

51. Roth, J. *Metabolism* 22:1059 (1973).
52. Cuatrecasas, P. *Ann. Rev. Biochem.* 43:169 (1974).
53. Freychet, P. *Diabetologia* 12:83 (1976).
54. Schimmer, B. P., K. Ueda and G. H. Sato. *Biochem. Biophys. Res. Comm.* 32:806 (1968).
55. Cuatrecasas, P. *Proc. Natl. Acad. Sci., U.S.* 63:450 (1969).
56. Lefkowitz, R. J., I. Pastan and J. Roth. in *The Role of Adenyl Cyclase and Cyclic 3', 5'-AMP in Biological Systems* (Bethesda, Md.: NIH Fogarty International Center Proceedings No. 4, 1969), pp.88-95.
57. Lefkowitz, R. J., J. Roth and W. Pricer. *Proc. Natl. Acad. Sci., U.S.* 65:745 (1970).
58. Lefkowitz, R. J., J. Roth and I. Pastan. *Ann. N. Y. Acad. Sci.* 185: 195 (1971).
59. Levey, G. S. *Biochem. Biophys. Res. Commun.* 38:86 (1970).
60. Levey, G. S. *Ann. N. Y. Acad. Sci.* 185:449 (1971).
61. Donta, S .T . *J. Infect. Dis.* 129:284 (1974a).
62. Ruben, M. S., N. I. Swislocki and M. Sonenberg. *Arch. Biochem. Biophys.* 157:252 (1973a).
63. Sonenberg, M. *Biochem. Biophys. Res. Comm.* 36:450 (1969).
64. Sonenberg, M. *Proc. Natl. Acad. Sci., U.S.* 68:1051 (1971).
65. Ruben, M. S., N. I. Swislocki and M. Sonenberg. *Arch. Biochem. Biophys.* 157:243 (1973b).
66. Bennett, V., E. O'Keefe, and P. Cautrecasas. *Proc. Natl. Acad. Sci., U.S.* 72:33 (1975).
67. Hardman, J. G., G. A. Robison and E. W. Sutherland. *Ann. Rev. Physiol.* 33:311 (1971).
68. Birnbaumer, L. and M. Rodbell. *J. Biol. Chem.* 244:3477 (1969).
69. Schreier-Muccillo, S., G. X. Niculitchelf, M. M. Oliveira, S. Shimuta and A. C. M. Paiva. *FEBS Lett.* 47:193 (1974).
70. Oliveira, M. M., S. Schreier-Muccillo, S. Shimuta, G. Niculitcheff and A. C. M. Paiva. in *Concepts of Membranes in Regulation and Excitation.* M. Rocha, E. Silva and G. Suarez-Kurtz, Eds. (New York: Raven Press, 1975), pp.167-180.
71. Bruce, D. L., M. J. Bach and J. Arbit. *Anesthesiology* 40:453 (1974).
72. Adam, N. *J. Comp. Physiol. Psychol.* 83:294 (1973).
73. Chang, L. W., A. W. Dudley, Jr., Y. K. Lee, and J. W. Katz. *Exp. Neurol.* 45:209 (1974).
74. Hinkley, R. E. and A. G. Telser. *J. Cell. Biol.* 63:531 (1974).
75. Trudell, J. R., W. L. Hubbell and E. N. Cohen. *Ann. N. Y. Acad. Sci.* 222:530 (1973).
76. Gause, E. M. and J. R. Rowlands. *Spectroscopy Ltrs.* 9:237 (1976).
77. DiPaolo, T. and C. Sandorfy. *Nature* 252:471 (1974).
78. Zimmerman, A. M., Ed. *High Pressure Effects on Cellular Processes.* (New York: Academic Press, 1970).
79. Sleigh, M. A. and A. G. McDonald, Eds. *The Effects of Pressure on Organisms.* (New York: Academic Press, 1972).
80. Lewis, R. W. *Comp. Biochem. Physiol.* 6:75 (1962).
81. Gause, E. M., V. M. Mendez and J. R. Rowlands. *Spectroscopy Ltrs.* 7:477 (1974).

82. Arioka, I. *Hakkaido Igaku Zasshi* 40:457 (1967); cf *Chem. Abst.* 58251c 68 (1968).
83. Symon, K. *Proc. Roy. Soc. Med.* 57:988 (1965).
84. Thomas, H. V., P. K. Mueller and R. Wright. *J. Air Pollution Control Assn.* 17:333 (1967).
85. Felmeister, A., M. Amanat and N. D. Wiener. *Environ. Sci. Technol.* 2:1 (1968).
86. Rowlands, J. R. and E. M. Gause. *Arch. Intern. Med.* 128:94 (1971).
87. Bielski, B. H. J. and J. M. Gebicki. *J. Phys. Chem.* 73:1402 (1969).
88. Jonkman, L., H. Muller, C. Kiers, *et al. J. Phys. Chem.* 74:1650 (1970).
89. Kon, H. *J. Biol. Chem.* 243:4350 (1968).
90. Gause, E. M., N. D. Greene, M. L. Meltz and J. R. Rowlands, "Review of Multidisciplinary Studies on 'Biological Effects of Sulfur Oxides.' " *Symposium on Biochemical Effects of Environmental Pollutants,* Cincinnati, Ohio (1976).
91. Gause, E. M. and J. R. Rowlands. *Environ. Ltrs.* 9:293 (1975).
92. Gunnison, A. F. and A. W. Benton. *Arch. Environ. Health* 22: 381 (1971).
93. Schneider, L. K. and C. A. Calkins. *Environ. Res.* 3:472 (1971).
94. Snipes, W. and A. Keith. *Res. Develop.* 21:22 (1970).
95. Rowlands, J. R., C. Allen-Rowlands and E. M. Gause. "Spin Label Study of the Effects of Peptide Hormone ACTH on the Plasma Membrane of Y-1 Adrenal Tumor Cells." Submitted for publication 1976b.
96. Donta, S. T. *Am. J. Physiology.* 227:109 (1974b).
97. Haksar, A., D. V. Maudsley, F. G. Peron and E. Bedigian. *J. Cell. Biol.* 68:142 (1976).
98. Uyesaka, N., K. Kamino, M. Ogawa, A. Inouye and K. Machida. *J. Membrane Biol.* 27:283 (1976).
99. Rowlands, J. R., Ca. J. Allen-Rowlands, E. M. Gause and M. L. Meltz. "Tier 2 Toxicological Studies of Environmental Agents." Submitted for publication 1976d.

CHAPTER 11

BIOCHEMICAL RESPONSES OF HUMANS TO GASEOUS POLLUTANTS

R.D. Buckley, J.D. Hackney, K. Clark, and C. Posin

USC-Rancho Los Amigos Hospital
7601 East Imperial Highway
Downey, California 90242

INTRODUCTION

The toxicology of inhaled gaseous and particulate substances has steadily gained the attention of investigators as the possible unfavorable health effects become known. This has not been an easy area in which to obtain reliable data, however, because of the wide variety of exposure methods employed. The biological effects of inhaled irritants depend upon the amount of substance absorbed, which is a function of the amount retained in the respiratory system rather than merely on the concentration in the inhaled air.[1] The effective dose is frequently difficult or impossible to measure and is usually ignored. One of the most critical variables to control is exercise since this parameter has a direct bearing on the minute volume of respiration and is known to increase the effective toxicity of inhaled irritants.[2]

Among the most thoroughly studied inhaled toxicants is the oxidant gas ozone (O_3), which is found in significant amounts in many urban and industrial areas. Extensive studies have shown that this oxidant is highly cytotoxic at high levels, and also produces a stimulation in lung cell metabolism at lower (ambient) concentrations.[3] Glycolytic and pentose pathways, glutathione peroxides (GSHpase) and glutathione reductase (GSS-Gase), as well as lysozome enzymes are stimulated.[3,4] These irritant-induced biochemical changes persist for some time and have been correlated with the increased tolerance to high levels of oxidant after previous

247

potentiation with exposure to a lower dose.[2,5] The stimulation is also thought to extend to proliferation of Type II cells to replace the more vulnerable Type I cells killed by the oxidant.[6] These data, along with the stimulation of the pentose pathway from which pentose sugars can be obtained for DNA synthesis, suggest that an increase in the rate of cell division is an important response to oxidant injury.

Many believe that the major pathway for the toxicity of O_3 involves oxidation of membrane unsaturated fatty acids (UFA) to produce ozonides, hydroperoxides, and other long-lived free radicals. These free radicals undergo chain reactions by which additional free radicals are produced to cause further cell damage. *In vitro* studies have shown that UFAs are readily attacked by low levels of O_3 and NO_2 to produce a variety of free radical products.[7] The products are not the same when O_3 and NO_2 are employed as individual oxidants, suggesting that the mechanism of peroxidation is different with the two gases. Roehm *et al.*[7] have also shown that the protection given by phenolic antioxidants is much greater when NO_2 is used, compared to O_3, again suggesting a different biochemical mechanism. Intravenous injections of hydroperoxides were found to be extremely toxic to rats, producing many changes in lung tissue resembling those found after acute O_3 or NO_2 exposure.[8] Additional studies have shown that the toxicity of injected hydroperoxides and ozonides is greater in vitamin E-deficient rats and that the serum levels of lecithin-cholesterol acyl transferase are depressed both by vitamin E-deficiency and by hydroperoxide injection.[9]

An important reason for toxicological studies of inhaled irritants in animals is to make inferences about possible short- and long-term effects on man. Biochemical measurements are now being made on blood and lung tissues of laboratory animals and on the blood of men exposed under similar conditions.[10-12] If the blood biochemical responses of animals (squirrel monkeys) and man are similar, indirect evidence will then exist for possible response of human lungs. Biochemical changes in blood of humans inhaling 0.5 ppm O_3 have been reported,[13] but such phenomena as adaptation and cross tolerance have not yet been convincingly demonstrated in man. Considerable attention has been given to experimental conditions in many studies and it has been found that the level of exercise during the exposure period has a great deal to do with the effects of O_3 in man,[14,15] in a manner similar to the responses seen in animals.

Another condition of considerable importance in studies of air pollution toxicity in humans is the dietary state of the subjects, especially with regards to the intake of such antioxidants as vitamin E. The biological role of vitamin E is uncertain,[16] but its deficiency has been shown in a variety of laboratory animals to result in an increased susceptibility to inhaled O_3 or NO_2.[17,18] Excess dietary vitamin E also appears to exert a protective effect, although even very high levels do not prevent a significant increase in thiobarbituric acid reactive substance from being produced in lung tissues after exposure.[19] A primary function of vitamin E appears to be as a tissue antioxidant, especially to terminate chain reactions by which free radicals are propagated.[16] Recent studies suggest that an interaction may also exist with vitamin A,[20] and in the mechanism(s) by which prostaglandins are generated.[21]

This chapter summarizes some of the human biochemical studies completed so far in this laboratory and discusses possible implications and some of the needs for further investigation.

MATERIALS AND METHODS

Healthy adult human volunteer subjects were exposed in an environmental chamber capable of maintaining predetermined atmospheric conditions. The facilities are described in detail elsewhere.[10-12] The temperature and relative humidity were maintained at 88°F and 40%, respectively, to simulate a typical summer day in Los Angeles. Each subject entered the chamber at least twice. The protocol called for intermittent exercise and pulmonary function tests during each session. Each period lasted from 2.5 to 3 hr. The subjects breathed only clean air during the first chamber period (sham control), and in subsequent periods breathed clean air to which a predetermined amount of O_3 had been added (exposure). Each subject could then serve as his own control. It was always necessary that the first day be a sham exposure because subjects did not always recover completely from an exposure period within 24 hours. Venous blood samples were obtained from the subjects after each exposure or sham period and experiments to detect biochemical changes performed. Clinical questionnaires were given to each subject so clinical, physiological, and biochemical data could later be correlated.

Biochemical changes were sought in blood erythrocytes (RBCs) and serum. Peroxidation-induced changes were thought to be the most likely to be detectable based upon the work of others in laboratory animals. Two observations were made of the RBC membrane. These included measurements of RBC susceptibility to hemolysis when challenged with 2% H_2O_2, and the activity of the RBC membrane enzyme acetylcholinesterase (AcChase). Other measurements include RBC-reduced glutathione (GSH), glutathione reductase (GSSGase), glucose-6-phosphate dehydrogenase, glutathione peroxidase (GSHpase) and thiobarbituric acid reactive substance (lipid [0]). Serum vitamin E and GSSGase were also measured. The methods were more thoroughly discussed in a previous report.[13]

Some studies were designed to detect significant differences in the clinical, physiological, and biochemical responses of people living in Los Angeles during the smoggy season, as compared to those of people living in cleaner atmospheres. Nonresident subjects were brought to the environmental chamber facility and studied immediately upon arriving in the area, and before adaptation or tolerance could develop. Studies were planned so that Los Angeles residents and out-of-area residents were studied within one week.

Subjects were exposed to 0.5 ppm and 0.4 ppm O_3. Dose-response relationships between biochemical responses and oxidant levels were sought as well as the comparison of exposed and control values. Paired group statistical analyses were employed, with the critical alpha of 0.05 being the accepted significance level.

RESULTS

Means, standard deviations and p values of biochemical measurements made on blood of humans exposed to 0.5 ppm O_3 x 2.5 hr are given in Table 11.1. This level of O_3 is the highest employed by us but is by no means unrealistic since it is below the third stage alert level for California (0.6 ppm x 1 hr), and is achieved yearly in the Los Angeles area. Efforts were also made to simulate a smoggy summer day in Los Angeles by controlling the temperature and humidity of the chamber and by instructing the subjects to perform intermittent light exercise.

Additional experiments with O_3 exposure were done in the same manner as above except a 0.4 ppm O_3 concentration was employed. These data are shown on Table 11.2. The subjects entered the chamber on four successive days in these experiments, breathing only clean air the first day (sham), and inhaling 0.4 ppm on days 2, 3, and 4. Statistically significant biochemical changes were observed but the extent of the response to O_3 challenge did not seem as marked as with 0.5 ppm.

Data from the comparisons of biochemical changes in blood samples of Los Angeles residents and nonresidents (Canadians) following O_3 exposure are listed on Table 11.3. Evidence was sought for the indications that a difference exists between the two groups' reactions to the inhaled oxidant. The sample size is small (four Canadians and four Los Angeles residents) but the available evidence suggests that the daily challenge of an atmosphere relatively high in oxidants does result in an increase in the resistance of Los Angeles residents.

Table 11.1   Human Blood Response to 0.5 ppm O_3 x 2.5 hour

| Measurement | $\bar{X} \pm S.D.$[a] | | p[b] |
	Sham	Exposure	
RBC fragility (% hem.)	29.81±1.48	37.74±2.60	< 0.001
AcChase (mM/ml/min)	18.03±1.80	15.27±1.09	< 0.001
GSH (mg %)	30.79±4.44	26.05±5.63	< 0.001
G6PDH (U/gmHb/min)	4.33±0.50	5.51±0.61	< 0.001
LDH (U/gmHb/min)	105.40±6.50	118.09±7.75	< 0.001
Lipid peroxidation (μgm/ml)	0.070±0.008	0.139±0.044	< 0.01
GSSGase, serum (mU/ml/min)	16.50±1.11	13.82±2.35	N.S.
Vit E (mg %)	0.711±0.143	0.932±0.180	< 0.025

[a]Group data, n = 6
[b]Computed from paired-group data

RBC fragility–erythrocyte hemolysis
  in presence of 2% H_2O_2
AcChase–acetylcholinesterase
GSH–reduced glutathione
G6PDH–glucose-6-phosphate dehydrogenase

LDH–lactate dehydrogenase
Lipid peroxidation–thiobarbituric
  acid positive substances
GSSGase–glutathione reductase
Vit E–d, alpha tocopherol

DISCUSSION

Inhaled O_3 is known to cause significant changes in the biochemistry of lung tissues of experimental animals.   Immediate responses are probably due to oxidation toxicity but other changes develop in a few days that increase the tolerance of the animals to subsequent O_3 challenge. It has been postulated that the initial cell damage elicits changes in lung metabolism, increasing the tissue's capacity to neutralize toxic free radicals produced by the attack of unsaturated fatty acids by O_3.[3,16]   Similar blood biochemical changes were seen in this study to occur at levels of O_3 found in the Los Angeles area.   The RBC Fragility and AcChase measurements detect changes in the red cell membrane while the remainder reflect changes occurring in the cell cytoplasm.   These two tests have shown a good dose-related reaction to O_3[12] with no-response intercepts at about 0.25 ppm concentration.

The AcChase assay has proven to be the most sensitive and reproducible

Table 11.2 0.4 ppm O_3 Exposure of Humans

Observation	$\bar{X}\pm$S.D.			
	Sham	Exposure 1	Exposure 2	Exposure 3
RBC fragility (% hemolysis)	23.47±2.78	25.52±4.18	24.68±3.77	26.96±4.12
AcChase (mM/ml/min)	20.98±3.14	20.36±2.77	18.83±2.56	18.57±2.46
RBC-GSH (mg %)	38.05±5.14	29.63±3.91	29.73±4.42	28.00±3.84
G6PDH (U/gmHb/min)	3.35±0.94	3.37±0.70	3.63±0.87	3.26±1.37
LDH (U/gmHb/min)	101.47±19.62	112.18±11.75	108.32±13.62	106.20±23.19
GSSGase, blood (U/ml/min)	2.61±0.45	2.70±0.46	2.73±0.43	2.67±0.43
Vit E (mg %)	1.33±0.12	1.36±0.18	1.36±0.11	1.34±0.13
Lipid peroxidation (µgm/ml)	0.185±0.036	0.254±0.034	0.249±0.017	0.254±0.019

RBC fragility–erythrocyte fragility to 2%H_2O_2 ——————— $p < 0.05$
AcChase–acetylcholinesterase ---- x ------ x -- $p < 0.025$
RBC-GSH–erythrocyte reduced glutathione ——— x ——— $p < 0.01$
G6PDH–glucose-6-phosphate dehydrogenase
LDH–lactate dehydrogenase -------------- $p < 0.001$
GSSGase–glutathione reductase
Vit E–serum vitamin E $n = 6$

indicator of oxidant-induced damage in human erythrocytes. Considerable variability in blood values for the AcChase exists among individuals (55-60%), but the day-to-day variance for an individual is much smaller (±8%). This day-to-day constancy of AcChase activity in individual subjects results in a very small standard deviation of the differences mean when paired group methods are used, thereby greatly increasing the discriminatory ability of the test. The RBC Fragility test is not as reproducible as the AcChase assay and may be influenced by red cell membrane vitamin E levels, membrane fatty acid and cholesterol composition, or other factors. Experiments are now planned that will attempt to correlate RBC membrane vitamin E levels with hemolysis values.

Increased levels of malonaldehyde-like substances in red cells following O_3 inhalation suggests that unsaturated lipid peroxidation is occurring

Table 11.3 O_3 and Human Blood: Canadians vs. Los Angeles Residents

Measure		$\bar{X}\pm$S.D.		p^c
		Sham	Exposure	
RBC fragility	Res.[a]	18.58±1.88	19.12±1.61	N.S.
(% hem)	Can.[b]	15.31±0.59	24.21±2.44	<0.005
AcChase	Res.	21.02±0.49	18.86±1.16	<0.005
(mM/ml/min)	Can.	22.34±0.72	18.78±1.18	<0.005
G6PDH	Res.	7.02±0.05	6.59±0.18	N.S.
(U/gmHb/min)	Can.	6.43±0.24	7.09±0.39	<0.10
LDH	Res.	113.0±4.4	127.0±2.3	<0.05
(U/gmHb/min)	Can.	131.7±4.1	158.8±5.6	<0.01

n = 4 residents and 4 Canadians

[a]Los Angeles residents
[b]Canadians
[c]paired t test

beyond the lung. The sequences of chemical reaction resulting from inter-action of O_3 with susceptible substances such as unsaturated fatty acids are known to be very complicated and are poorly understood.[7,16] We do not know if O_3 is present in blood to initiate free radical formation or if the chain reaction begins in the lung and extends to other tissues. The presence of large amounts of oxidizable substances in lung, coupled with the high oxidation potential of O_3, would suggest that the gas would not survive past the air-blood barrier. The actual fate of inhaled O_3 is, however, still unknown. Serum vitamin E levels are elevated following inhalation of the higher level of O_3 but not when a lower level challenge is employed. It is presumed that the vitamin is mobilized from liver and lipid stores and it is tempting to assume that the change will provide some added protection against subsequent exposures to oxidants. The assumption will need to be tested by determining if the serum levels remain elevated for any appreciable time, and also by performing vitamin E analyses of erythrocyte membranes to determine if any change occurs in the membrane levels corresponding to the changes in serum levels.

The significant reduction in GSH after O_3 inhalation could well be attributed to the presence in the cells of free radicals or O_3, whose high oxidation potential would readily oxidize GSH. The apparent increase in G6PDH and LDH enzyme activity levels is not so easily explained since erythrocytes lack a nucleus, microsomes, and other machinery necessary for enzyme induction. It is known that the activity of most erythrocyte enzymes decreases with the age of the cell, so it is possible that the

increase in the activity of these enzymes could result from a selective removal of older erythrocytes from circulation by sequestration in the spleen
or by hemolysis and subsequent removal by spleen and liver. Experiments
are now in progress to test these hypotheses. The concept of an O_3 -in-
duced aging of the erythrocyte might explain the increased activity of
cytoplasmic enzymes but would hardly explain the significant decrease
observed in membrane AcChase. This enzyme, however, resides in the
red cell membrane and would possibly be more directly exposed to O_3
or to free radicals. Acetylcholinesterase is also known to be very vulnerable to inactivation by oxidation of the serine group at the active site,
while G6PDH and LDH are not known to be so susceptible to similar
attack.

The capacity of laboratory animals to develop an increased tolerance
to inhaled oxidants following brief exposure to O_3, or a similar oxidant,
has been well documented. Data from Table 3 suggest that humans also
develop an increased adaptation by breathing air containing normal oxidant
levels found in urban atmospheres where photochemical smog exists.
The numbers of subjects studied are small but the tentative data suggests
that residence of a locality in which appreciable atmospheric oxidant levels
prevail show less biochemical change when challenged by O_3. Los Angeles
residents also showed fewer pulmonary physiological and clinical changes
than the Canadian residents when all were exposed to the same conditions.[12]

The adaptation of humans to acute or chronic inhalation of toxic inhalants such as O_3 needs to be more thoroughly studied and characterized.
It would be important to know the length of time the biochemical adaptation persists, and if it fails to occur in people with such biochemical
conditions as G6PDH deficiency. There has also been relatively little
oxidant effect research with asthmatics and subjects with other types of
chronic pulmonary disease. The apparent O_3-induced increase in erythrocyte G6PDH and LDH also needs to be explained. Tentative data (unpublished) indicates that an increased splenic sequestering of erythrocytes
following acute O_3 exposure does occur, suggesting that the cell membranes
are "aged" by the exposure and subsequently sequestered by the spleen.
If sequestered cells are the older cells, those remaining in the circulation
would be "younger" and possess higher enzymatic activity.

REFERENCES

1. MacFarland, H.N. "Inhalation Toxicology," *J. Assoc. Offic. Anal.
   Chem.* 58(4): 689 (1975).
2. Stockinger, H.E., W.D. Wagner, and P.G. Wright. "Studies of Ozone
   Toxicity Potentiating Effects of Exercise and Tolerance Development,"
   AMA Arch. Indust. Health, 14: 158 (1956).

3. Chow, C.K., and A.L. Tappel, "Activities of Pentose Shunt and Glycolytic Enzymes in Lungs of Ozone-Exposed Rats," *Arch. Environ. Health,* 26:205 (1973).
4. Chow, C.K., C.J. Dillard, and A.L. Tappel, "Glutathione Peroxidase System and Lysozyme in Rats Exposed to Ozone or Nitrogen Dioxide," *Environ. Res,* 7:311 (1974).
5. Chow, C.K. "Biochemical Responses in Lungs of Ozone-Tolerant Rats," *Nature,* 260(553):721 (1976).
6. Stephens, R.J., M.F. Sloan, M.J. Evans, and G.F. Freeman, "Alveolar Type I Cell Response to Exposure to 0.5 ppm O_3 for Short Periods," *Exp. Mol. Pathol,* 20:11 (1974).
7. Roehm, J.N., J.G. Hadley, and D.B. Menzel, "Oxidation of Unsaturated Fatty Acids by Ozone and Nitrogen Dioxide," *Arch. Environ. Health,* 23:142 (1971).
8. Anderson, W.R., W.C. Tan, T. Takatori, and O.S. Privett, "Toxic Effects of Hydroperoxide Injections on Rat Lung," *Arch. Pathol. Lab. Med,* 100(3):154 (1976).
9. Takatori, T., and O.S. Privett, "Studies of Serum Lecithin-Cholesterol Acyl Transferase Activity in Rat: Effect of Vitamin E Deficiency, Oxidized Dietary Fat, or Intravenous Administration of Ozonides or Hydroperoxides," *Lipids,* 9(12):1018 (1974).
10. Hackney, J.D., W.S. Linn, R.D. Buckley, *et al.* "Experimental Studies on Health Effects of Air Pollutants. I Design Considerations," *Arch. Environ. Health,* 30:373 (1975).
11. Hackney, J.D., W.S. Linn, J. Mohler, *et al.* "Experimental Studies on Human Health Effects of Air Pollutants. II. Four-Hour Exposure to Ozone Alone and in Combination with Other Pollutant Gases," *Arch. Environ. Health,* 30:379 (1975).
12. Hackney, J.D., W.S. Linn, D.C. Law, *et al.* "Experimental Studies on Human Health Effects of Air Pollutants. III. Two-Hour Exposure to Ozone Alone and in Combination with Other Pollutant Gases," *Arch. Environ. Health,* 30:385 (1975).
13. Buckley, R.D., J.D. Hackney, K. Clark, and C. Posin. "Ozone and Human Blood," *Arch. Environ. Health,* 30:40 (1975).
14. Kagawa, J., and T. Toyama. "Effects of Ozone and Brief Exercise on Specific Airway Conductance in Man," *Arch. Environ. Health,* 30(1):36 (1975).
15. Folinsbee, L.J., F. Silverman, and R.J. Shephard. "Exercise Responses Following Ozone Exposure," *J. Appl. Physiol,* 38(6):996 (1975).
16. Menzel, D.B. "Oxidants and Human Health," *J. Occup. Med,* 18(5):342 (1976).
17. Menzel, D.B., J.N. Roehm, and S.D. Lee. "Vitamin E: The Biological and Environmental Antioxidant," *J. Agric. Food. Chem,* 20(3):481 (1972).
18. Schatte, C., and A. Swansinger. "Effect of Dietary 'Antioxidant' Supplementation on the Susceptibility to Oxygen Toxicity in Mice." *Aviation, Space, Environ. Med,* 47(2):147 (1976).
19. Fletcher, B.L., and A.L. Tappel. "Protective Effects of Dietary α-Tocopherol in Rats Exposed to Toxic Levels of Ozone and Nitrogen Dioxide," *Environ. Res,* 6:165 (1973).

20. Jenkins, M.Y., and G.V. Mitchell. "Influence of Excess Vitamin E on Vitamin A Toxicity in Rats,"*J. Nutr,* 105(12): 1600 (1975).
21. Hope, W.C., C. Dalton, L.J. Machling, *et al.* "Influence of Dietary Vitamin E on Prostaglandin Biosynthesis in Rat Blood," *Prostaglandins,* 10(4): 557 (1975).

CHAPTER 12

SHORT-TERM EFFECTS OF SULFURIC ACID AEROSOLS ON THE RESPIRATORY TRACT. A MORPHOLOGICAL STUDY IN GUINEA PIGS, MICE, RATS AND MONKEYS

L. W. Schwartz, P. F. Moore, D. P. Chang, B. K. Tarkington, D. L. Dungworth and W. S. Tyler

California Primate Research Center and
Department of Veterinary Pathology
University of California
Davis, California 95616

INTRODUCTION

Health effects of industrial smogs composed mainly of sulfur compounds and particulates are of current concern since the present energy situation will require an increasing use of fossil fuels containing high concentrations of sulfur. The contribution of gasoline combustion to ambient sulfate levels in major urban areas is also of interest since some reports indicate that sulfur-containing components of gasoline are generally converted to droplets of sulfuric acid by automobile oxidation catalysts.[1,2] Sulfate atmospheric contamination, however, is primarily from sources other than the combustion of gasoline.

The purpose of this study was to reevaluate the morphological influence of sulfuric acid droplets on the respiratory system. Particular emphasis was placed on the use of acid droplets in the submicron range and the use of modern morphological techniques to provide a critical evaluation of multiple sites along the respiratory tract. This study is part of a larger study to investigate the pulmonary effects of sulfates using morphological, biochemical, and physiological parameters.

METHODS AND PROCEDURES

Male Sprague-Dawley and Long-Evans rats ± 3.5 days of age were obtained from colonies free of chronic respiratory disease (Hilltop Laboratory Animals, Inc., Chatsworth, Pa., and Blue Spruce Farms, Inc., Altamont, N. Y., respectively).   They were housed under microbiologic filters prior to exposure.   Conventional and SPF albino Hartley male guinea pigs (Charles Rivers, Wilmington, Mass.) weighing 400 to 800 gm were obtained and housed in stainless steel wire mesh cages within exposure chambers prior to exposure.   Male Swiss-Webster mice 60 ± 3.5 days of age, free of chronic respiratory diseases (Hilltop Laboratory Animals, Inc., Chatsworth, Pa.) were housed six to eight per cage and handled similarly to the rats. Rodents were provided free access to water and the appropriate Purina Lab Chow.   Six female rhesus monkeys (*Macaca mulatta*), all wild-caught and housed individually indoors at the California Primate Research Center for a minimum period of 90 days prior to exposure, were determined to be clinically free of active spontaneous disease processes prior to exposure.   During exposure, all animals were housed within either a 93 ft^3 or 113 ft^3 Hinners-type chamber.[3]   The temperature was controlled 23 ± 2°C, and the relative humidity never exceeded 60%.

The sulfuric acid aerosol generation system has been described in detail elsewhere.[4]   Briefly, the sulfuric acid aerosol is produced by bubbling a stream of dry high purity N_2 gas through a vessel of liquid sulfur trioxide, SO_3.   The vapor is further diluted with N_2 to prevent crystallization.   The stream of gas bearing SO_3 vapor is introduced at the turbulent entry point of air supplied to the chamber.   The SO_3 combines with ambient water vapor, and immediate condensation of sulfuric acid aerosol occurs.   Excessive coagulation is minimized by rapid dilution from the high chamber air flow rate.   Figure 12.1 further illustrates the generation system.

The mass distribution was determined using a seven-stage impactor (ARIES Model 07-001).   The MMAD was determined to be 0.3 to 0.6 μm with a mean of 0.38 μm.   Optical particle counters (Royco 225 and Climet 201) indicated that the peak particle size was below 0.5 μm in diameter.

Sulfate concentration was determined by collecting the sulfuric acid aerosol from known volumes of air on polytetrafluorethylene membrane filters having a pore size of 0.2 μm.   The sulfate was eluted with an aliquot of 80% spectrograde isopropanol, and the sulfate concentration was determined with the barium chloranilate procedure.[4]   In addition, the average mass concentration was calculated by determining the weight loss from the SO_3 vessel during a timed exposure interval and dividing by the chamber air flow rate.

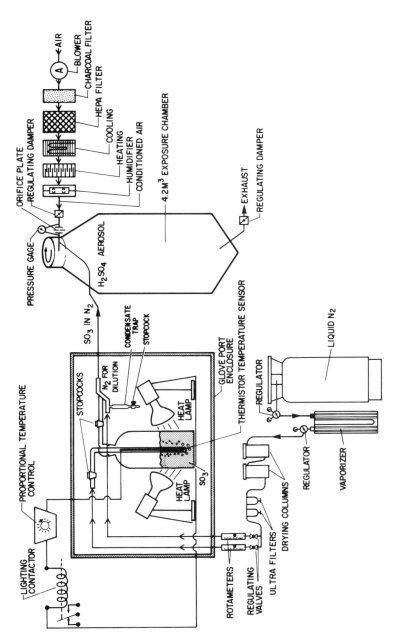

Figure 12.1. Schematic of the sulfuric acid aerosol generation and exposure system.

Details of each exposure are summarized in Table 12.1. Equal num-bers of control animals were housed identically to exposed animals for similar periods of time. Controls breathed air passed through a chemical, bacteriological and radiological filter. Control animals were used in all studies except those involving nonhuman primates. Expense and availa-bility of these animals is such that it was only practical to compare ex-posed rhesus monkeys with control rhesus monkeys used in other studies[5] but housed and handled in a similar fashion.

Methods of lung fixation and evaluation have been described previously in detail.[6] The thoracic viscera were removed from a deeply anesthetized animal, the trachea was cannulated, and the lungs were fixed by airway perfusion with modified Karnovsly's fixative at 30 cm of water pressure. To achieve maximum perfusion of guinea pig lungs, the fixative was warmed to 37°C. Tissues were selected for light microscopy (LM) and scanning electron microscopy (SEM). Tissues examined included nasal septum, trachea, major bronchi, and terminal respiratory units. The right apical and diaphragmatic lobes were generally sampled. A group of tissues including nasal septa, trachea, and major bronchi were chosen from rats and nonhuman primates for subjective evaluation following the application of the periodic acid-Schiff reaction-alcian blue sequence or the high iron diamine-alcian blue sequence to determine characteristics of airway muco-substance.[7]

Table 12.1 Exposure Data Summary

Animals	Numbers	Aerosol Size (μm)	Sigma g	Mass Concen-tration mg/m^3	Exposure Length Days
Rats	6	0.52 (CMD)[a]	N.D.[d]	45	11
Rats	10	0.4 (MMAD)[b]	N.D.	68	6
Rats	18	0.45 (CMD)[c]	N.D.	172	7
Guinea Pigs	5	0.31 (MMAD)	1.6	30	7
Guinea Pigs	6	0.31 (MMAD)	1.5	38	7
Guinea Pigs	2	0.52 (CMD)[a]	N.D.	71	4
Mice	45	0.32 (MMAD)	1.4	140	14
Mice	8	0.62 (MMAD)	1.7	170	10
Rhesus Monkeys	2	0.3-0.5 (CMD)	N.D.	150	3
Rhesus Monkeys	2	0.43 (MMAD)	1.6	361	7
Rhesus Monkeys	2	0.48 (MMAD)	1.5	502	7

[a]A condensation nuclei generator using pure H_2SO_4 as described by Liu, Whitby, and Yu[31] was used for these early exposures.
[b]Mass median aerodynamic diameter.
[c]Count median diameter determined by optical particle counting.
[d]Not determined.

RESULTS

Light microscopic examination of rats exposed to various levels of acid aerosol as summarized in Table 12.1 failed to demonstrate morphological evidence of pulmonary damage. This included examination of nasal septum, trachea, and pulmonary parenchyma. Selected regions were examined by SEM; exposed rats were indistinguishable from controls. Rhesus monkeys after exposure to extremely high levels also failed to demonstrate morphological alterations. Changes in histochemical characteristics of airway mucosubstance were not observed.

Exposure of guinea pigs to 71 mg/m^3 produced the most dramatic lesions. Both bronchial and alveolar levels were focally damaged. Regions of edema, fibrinoid necrosis of alveolar septae, and inflammatory cell infiltration were present extending to the pleural surface (Figure 12.2).

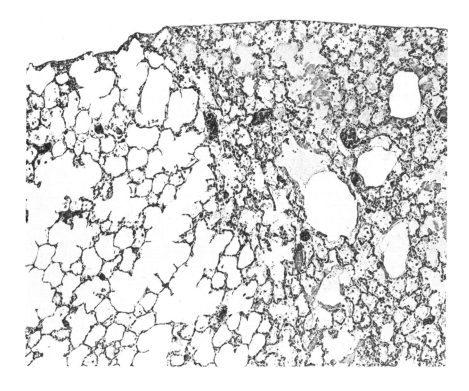

Figure 12.2 Guinea pig lung following exposure to 71 mg/m^3 H$_2$SO$_4$. Alveolar regions were focally edematous and alveolar septae necrotic. X 41, H&E.

Occasionally, bronchioles communicating with these alveolar regions were observed and were partially occluded with edema fluid, necrotic debris, and inflammatory cells. The bronchiolar epithelium also appeared involved in a necrotizing process. Damage to large conducting airways was distributed randomly throughout the lung lobes, although airways containing cartilage were more frequently involved. Light microscopy demonstrated complete ulceration of the epithelial surface and residual necrotic debris. The underlying connective tissue stroma, smooth musculature, and cartilage focally lacked detail and stained uniformly eosinophilic. Immediately adjacent tissue appeared viable and unaltered (Figure 12.3). Inflammatory cells adjacent to the necrotic regions were limited in number.

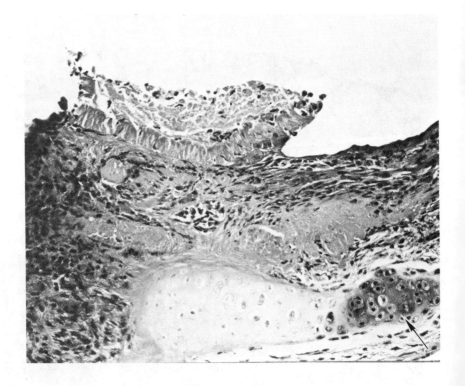

Figure 12.3 Bronchus from a guinea pig exposed to 71 mg/m^3 H$_2$SO$_4$ with focal epithelial necrosis and ulceration. The necrosis extends through the smooth muscle and cartilage of the airway wall. A portion of the cartilaginous plate remains viable (arrow). X 155, H&E.

Similar focal areas of damage to bronchi were observed by SEM. The usual ciliated, nonciliated cell pattern of bronchi was focally interrupted and associated with a surface accumulation of granular cell debris and inflammatory cells. The surface epithelium assumed a smooth, flattened appearance with clusters of cells adjacent to the granular debris (Figure 12.4).

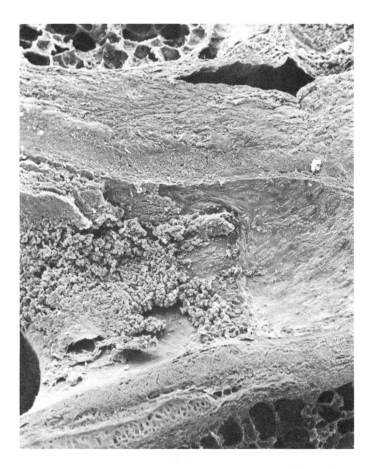

Figure 12.4 Scanning electron micrograph of an area comparable to that present in Figure 12.3. The airway surface adjacent to the inflammatory cell infiltrates has a smooth appearance and ciliated cells are not observed. X 274.

These lesions were only observed in the guinea pigs exposed to the highest level of acid aerosol. Changes were not observed by LM within the trachea or nasal septum. Guinea pigs exposed to 30 to 38 mg/m^3 contained minimal changes, which consisted of variability in density and length of cilia (Figure 12.5). Changes of cilia were randomly distributed but appeared more frequently at sites of airway bifurcation. This relatively subtle surface variation was observed in six of nine exposed guinea pigs but was also observed in one control animal.

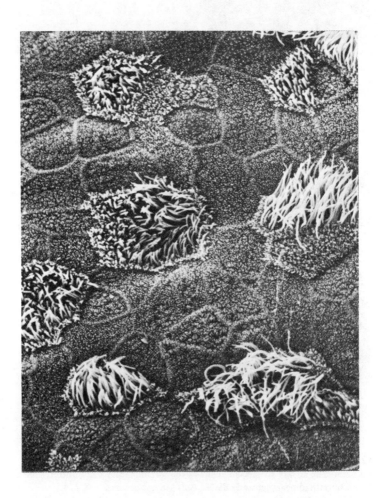

Figure 12.5 Scanning electron micrograph of a guinea pig main bronchus after exposure to 30 mg/m^3 H$_2$SO$_4$. Variability in height and density of cilia can be observed. X 4857.

After exposure of mice to 140 or 170 mg/m^3 for 1 to 14 days, lesions were observed only within the larynx and upper trachea. The lesions were generally confined to the posterior and ventral portion of the larynx and extended no further than 2-3 mm into the trachea. The surface epithelium was ulcerated and the adjoining connective tissue stroma was edematous and heavily infiltrated with neutrophils (Figure 12.6). Adjacent cartilage did not appear to be affected. This focal necrotizing laryngitis was observed as early as 24 hr after the initial acid exposure and persisted throughout a 7-day exposure period. Cellular components of the inflammatory response became spindloid and fibrous in character with increasing length of exposure, but regions of ulceration persisted (Figure 12.7). Lesions within the upper trachea were similar in nature to those of the larynx and were characterized by ulceration, accumulation of cellular debris, and inflammatory cell infiltrates.

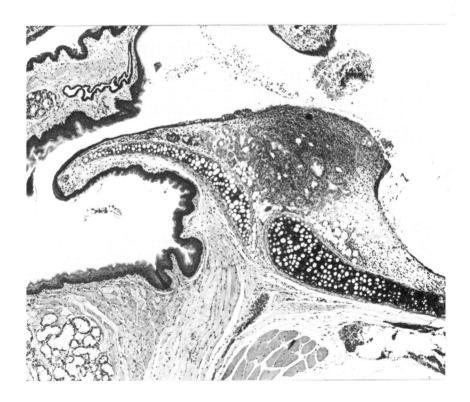

Figure 12.6 Larynx of a mouse after exposure to 140 mg/m^3 H$_2$SO$_4$ for 1 day. The posterior surface of the epiglottis is densely infiltrated by inflammatory cells, and debris is present within the airway lumen. X 38, H&E.

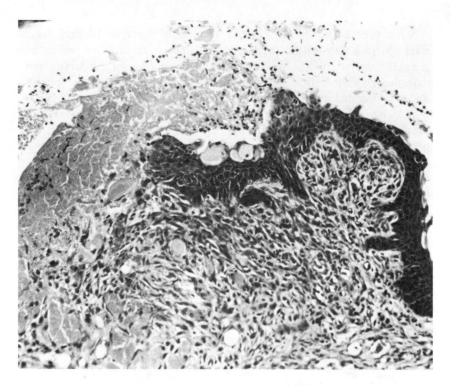

Figure 12.7 Larynx of a mouse after exposure to 140 mg/m^3 H$_2$SO$_4$ for 7 days. The ulceration persists and spindle cells (fibroblasts) are the primary cell within the inflammatory lesion. X 148, H&E.

DISCUSSION

Increased incidence of acute respiratory disease has been associated with environments heavily polluted with sulfur dioxide and suspended sulfates.[8,9] Altshuller has recently summarized air surveillance measurements of sulfur dioxide and suspended water-soluble sulfates.[10] This summary indicates that sulfate-containing aerosols are broadly distributed throughout large regions of the eastern and midwestern U. S. Amdur, in a series of studies including both animals and man, has examined effects of sulfuric acid mist on structural and functional characteristics of the respiratory system.[11-16] In a review of the toxic effects of sulfate aerosols, she specifically emphasized that particle size was extremely important in producing pulmonary effects. Particles in the submicron range produced the greatest alteration in air flow resistance. Additionally, differences in species sensitivity were recognized; LD$_{50}$ data indicated that the order of increasing sensitivity was rabbit, rat, mouse, and guinea pig.[17] Fairchild *et al.*[18] recently reported a reduction in clearance rates of nonviable streptococci from lungs and noses of mice exposed to relatively large aerosols of H_2SO_4 (15 mg/m^3). They also observed a greater total deposition rate of radiolabeled streptococcus aerosols and a proximal shift in the regional pattern of deposition to the nasopharynx after exposure of guinea pigs to H_2SO_4.[19]

Results of this study confirm and extend observations of others. Amdur indicated that a particle size of 0.8 μm was the most effective in increasing air flow resistance when 7 μm, 2.5 μm, and 0.8 μm droplets were compared.[11] We are unaware of studies, other than ours, that have concentrated on species sensitivity and morphological changes after exposure to acid droplets in the 0.3 to 0.6 μm range. Generation of an aerosol with narrow size distribution in this range was made possible by the development of the above described acid generation system.

Since the objective of most laboratory animal exposures has been to extrapolate results to man, the exposure of nonhuman primates was a major goal of this study. The use of the rhesus monkey in this study provides broad phylogenetic and anthropomorphic similarities relating nonhuman primates to man, thus providing a more confident extrapolation of the data to human exposures. Morphological features of rat,[6] mouse,[20] and nonhuman primate[21] have been described, and of these species the nonhuman primate certainly has a lung structure most comparable to that of humans. Exposure of rhesus monkeys to levels as high as 502 mg/m^3 of sulfuric acid for periods of up to seven days with no discernible respiratory system structural change attests to the resistance of this species. Our results concur with the observations that the guinea pig and mouse are the more sensitive species, even with exposure to acid droplets in the submicron range of 0.3 to 0.6 μm. In addition, our data indicate that rhesus monkeys are at least as resistant as rats.

Previous studies that have used microscopic evaluation to define the scope of sulfuric acid aerosol damage have confined observations to the light microscopic level. The development of procedures to evaluate biological specimens by SEM has provided an extremely effective method to detect subtle surface changes within the respiratory system. The advantages of SEM are rapid observation of large surface areas, great depth of field, and magnification overlapping light and transmission electron microscopy. SEM has allowed the detection of subtle alterations of cilia; however, the variation of this change between similar animals at similar exposure levels leaves doubt as to whether this lesion is related to acid exposure.

Sulfuric acid-induced lesions in the guinea pig and mouse were similar in nature but distinctly different in location. Edema and atelectasis were features previously described for the guinea pig.[22] The focal necrotizing bronchiolitis was observed only in two guinea pigs and was interpreted as focal ischemia or an infarctive type of lesion. Alveolar lesions appeared to extend from damaged airways and may have resulted from obstruction of main bronchi.

The pathogenesis of these airway changes is unknown, but recent evidence reported by Charles and Menzel indicates that the irritating characteristics of certain sulfates may be associated with their ability to release histamine, at least in *in vitro* situations.[23] The guinea pig lung is consistently high in histamine; endogenous levels are 10 to 20 times levels observed in the rat, rabbit, or monkey lung.[24-26] Mast cells, as a major source of histamine, are generally located in strategic peribronchiolar and perivascular locations. This combination of features including high tissue histamine levels, mast cells in peribronchiolar regions, and histamine-releasing potential of sulfate most likely contribute to the airway hyperreactivity of guinea pigs during sulfuric acid aerosol exposure. The focal nature of the bronchiolar lesions in the absence of tracheal damage suggests that the lesions are not the direct effect of sulfuric acid on surface epithelium.

Pattle *et al.* observed that as the particle size decreased, the mass concentration necessary to produce an LD_{50} increased.[27] Their early studies using acid droplets of 2.7 μm produced an LD_{50} in 200- to 250-g guinea pigs at a mass concentration of 27 mg/m^3, but acid droplets of 0.8 μm required a mass concentration of 60 mg/m^3 to produce an LD_{50}. Currently we are establishing the LD_{50} for SPF guinea pigs for acid droplets of 0.3 to 0.4 μm; preliminary results indicate that the mass concentration will be above 62 mg/m^3.

This study provides initial information relative to pulmonary morphological changes in guinea pig, mouse, rat and monkey following short-term high-level exposures to submicron droplets of sulfuric acid. The guinea pig and mouse are the most sensitive species. Both provide poor laboratory animal models for extrapolating results to human exposures because of lung structural and pharmacological differences. The guinea pig is notorious for its hyperreactive airways and perhaps more closely represents the human individual already compromised with chronic bronchitis or other airway-associated diseases. Increasing levels of sulfuric acid failed to induce pulmonary damage in nonhuman primates even after exposure to levels in excess of four orders of magnitude over environmental levels reported during periods of industrial type smog. Functional changes will occur at levels below those used in this study, but indications are that irreversible structural change does not occur in the nonhuman primate lung after short-term exposures. Evidence presented by Hyde *et al.* from a study of chronically exposed beagle dogs (68 months exposure, 36 months postexposure recovery) points to the difficulties in extrapolation from short-term high-level effects to the more realistic long-term low-level types of exposure.[28] Their results indicate that oxides of sulfur can induce centriacinar emphysema and hyperplastic changes of bronchiolar cells. Other studies involving exposures of 1 to 1.5 years have reported minimal changes.[29,30] The respiratory system appears to be well shielded against sulfuric acid induced structural damage, but this short-term resistance should not be extended to include persistent low-level exposures; more importantly, it should not be assumed to function in environmental situations where various metallic sulfates are present in addition to solid particulates and gaseous pollutants since synergy may amplify pulmonary effects.

ACKNOWLEDGMENTS

This study was supported by Contract No. 68-02-1732 from the Environmental Protection Agency and Grant No. RR00169 from the National Institutes of Health.

The authors wish to acknowledge the support and assistance of Mr. Philip Chiu, Ms. Margaret Brummer and Ms. Nancy McQuillen.

This work was presented in part at the 172nd National Meeting of the American Chemical Society, Division of Environmental Chemistry, September 1976.

REFERENCES

1. Somers, J. H. "Automotive Sulfate Emission Data," *Environ. Health Perspect.* 10:15 (1975)
2. Pierson, W. R., R. H. Hammerle and J. T. Kummer. "Sulfuric Acid Aerosol Emissions from Catalyst-Equipped Engines," *SAE Paper 740287,* SAE Meeting, Detroit, Michigan, February 25-March 1, 1974, p. 1233.
3. Hinners, R. G., J. K. Burkart and C. L. Punte. "Animal Inhalation Exposure Chambers," *Arch. Environ. Health* 16:194 (1968).
4. Chang, D. P. Y. and B. K. Tarkington. "Experience with a High Output Sulfuric Acid Aerosol Generator," *J. Am. Ind. Hyg. Assoc.,* submitted for publication (1976).
5. Mellick, P. W., D. L. Dungworth, L. W. Schwartz and W. S. Tyler. "Short-Term Morphologic Effects of High Ambient Levels of Ozone on Lungs of Rhesus Monkeys," *Lab. Invest.,* 36(1):82 (1977).
6. Schwartz, L. W., D. L. Dungworth, M. G. Mustafa, B. K. Tarkington and W. S. Tyler. "Pulmonary Responses of Rats to Ambient Levels of Ozone," *Lab. Invest.* 34(6):565 (1976).

7. Spicer, S. S., R. G. Horn and T. J. Leppi. "Histochemistry of Connective Tissue Mucopolysaccharides," *Monogr. Pathol.* 7:251 (1967).
8. French, J. G., G. Lowrimore, W. C. Nelson, J. F. Finklea, T. English and M. Hertz. "The Effect of Sulfur Dioxide and Suspended Sulfates on Acute Respiratory Disease," *Arch. Environ. Health* 27:129 (1973).
9. Shy, C. M. and J. F. Finklea. "Air Pollution Affects Community Health," *Environ. Sci. Technol.* 7(3):204 (1973).
10. Altshuller, A. P. "Atmospheric Sulfur Dioxide and Sulfate Distribution of Concentration at Urban and Nonurban Sites in United States," *Environ. Sci. Technol.* 7(8):709 (1973).
11. Amdur, M. O. "Aerosols Formed by Oxidation of Sulfur Dioxide," *Arch. Environ. Health* 23:459 (1971).
12. Amdur, M. O. "1974 Cummings Memorial Lecture. The Long Road from Donora," *J. Am. Ind. Hyg. Assoc.* 35:589 (1974).
13. Amdur, M. O. "The Impact of Air Pollutants on Physiologic Responses of the Respiratory Tract," *Proc. Am. Philos. Soc.* 114(1):3 (1970).
14. Amdur, M. O. "The Respiratory Response of Guinea Pigs to Sulfuric Acid Mist," *Arch. Ind. Hyg. Occup. Med.* 18:407 (1958).
15. Amdur, M. O., L. Silverman and P. Drinker. "Inhalation of Sulfuric Acid Mist by Human Subjects," *Arch. Ind. Hyg. Occup. Med.* 6:305 (1952).
16. Amdur, M. O., R. Z. Schulz and P. Drinker. "Toxicity of Sulfuric Acid Mist to Guinea Pigs," *Arch. Ind. Hyg. Occup. Med.* 5:318 (1952).
17. Treon, J. F., F. R. Dutra, J. Cappel, H. Sigmon and W. Younker. "Toxicity of Sulfuric Acid Mist," *Arch. Ind. Hyg. Occup. Med.* 2:719 (1950).
18. Fairchild, G. A., P. Kane, B. Adams and D. Coffin. "Sulfuric Acid and Streptococci Clearance from Respiratory Tracts of Mice," *Arch. Environ. Health* 30:538 (1975).
19. Fairchild, G. A., S. Stultz and D. L. Coffin. "Sulfuric Acid Effect on the Deposition of Radioactive Aerosol in the Respiratory Tract of Guinea Pigs," *J. Am. Ind. Hyg. Assoc.* 36:584 (1975).
20. Karrer, H. E. "Electron Microscopic Study of Bronchiolar Epithelium of Normal Mouse Lung," *Exp. Cell Res.* 10:237 (1956).
21. Castleman, W. L., D. L. Dungworth and W. S. Tyler. "Intrapulmonary Airway Morphology in Three Species of Monkeys: A Correlated Scanning and Transmission Electron Microscopic Study," *Am. J. Anat.* 142:107 (1975).
22. Thomas, M. D., R. H. Hendricks, F. D. Gunn and J. Critchlow. "Prolonged Exposure of Guinea Pigs to Sulfuric Acid Aerosol," *Arch. Ind. Health* 17:70 (1958).
23. Charles, J. M. and D. B. Menzel. "Ammonium and Sulfate Ion Release of Histamine from Lung Fragments," *Arch. Environ. Health* 30:314 (1975).
24. Schwartz, L. W., B. I. Osburn and O. L. Frick. "An Ontogenic Study of Histamine and Mast Cells in the Fetal Rhesus Monkey," *J. Allergy Clin. Immunol.* 56(5):381 (1975).

25. Cowan, A. and N. G. Waton. "Distribution of Free Histamine and Histamine-Forming and Destroying Activities in Animal Tissue," *Comp. Gen. Pharmacol.* 3:75 (1972).

26. Shore, P. A., A. Burkhalter and V. H. Cohn, Jr. "A Method for the Fluorometric Assay of Histamine in Tissues," *J. Pharmacol. Exp. Ther.* 127:182 (1959).

27. Pattle, R. E., F. Burgess and H. Cullumbine. "The Effects of a Cold Environment and of Ammonia on the Toxicity of Sulfuric Acid Mist to Guinea Pigs," *J. Pathol. Bacteriol.* 72:219 (1956).

28. Hyde, D. M., N. E. Robinson, J. R. Gillespie and W. S. Tyler. "Morphometry of the Distal Air Spaces in Lungs of Aging Dogs," *J. Appl. Physiol.* in press (1977).

29. Alarie, Y., W. M. Busey, A. A. Krumm and C. E. Ulrich. "Long-Term Continuous Exposure to Sulfuric Acid Mist in Cynomolgus Monkeys and Guinea Pigs," *Arch. Environ. Health* 27:16 (1973).

30. Alarie, Y. C., A. A. Krumm, W. M. Busey, C. E. Ulrich and R. J. Katz. "Long-Term Exposure to Sulfur Dioxide, Sulfuric Acid Mist, Fly Ash, and Their Mixtures. Results of Studies in Monkeys and Guinea Pigs," *Arch. Environ. Health* 30:254 (1975).

31. Liu, B. Y. H., K. T. Whitby and H. H. S. Yu. "A Condensation Aerosol Generator for Producing Monodispersed Aerosols in the Size Range from 0.0036 μm to 1.3 μm," *Recherches Atmospheriques* 2:397 (1966).

CHAPTER 13

IN VIVO AND *IN VITRO* EFFECTS OF SULFUR DIOXIDE UPON BIOCHEMICAL AND IMMUNOLOGICAL PARAMETERS

E. M. Gause, N. D. Greene, M. L. Meltz and J. R. Rowlands

Southwest Foundation for Research and Education
P.O. Box 28147 (8848 West Commerce Street)
San Antonio, Texas 78284

The biological effects of exposure of the human population to atmospheres containing oxides of sulfur have been a subject of concern in recent years. As a result of research activity involving exposure of many different animal species to atmospheres containing known concentrations of the oxides of sulfur, it is generally accepted that sulfuric acid and certain metal sulfate-containing atmospheres cause significantly more lung damage than atmospheres containing corresponding concentrations of sulfur dioxide. These conclusions have been reached as a result of relatively short-term exposures to relatively high concentrations of the sulfur oxides. Biological effects have, in general, been judged by the occurrence of morphological change in lung ultrastructure.

Specific properties of the SO_2 molecule not shared by sulfuric acid lead to the distinct probability that toxicological effects of sulfur dioxide exposure might be of a more subtle nature than those observed with H_2SO_4. However, SO_2 effects remain an important factor to be considered in establishing criteria for a safe environment.

In order to properly understand the specific biological effects that might be attributable to SO_2 exposure, it is necessary to study the chemistry of the SO_2 molecule in defined molecular environments. This chapter will present discussions of the photochemical events that lead to the photooxidation of SO_2 to sulfuric acid and show that similar reactions can take place under *in vivo* conditions leading to the biotransformation

273

of SO_2 to sulfate salts. The results of *in vivo* exposures of rats to SO_2 upon alveolar macrophages and *in vitro* exposures of baboon alveolar macrophages to SO_2 will also be discussed, and an attempt made to relate some of these observations to the molecular properties of the SO_2 molecule.

Sulfur dioxide remains in the atmosphere for 1-7 days[1] and is known to be subject: (1) to oxidation by light and by oxidant species such as O_3 and NO_2 and (2) to various reactions rather vaguely described as "catalyzed by particulates." In atmospheric chemistry and health hazard studies, attention appears to have been devoted entirely to oxidation products of SO_2, such as H_2SO_4 and particulate sulfates, to products formed by the interaction of SO_x with hydrocarbons, or to reactions of HSO_3^- with biochemical electrophilic reagents. In all of these reactions, SO_2 or bisulfite has been considered to act as an electron *donor*.

Sulfur dioxide is also an extremely efficient electron *acceptor*, and this molecular property has very significant implications. In three papers, published sequentially in *Environmental Letters* during 1975,[2-4] we described studies on two different aspects of the behavior of SO_2 as an electron acceptor. To summarize briefly, the first paper reported on fluorescence and optical studies of buffered aqueous SO_2 and HNO_3^- solutions. Evidence was presented that enough SO_2 exists at pH 7.4 to form molecular complexes with compounds containing indole rings; further, the nature of this complex is that of charge-transfer from the indole ring acting as electron *donor* to an excited SO_2 molecule acting as electron *acceptor*.

In these studies, the effects of equimolar solutions of SO_2, $NaHSO_3$, H_2SO_4 and HCl on both the fluorescence of tryptophan residues of albumin and on the efficiency of energy transfer from the excited tryptophan residues into a covalently attached fluorescent probe were compared. Figure 13.1 illustrates the room temperature fluorescence spectrum of a solution (in modified Hanks BSS, pH 6.2) of human albumin labeled with the fluorescent probe, N-(3-pyrene) maleimide. Tryptophan emission was excited at 290 nm, and corresponding fluorescence appeared as a broad peak maximized at approximately 360 nm (curve 1a). The shoulders superimposed on the long wavelength side of the tryptophan band are fluorescence peaks of the label (375, 385, 395, and 404). The maleimide label is excited at 340 nm and the substantial tryptophan emission at this wavelength provides for energy transfer to the label.

The effects on this fluorescence spectrum of four reagents (SO_2, $NaHSO_3^-$, H_2SO_4 and HCl) were tested at the molarities and pH values indicated in Table 13.1. Hydrochloric acid was included as a monitor for possible pH effects. The results, illustrated in Figure 13.2, show a sharp contrast in the response of the system to SO_2 addition as opposed

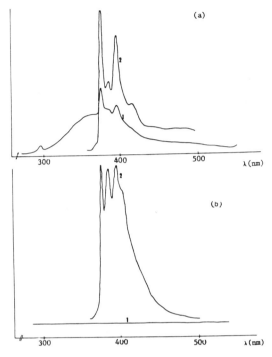

Figure 13.1 Fluorescence spectra of a 0.5 mg/ml solution of human albumin in Hanks BSS, labeled with 0.006 mg/ml N-(3-Pyrene) maleimide. In each case, curve 1 represents excitation at 290 nm (tryptophan excitation), and curve 2 represents excitation at 340 nm (maleimide excitation). All spectra were run at room temperature. Figure (a) exhibits the original spectra with no SO_2 addition. Figure (b) shows them with SO_2 added to a concentration of 0.06 M.

Table 13.1 pH Values for SO_2, $NaHSO_3$, H_2SO_4 and HCl Dissolved to the Indicated Molarities in Modified Hanks Balanced Salt Solution (Room Temperature)

| Molarities | Reagents | | | |
	SO_2	$NaHSO_3$	H_2SO_4	HCl
0	6.16	6.16	6.16	6.16
0.002	2.78	5.77	2.26	2.57
0.005	2.30	5.47	1.87	2.08
0.01	1.94	5.15	1.51	1.73
0.02	1.73	4.80	1.21	1.39
0.06	1.32	3.93	0.76	0.87
0.10	1.13	3.69	0.55	0.63

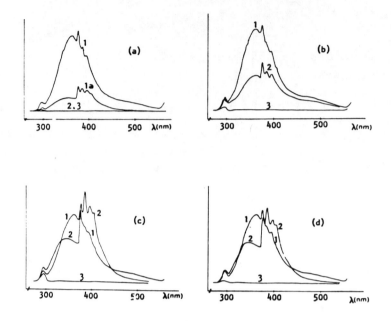

Figure 13.2   Fluorescence spectra of a 0.5 mg/ml solution of human albumin in Hanks BSS, labeled with 0.006 mg/ml N-(3-Pyrene) maleimide. Excitation wavelength was 290 nm, and spectra were run at room temperature. Each figure indicates the effect on the spectrum of addition of a particular reagent. The reagents are (a) SO_2, (b) $NaHSO_3$, (c) H_2SO_4, and (d) HCl. In each case, curve 1 is labeled albumin spectrum without reagent addition, curve 2 is the spectrum at reagent molarity of 0.06 M, and curve 3 is the Hanks BSS baseline. In the first figure, curve 1a represents a 0.01 M SO_2 concentration.

to its response to either HSO_3^- or H_2SO_4. In each figure, curve 2 represents a reagent molarity of 0.06 M, at which concentration the fluorescence in the SO_2 case is completely obliterated, while appreciable intensity remains in the other cases.

Similar results were obtained for the fluorescence and phosphorescence of tryptophan residues in lysozyme at $77°K$. The protein was dissolved to a concentration of 0.2 mg/ml in 0.09 M phosphate buffer (pH 6.2); fluorescence at 343 nm and phosphorescence at 425, 451 and 478 nm were observed upon irradiation at 296 nm. Again, SO_2 quenched these emission bands strongly and although HSO_3^- and H_2SO_4 quenched the emission slightly, their effects were not comparable with that of SO_2. No significant changes were noticed in any case for the structure of the emission or for fluorescence/phosphorescence intensity ratios.

Characterization of the SO_2 reaction with tryptophan was accomplished by studying the reactions with other indole systems. It was found that SO_2 quenches the fluorescence of these compounds in general, this being verified for tryptophan, indole (Figure 13.3), 3-indoleacetic acid, and N-methylindole. In all cases measured quantitatively, the Stern-Volmer quenching law was obeyed up to concentrations of around 0.005 to 0.01 M SO_2, above which deviations occurred toward greater quenching. Thus the quenching of protein fluorescence is due to direct interaction of SO_2 with the tryptophan residues rather than conformational or structural alterations elsewhere. The observed fluorescence quenching can be explained through an excited state charge-transfer intermediate with partial electron donation from its pyrrole system to the SO_2 molecule.

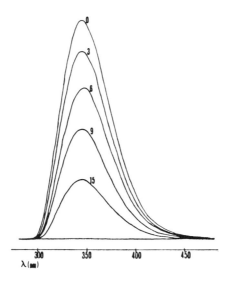

Figure 13.3 Fluorescence spectra of indole (0.01 M in H_2O) exhibiting the quenching effect of SO_2 addition. Excitation wavelength was 302 nm. The number on each curve represents the millimolar concentration of SO_2. The unlabeled curve at the bottom is the solvent baseline.

In other experiments, difference spectroscopy was employed to observe a broad charge-transfer absorbance resulting from the interaction of SO_2 with tryptophan. The charge-transfer band extends from about 325 nm up to over 450 nm, and is shown in Figure 13.4.

In the second paper of this series, evidence of another molecular species formed by SO_2 acting as an electron acceptor was presented. This species is a persistent, free-radical form of SO_2 that exists in aqueous environments.

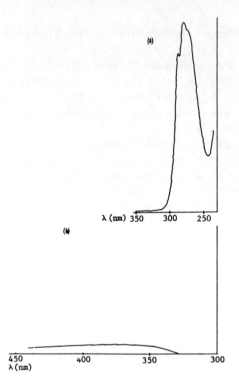

Figure 13.4 Optical absorption spectra of (a) 1-tryptophan, and (b) its complex with SO_2. Figure (b) is a spectrum of the charge transfer complex obtained as follows: in the sample beam were a 1-mm cuvette containing a water solution of 0.1 M tryptophan and 0.1 M SO_2 M SO_2, and a 10-mm cuvette containing water. In the reference beam were a 2-mm cuvette containing a 0.1 M SO_2 solution in water, and a 10-mm cuvette containing a 0.01 M solution of tryptophan in water.

This free radical, formed by the transfer of one electron to a molecule of SO_2, producing the negative ion radical of SO_2, $SO_2^{\cdot}$, is produced in aqueous SO_2 solutions by the action of light, chemical-reducing agents or biochemical-reducing agents.

Considering first the photochemical production of this radical, we observed by means of ESR that when aqueous solutions of SO_2 were irradiated with UV light, a free radical was produced that was extremely slow to disappear. We identified this radical as $SO_2^{\cdot}$, and immediately began to consider the implications of the existence and persistence of this species for environmental studies. The SO_2^{-} radical anion has been previously characterized, both in ionizing radiation studies and in dithionite reduction reactions as a rapidly disappearing intermediate.

The first question was whether the $SO_2^{\cdot}$ radical could be produced by light of wavelengths corresponding to that actually entering the atmosphere, *i.e.*, greater than 300 nm. We found that when aqueous solutions of SO_2 were irradiated with light in the 300-340 nm range (and of moderate to low intensity), the same radical was again produced with no difficulty. The ESR spectrum of the radical and the relative rate of decay are shown in Figure 13.5.

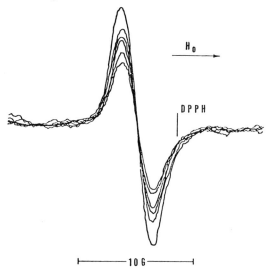

Figure 13.5   Room temperature ESR spectra of a 1.0 M solution of SO_2 in H_2O, after irradiation for 2.5 hr at 3000 Å.   The largest signal is that observed immediately after irradiation.   Successively smaller signals were recorded at 30-min intervals, so the signal of least amplitude shown was recorded 2.5 hr after irradiation. All spectral parameters were kept constant.

Before considering the mechanism by which this radical is produced, we will briefly survey the optical properties of SO_2. The optical spectrum of SO_2 in aqueous solution exhibits two absorption maxima—a strong band in the UV region extending from *ca.* 240 nm up to *ca.* 350 nm, peaking at 280-290 nm, and a much weaker band in the visible region peaking *ca.* 340-350 nm and extending up above 400 nm as shown in Figure 13.6.

Absorption of light of any wavelength from 240-350 nm produces the lowest excited singlet state of SO_2 ($^1SO_2^*$), while the weak absorption band from around 350 to over 400 nm represents the first excited triplet state of SO_2 ($^3SO_2^*$). Production of this triplet state by direct

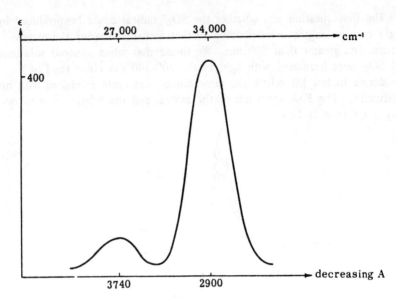

Figure 13.6   The absorption spectrum of the SO_2 molecule.

irradiation with light of this wavelength is a low-probability process; however, significant quantities of this triplet state species can be produced by intersystem crossing from the excited singlet state. (Indeed, emission from the triplet state can be observed readily by fluorescence spectroscopy when excitation is into the 290 nm band.)

In studying the mechanism of photochemical generation of the radical, we carried out both the irradiation and the ESR spectral measurements at 77°K for H_2O and D_2O solutions of SO_2. Under these conditions, we were able to observe another free radical species that decays upon warming to -130 to -115°C. We have identified this second transient radical species as the hydroxyl radical, shown in Figure 13.7.

Our results are consistent with photochemical reduction of SO_2 via: (1) production of an excited singlet state of SO_2 by irradiation into any portion of the broad singlet absorption band (from 240 nm-350 nm) (2) intersystem crossing yielding an excited triplet state species, which in the presence of hydroxyl ions from H_2O decays with (3) production of SO_2^- radicals and hydroxyl radicals, the scheme for which is shown in Figure 13.8. Incidentally, the hydroxyl free radical is considered one of the primary biologically reactive species involved in ionizing radiation damage.

One point that is particularly important is the extreme persistence of the SO_2^- radical, that is, its apparent very slow rate of decay in the

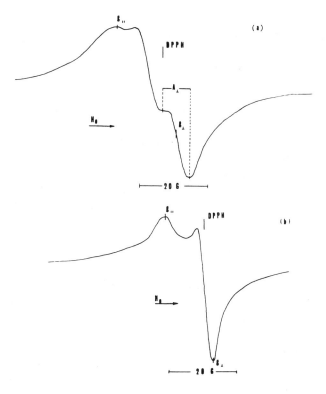

Figure 13.7   ESR spectra ($77°$K) of approximately 1 M solution of SO_2 in (a) H_2O, and (b) D_2O, each irradiated at $77°$K under a mercury arc for 2 hr.

Proposed Mechanism

$$^1SO_2^* + OH^- \longrightarrow SO_2^{\bar{}} + OH^{\cdot}$$

$$^1SO_2^* \longrightarrow {}^3SO_2^*$$

$$^3SO_2^* + OH^- \longrightarrow SO_2^{\bar{}} + OH^{\cdot}$$

Figure 13.8   Mechanism proposed for the photochemical production of SO_2 radical anion and hydroxyl atom by light entering earth's atmosphere.

aqueous systems we have studied, particularly in comparison to the rapid disappearance of this radical as reported from dithionite reduction reactions. We believe the slow rate of decay in our systems to be attributable to an exchange between two molecular species, specifically $SO_2^{\cdot}$ in the presence of a large excess of dissolved molecular SO_2:

$$SO_2^{\cdot} + SO_2 \rightleftharpoons SO_2 + SO_2^{\cdot}$$

Without irradiation, $SO_2^{\cdot}$ can be produced with chemical reducing agents such as borohydride, and, notably, metals such as zinc dust. Therefore, in the atmosphere a combination of metal particulates, SO_2 and high ambient relative humidity would tend to optimize conditions for maximum concentrations and maximum persistence times of the $SO_2^{\cdot}$ radical, even in the dark or under conditions of low light intensity; at the same time conditions of water aerosols, or water vapor on inert particulates, SO_2, and strong sunlight would also maximize $SO_2^{\cdot}$ concentrations in the absence of metal particulates.

In short, atmospheric chemistry appears to have considered sulfur dioxide entirely as an electron donor, *i.e.*, being oxidized by taking on more electronegative elements but not capable of accepting electrons to be reduced. However, SO_2 in aqueous media obviously *does* accept electrons from other components of the aqueous medium, as in photoreduction, or from other chemical reducing agents. This observation suggests many other specific molecular interactions that might occur in polluted atmospheres and in drug and food formulations in which SO_2 is used as a preservative.

Is the $SO_2^{\cdot}$ radical species biologically relevant? Two questions immediately come to mind: (1) What is the fate of the radical upon inhalation? and (2) Is this radical species produced *in vivo*? We will discuss the second question first.

It would seem logical that since we have been talking about electron transfer to the SO_2 molecule in the presence of excess SO_2 and in acidic media there would be no basis for suspecting the existence of the $SO_2^{\cdot}$ radical in biological systems, especially if we accept the common assumption that SO_2 exists only as bisulfite or sulfite ions *in vivo*.

However, when we prepared 10^{-4} M solutions of SO_2 in phosphate buffer, pH 6.25 to 6.4 (pH adjusted with NaOH or KOH) and added micromolar to millimolar amounts of NADH or NADPH, the $SO_2^{\cdot}$ radical was again observed and the free radical concentrations continued to increase for hours to days. The same result was observed when ascorbic acid was added to SO_2 in phosphate buffer at pH 7.4-7.6 (Figure 13.9). In both of these systems it made no difference whether the starting

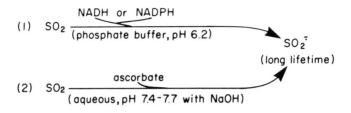

Figure 13.9 Summary of interactions of SO_2 molecule with biochemical reducing agents to produce SO_2^- free radical.

material was buffered SO_2 or buffered $NaHSO_3$ or $KHSO_3$; the free radical was produced and continued to grow for long periods. The reactive species and the mechanisms of interactions we believe to be involved are summarized in Figures 13.10 and 13.11. As postulated, the chemical oxidation of NADH or NADPH by aqueous SO_2 to produce SO_2^- also produces H atoms. Hydrogen atoms are extremely mobile reactive free radicals and another species responsible for much of the damage associated with ionizing radiation.

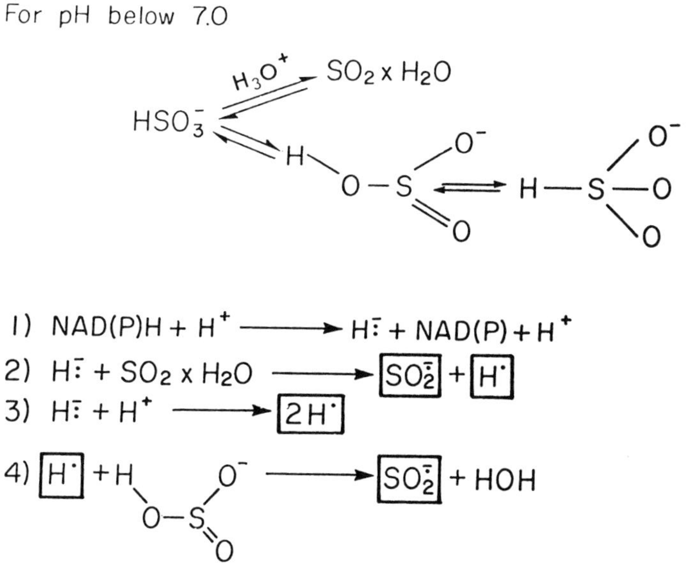

For pH below 7.0

1) $NAD(P)H + H^+ \longrightarrow H^{\overline{\cdot}} + NAD(P) + H^+$

2) $H^{\overline{\cdot}} + SO_2 \times H_2O \longrightarrow \boxed{SO_2^{\overline{\cdot}}} + \boxed{H^{\cdot}}$

3) $H^{\overline{\cdot}} + H^+ \longrightarrow \boxed{2H^{\cdot}}$

4) $\boxed{H^{\cdot}} + H\,O\!-\!S \longrightarrow \boxed{SO_2^{\overline{\cdot}}} + HOH$

Figure 13.10 Reaction scheme for the observed production of SO_2^- free radical from HSO_3^- at pH slightly below 7.0.

For pH above 7.0

1) ascorbic acid $\rightleftharpoons$ $2e$ + dehydroascorbate
   pH>7

2) $HSO_3^- + H_3O^+ \rightleftharpoons SO_2 x\ H_2O$
   pH 7.4-7.6

3) $SO_2 x\ H_2O + e \rightleftharpoons \boxed{SO_2^-} + H_2O$

Figure 13.11 Pathway for the observed production of SO_2^- free radical from HSO_3^- at pH above 7.0

Under conditions of pH existing in the cytoplasm, two free radical species are produced, one of which $(SO_2^{\cdot})$ is effectively sequestered in a matrix of other SO_2 molecules, leaving the highly mobile H atom free to find and interact with any nearby molecule instead of recombining with the $SO_2^{\cdot}$. If the target molecule is a peptide containing disulfide linkages, then the series of reactions outlined in Figure 13.12 might occur. Note that (1) the overall reaction involves bisulfite ion, hydride ion from NADH or NADPH, and a disulfide bond, (2) two new sulfhydryl sites are produced, and (3) SO_2 is recycled to react with more reduced pyridine coenzyme.

1) $HSO_3^- + H_3O^+ \rightleftharpoons SO_2 x\ H_2O$

2) $NAD(P)H + H^+ \longrightarrow NAD(P) + H^{\bar{:}} + H^+$

3) $SO_2 x H_2O + H^{\bar{:}} \longrightarrow SO_2^- + H^{\cdot}$

4) $R-S-S-R' + H^{\cdot} \longrightarrow R-SH + {}^{\cdot}S-R'$

5) $SO_2^{\cdot} + {}^{\cdot}S-R' \longrightarrow SO_2^- -S-R'$

6) $SO_2^- -S-R' \xrightarrow{H^+} SO_2 + HS-R'$

Overall:
$HSO_3^- + H^{\bar{:}} + R-S-S-R' \longrightarrow R-SH + R'-S-H$

Figure 13.12 Reaction scheme suggested for the interaction of HSO_3^- with disulfide bonds *in vivo*.

Obviously, the investigation of the role of the free radical SO_2^{-} in biochemical systems is just beginning. What we do know at this point suggests that the continuing *in vivo* generation of the radical provides, at the least, an artificial drain of essential reducing power in the form of NADH/NADPH, especially if SO_2 is recycled as we have suggested. In this sense, SO_2 or bisulfite would compete for NAD(P)H with over 200 enzymes that require one or the other of the reduced pyridine coenzymes. That other biological reducing agents may also reduce SO_2/HSO_3^{-} non-enzymatically is apparent from the effect of ascorbic acid; therefore the reducing power of agents such as $FMNH_2$, $FADH_2$, tetrahydrofolate and reduced gluthathione may also be depleted by interaction with SO_2/HSO_3^{-}.

In addition to the implications of persistent competition with a multitude of enzymatic pathways for their natural reducing agents, the subsequent reactions by which the free radical SO_2^{-} interacts with biologically important molecules must be considered significant. Here we would like to propose that the SO_2^{-} species is the long-postulated reducing agent form of SO_2; SO_2^{-} would be expected to readily donate its electron to any nearby electrophilic molecule.

We have also obtained preliminary evidence that SO_2^{-} reacts with molecular oxygen to produce SO_4^{-}. This evidence was obtained by irradiation of SO_2 solutions in water (pH 6.2) with visible light. In the absence of oxygen when such solutions are irradiated with light of 300 nm, *i.e.*, into the low energy tail of the first excited singlet state, an emission can be observed that peaks at 380 nm. This emission corresponds to the emission from the first excited triplet state. When the solutions are oxygenated, the low energy side of this emission is found to broaden and extend to *ca.* 500 nm, consistent with the development of a new emission centered at *ca.* 450 nm. The free radical HSO_4, which is the protonated form of SO_4^{-} produced in radiolysis studies of ceric sulfate solutions, has been shown previously to give rise to an absorption centered at this wavelength. The species HSO_4 would need only a single electron from any source to produce HSO_4^{-}, which is the product of the first dissociation of H_2SO_4.

This reaction scheme, which is shown in Figure 13.13, provides a pathway for the nonenzymatic conversion of SO_2 or bisulfite to sulfate. The electron required could be supplied in the atmosphere by metals in particulates. In biological systems, the electron could come from ascorbate, quinones, or any compound capable of one-electron transfer redox reactions. It could also come from ever-present hydroxyl ions, which reaction would again be a source of hydroxyl atoms (OH·).

Finally, before moving from the discussion of SO_2^{-}, let us consider the implications of the reaction of a hydride ion from NAD(P)H with

$$SO_2^* + OH^- \rightarrow SO_2^{\cdot} + OH \cdot$$

$$SO_2^{\cdot} + O_2 \rightarrow SO_4^{\cdot}$$

$$H^+ + SO_4 \rightarrow HSO_4^{\cdot}$$

$$HSO_4^{\cdot} + e \rightarrow HSO_4^-$$

$$\lambda_{max} (HSO_4^{\cdot}) = 450 \text{ nm}$$

Figure 13.13   Proposed photochemical conversion of SO_2 to $HSO_4^{\cdot}$.

hydrated SO_2 to produce $SO_2^{\cdot}$ and a hydrogen atom ($H \cdot$). Since the $SO_2^{\cdot}$ concentration continues to increase almost indefinitely, $H \cdot$ does not decay by recombination with the other half of the radical pair ($SO_2^{\cdot}$); hence, it must "hit" some proximate biomolecule. This situation provides a striking analogy to that characteristic of ionizing radiation, which would make SO_2/HSO_3^- radiomimetic. Perhaps prolonged exposure to atmospheric SO_2 can produce long-term damage similar to exposure to radioactivity in the environment.

Another facet of our concern with effects of SO_2 at the molecular level has been documentation of biochemical systems sensitive to exposure to SO_2 *in vivo*. We are currently surveying the effects of SO_2 inhalation upon biochemical parameters of alveolar macrophages, with emphasis upon those parameters involved in plasma membrane activity.

The bulk of our data is from rats exposed to 5 and 0.5 ppm SO_2, although we have also exposed baboon alveolar macrophages *in vitro*. In general, we have seen effects upon a plasma membrane enzyme, ATPase, and upon another enzyme, lysozyme, the secretion of which is associated with plasma membrane function, at doses of SO_2 below that at which effects upon intracellular biochemical parameters are detectable.

When inbred Fisher, adult, male rats are exposed to SO_2 for short periods of time and sampled immediately upon removal from the atmosphere, their alveolar macrophages consistently exhibit elevated levels of ATPase activity. This is summarized in Table 13.2.

We have also examined the effects of considerably higher concentrations of SO_2 upon baboon alveolar macrophages *in vitro* with the results shown in Table 13.3. It can be seen that immediately after exposure to 10^{-3} M SO_2, the cells were significantly depleted of ATP, while ATPase activity was elevated. We do not have any evidence as to whether this ATP depletion is due to (1) increased ATP utilization, which could be indicated because the much higher ATPase activity at the lower SO_2 concentration

Table 13.2 ATPase Activity of Alveolar Macrophages from Fisher Male Rats Exposed *in vivo* to SO_2 for 4 Hours and Terminated Immediately

SO_2 Level (ppm)	ATPase Activity as % of Controls
0.5	113.6
5.0	115.2

Table 13.3 Effect of *in vitro* Exposure of Baboon Alveolar Macrophages in Culture to SO_2

SO_2 Dose[a]	Recovery Time (hr)	ATPase Activity (μ mol P_i/ mg protein/hr)	% of Controls	ATP (femtomoles per mg protein)	% of Controls
None	0	1.69		1.88	
	20	1.83		2.03	
5×10^{-4}M	0	4.27	253	2.67	115
	20	2.39	131	3.28	116
1×10^{-3}M	0	2.19	130	1.27	25
	20	1.71	93	2.06	113

[a]Cells were incubated for 2 hr in medium without serum containing dissolved SO_2 at indicated concentrations. At end of 2 hr, cells were washed, given complete medium and sampled for 0 recovery time point.

has now subsided—perhaps due to substrate exhaustion, or (2) decreased ATP synthesis. For the 10^{-3} M level at 20 hr postexposure, ATP levels had increased to above controls, while ATPase activity had subsided to slightly below controls. The cells exposed to the 5×10^{-4} M level exhibited stimulation of both intracellular ATP and ATPase. In this experiment, even though SO_2 levels were high, viability at all times was greater than 99%, and the number of cells phagocytizing latex particles increased with time and was not adversely affected by SO_2 exposure. In addition, incorporation of RNA and DNA precursor molecules by the cells in this experiment was found not to be affected. The conclusions from Tables 13.2 and 13.3 are that there is a definite elevation of ATPase activity of alveolar macrophages, following both *in vivo* and *in vitro* exposure to SO_2.

The time course of macrophage ATPase activity subsequent to SO_2 exposure has been followed, with the results shown in Figure 13.14. Enzyme activity elevates immediately after exposure, falls to near control levels within 3 hr, rises briefly again to peak at 24-26 hr, and then falls and remains close to control values. The reason for the peak at 24-26 hr is presently not clear. Possible explanations include: (1) some phases of maturation activation requiring more nutrient uptake, (2) new stem cell population arriving from narrow, (3) bacterial invasion. We are presently reexamining this response. However, ATPase elevation during

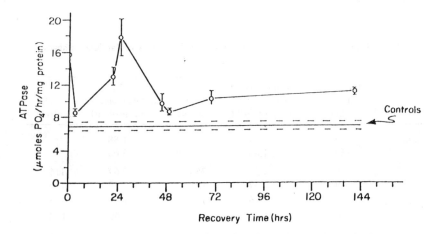

Figure 13.14 Fisher adult male rat alveolar macrophage ATPase activity as function of recovery time after exposure to 5 ppm SO_2 for 4 hr.

exposure, *i.e.*, at zero recovery time, might be due to enzyme activation. In duplicate experiments, macrophages from rats exposed *in vivo* to 5.0 ppm SO_2 exhibited lower energies of activation than did cells from controls as determined by Arrhenius plots. Ebel and Lardy[5] observed anion activation of liver mitochondrial ATPase (both purified and in submitochondrial particles). Of numerous anions examined, HCO_3^- exhibited pronounced activation but HSO_3^- was a better activator.

Thinking that alveolar macrophages might actually be in contact with HSO_3^- in the extracellular (surfactant) phase, we examined the effects of HSO_3^- upon ATPase of intact macrophages. As can be seen from Figure 13.15, intact macrophages do exhibit activation of ATPase activity when they encounter submillimolar concentrations of HSO_3^- in the environment, while at higher HSO_3^- concentrations enzyme activity is inhibited.

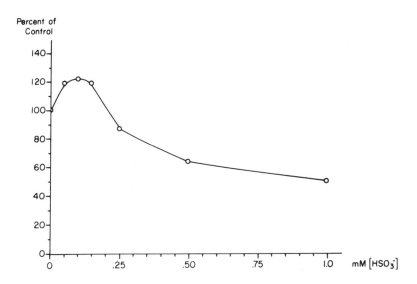

Figure 13.15 Effect of bisulfite ion upon ATPase activity of rat alveolar macrophages.

Lysozyme, an enzyme that acts to cleave a specific glycosidic linkage found in bacterial cell walls, is another enzymatic parameter of alveolar macrophages that is affected by *in vivo* exposures to SO_2. In rats exposed to both 0.5 and 5.0 ppm, macrophage lysozyme intracellular levels were markedly elevated, while extracellular levels remained relatively constant. This effect is shown in Figure 13.16. Lysozyme levels as a function of time of recovery were also measured in the same experiment and on the same animals as the ATPase recovery response. Results are shown in Figure 13.17. Intracellular lysozyme activity levels were clearly elevated throughout the observed recovery period of 144 hr. Whether this represents some form of activation of the enzyme or *de novo* protein synthesis is not known at this time. Enzyme activity continues to increase for at least 72 hr postexposure, after which time although levels decrease, they are still significantly higher than controls. Secreted lysozyme activity also increased after exposure, peaking at approximately 24 hr recovery. Levels were depressed somewhat at 48 hr, but elevated again at 72 hr and 144 hr. At 144 hr, greater variation between individual animals was encountered, which we interpret as some animals returning to essentially control status, while others still exhibited the effects of the exposure.

The peak of secreted lysozyme activity at 24 hr is interesting, coinciding as it does with the peak in ATPase activity. Since so little is

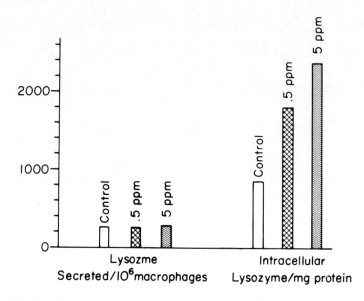

Figure 13.16   Effect of *in vivo* exposure to SO_2 for 4 hr upon rat alveolar macrophage lysozyme levels and secretion.

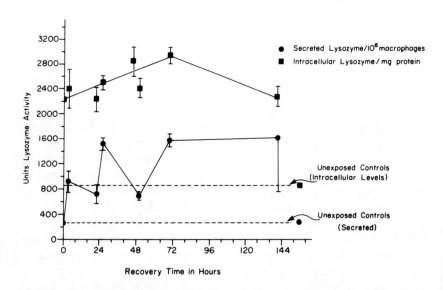

Figure 13.17   Effect of length of recovery period upon lysozyme intracellular levels and secretion; alveolar macrophages isolated from rats exposed *in vivo* to 5.0 ppm SO_2 for 4 hr.

known about regulation of lysozyme synthesis and secretion by alveolar macrophages, it is difficult to interpret this effect.

Lysozyme is apparently secreted continuously by macrophages separately and independently of the normal lysosomal enzymes such as acid phosphatase and β-glucuronidase. It is also secreted independently of phagocytosis and has been proposed as an extracellular marker specific for the presence of macrophages.[6] It is a small (m.w. 14,000), positively charged molecule due to the presence of a large number of basic amino acid residues. There is at least one exposed tryptophan residue (Trp-62 in egg white lysozyme) that is essential for activity and that can be inactivated by sulfonyl compounds. Another buried tryptophan residue (Trp-123 of egg white lysozyme) is susceptible to attack by 2,3-dioxo-5-indoline sulfonic acid, resulting in increased susceptibility of disulfide bonds to reduction.

Since lysozyme is secreted and may only function extracellularly, its location (lung surfactant) and its chemical structure suggest that it might be particularly susceptible to inhaled SO_2. As mentioned above, the observed stimulation of macrophage ATPase activity indicated that SO_2/HSO_3^- does reach the lung surfactant phase, which is the extracellular environment of the alveolar macrophage. Since this surfactant also contains the secreted lysozyme it is reasonable to assume that the SO_2/HSO_3^- present reacts with the surface tryptophan residue to inactivate lysozyme. Indeed, our data indicate that either (1) the secretion process itself is blocked by perturbation of the membrane, or (2) the enzyme that has been secreted is inactivated by direct molecular attack, thereby triggering some type of feedback mechanism and causing the cells to increase enzyme production to provide constant levels of extracellular lysozyme. We intend to pursue study of the mechanisms involved in lysozyme synthesis, secretion and degradation.

Inhalation of SO_2 during the course of ongoing bacterial infection could potentiate the infection by competing with bacteria for extracellular lysozyme. There may also be more long-term implications of chronic SO_2 inhalation if it results in chronic depression of extracellular lysozyme. For example, lysozyme may well act upon glycoproteins other than the N-acetyl glucosamine-N-acetyl muramic acid glycosidic linkage found in cell wall peptidoglycan of gram positive bacteria considered to be its natural substrate. Since glycoproteins are recognized as important features of mammalian cell membranes, lysozyme could act upon cell membranes. Indeed, there is some evidence to this effect and it has been suggested that lysozyme plays a key role in the antitumor activity of macrophages.[7] If lysozyme can act upon these glycoproteins, then it may also interact with viral membrane glycoproteins and play a role in host defense against viruses.

We have also been studying the response of baboon alveolar macrophages to MIF (macrophage inhibitory factor), a lymphokine produced by stimulated lymphocytes. Baboon alveolar macrophages do normally respond to MIF; however, after *in vitro* exposure to SO_2, these cells lose the ability to respond to MIF and, in fact, show increased migration over controls.

Considering other membrane surface receptors, we have also employed spin labeling to observe an SO_2-induced dose-dependent aggregation and internalization of human lymphocyte membrane proteins. This study is described in the third paper of the series mentioned earlier.[4]

ACKNOWLEDGMENTS

Work described in these studies was supported in part by the National Institutes of Health Grant #1-RO1-ESO1162-01 and in part by the Southwest Founcation for Research and Education, San Antonio, Texas.

REFERENCES

1. Rall, D. P. *Environ. Health Persp.* 8:97 (1974).
2. Eickenroht, E. Y., E. M. Gause and J. R. Rowlands. *Environ. Letters* 9:265 (1975).
3. Eickenroht, E. Y., E. M. Gause and J. R. Rowlands. *Environ. Letters* 9:279 (1975).
4. Gause, E. M. and J. R. Rowlands. *Environ. Letters* 9:293 (1975).
5. Ebel, R. E. and H. A. Lardy. *J. Biol. Chem.* 250:191 (1975).
6. Gordon, S., J. Todd and Z. A. Cohn. *J. Exp. Med.* 139:1228 (1974).
7. Osserman, E. F., M. Klockars, J. Halper and R. E. Fischel. "Studies of the Effects of Lysozyme on Mammalian Cells," In *Lysozyme*, E. F. Osserman, R. E. Canfield and S. Beychok, Ed. (New York: Academic Press, 1974), pp. 471-490.

CHAPTER 14

SULFUR DIOXIDE:
A VIEW OF ITS REACTIONS WITH BIOMOLECULES

D. H. Petering

Department of Chemistry
University of Wisconsin-Milwaukee
Milwaukee, Wisconsin 53201

Sulfur dioxide is a combustion product of the burning of fossil fuels. Concern about its possible adverse health effects stem initially from the epidemiological correlation of respiratory ailments with air pollution and with the presence of SO_2 in the atmosphere.[1-4] Efforts to define the nature of the physiological impact of SO_2 upon humans have relied upon model studies in which test animals are exposed to SO_2 under controlled conditions. Its proximate effects upon the lung have been the subject of a number of experiments.[5-10] Although SO_2 is lethal at high concentrations, long-term exposure of animals to levels that more closely approximate conditions in the urban environment seem much less harmful. These results show that SO_2 is not an acute toxin when present at low concentrations in the environment of healthy, well-fed, hygenically kept animals. Hence, single variable, controlled experiments do not reveal SO_2 to be a major health hazard in the urban atmosphere.[11]

It is entirely possible that this approach to the definition of the harmful components of air pollution will be unable to elucidate the causal associations seen in epidemiological studies. Cassell has written that in chronic, low-level exposure to air pollution, one must think of the problem of cause and effect in terms of a complex or network of variables acting in concert on the organism and not in terms of single cause-single effect interactions.[12] That is, SO_2 may be only one of several contributing causes to a resultant effect. It may be a permissive cause, allowing for a greatly enhanced effect of another agent. Or it may damage the system significantly only under certain predisposing conditions.[13] Certainly, a few studies with sulfur dioxide point to the validity of this view and support the necessity of doing multivariable studies.[14-16]

The question arises as to which variables among the myriad that exist should be included in multivariable animal studies. Suggestions, of course, come from the epidemiology and pathology of respiratory disease associated with breathing polluted air containing SO_2. In addition, it is argued here that a knowledge of the chemical and biochemical reactivity of SO_2 is a necessary, useful foundation for the design of animal experiments relevant to the problem of health effects of chronic exposure to sulfur dioxide. If one has a picture of the potential modes of reaction of SO_2 with biomolecules—what can occur, what is likely to occur—rational animal experimentation can then be undertaken because hypotheses that are chemically sound can be developed and tested. The following review of the reactions of sulfur dioxide with biomolecules is presented to support this viewpoint.

Sulfur dioxide is hydrated very rapidly according to the following equation:

$$SO_{2g} + H_2O \underset{k_{-1}}{\overset{K_{eq} \; k_1}{\rightleftharpoons}} HSO_3^- + H^+ \tag{14.1}$$

The rate constants for this reaction are quite large, $k_1 = 3.4 \times 10^6 \; M^1 \; sec^{-1}$ and $k_{-1} = 2 \times 10^8 \; M^1 \; sec^{-1}$ at $20°C$.[17] Given $K_{eq} = 1.7 \times 10^{-2}$ for this reaction, at pH 7 the equilibrium constant between bisulfite and dissolved SO_{2g} is 1.7×10^5. Hence, upon contact with water SO_2 is quickly and completely converted to bisulfite.

Bisulfite is a weak acid having an acid dissociation constant of $6.24 \times 10^{-8} \; M$ at $25°C$.[18,19]

$$HSO_3^- + H_2O \rightleftharpoons SO_3^{2-} + H_3O^+ \tag{14.2}$$

Hence both sulfite and bisulfite are present in solutions near pH 7. Bisulfite* can also dimerize with an equilibrium constant of $0.076 \; M^{-1}$ at $25°C$.[20] Since this is small, the contribution

$$2HSO_3^- \overset{K}{\rightleftharpoons} S_2O_5^{2-} + H_2O \tag{14.3}$$

---

*The terms bisulfite and sulfite will be used to indicate the total concentration of HSO_3^- and SO_3^{2-} in solution.

of this reaction to the solution biochemistry of bisulfite will be neglected.

The sulfite ion has a lone pair of electrons on the sulfur, which is favorably disposed in the pyrimidyl structure of the ion for nucleophilic attack on electron-deficient sites. This property of bisulfite accounts for much of its reactivity with biomolecules.

$$^-O{-}\ddot{S}{-}O^- \qquad\qquad \ddot{S}$$
$$O \qquad\qquad O\ O\ O$$

In the following reactions, rate and equilibrium data are provided for use in the analysis of their potential significance. To approximate the biological system the preferred reaction conditions are pH 7 and 37°C. Constants have been calculated as follows: for any site of attack, X, in which $[X \cdot SO_3^-]$ and $[X]$

$$X + SO_3^{2-} \underset{k_{-1}}{\overset{k_1}{\rightleftharpoons}} X{\cdot}SO_3^- \qquad\qquad (14.4)$$

$$\updownarrow$$

$$HSO_3^- \qquad K_{eq}$$

$$K_{eq}(pH) = \frac{[X{\cdot}SO_3^-]}{[X]\left\{[SO_3^{2-}] + [HSO_3^-]\right\}} \qquad\qquad (14.5)$$

represent the sum of all forms of the component at the given pH.

Besides nucleophilic addition or substitution reactions, bisulfite can also be readily oxidized according to the chain reaction, which can be initiated by Equation 14.6 or 14.7.[21,22]

$$HSO_3^{1-} + O_2 \xrightarrow{Mn^{2+}} HSO_3 + O_2^- \qquad\qquad (14.6)$$

$$SO_3^{2-} + O_2^- + 3H^+ \longrightarrow HSO_3 + 2OH \qquad\qquad (14.7)$$

$$HSO_3 + O_2 \rightarrow SO_3 + O_2^- + H^+ \qquad\qquad (14.8)$$

$$HSO_3 + OH \rightarrow SO_3 + H_2O \qquad\qquad (14.9)$$

$$2HSO_3 \longrightarrow SO_3 + SO_3^{2-} + 2H^+ \qquad\qquad (14.10)$$

$$SO_3 + H_2O \rightarrow SO_4^{2-} + 2H^+ \qquad\qquad (14.11)$$

DISCUSSION

The nucleophilic reaction of bisulfite with biomolecules will be considered first and is shown in Table 14.1, reactions 14.12-14.21. It is clear that HSO_3^- is a highly reactive, versatile nucleophile. Considering

Table 14.1   Reactions of Bisulfite

Reaction		Reference
14.12	RS-SR + HSO_3^- $\xrightleftharpoons{\substack{K \\ K = 8.9 \times 10^{-2}}}$ $RSSO_3^-$ + RSH Cystine $\quad\quad$ pH 7.75, 37°C	23

14.13 $\underset{/\;\backslash}{\overset{O}{\underset{\quad}{\overset{\|}{C}}}}$ + HSO_3^- $\xrightleftharpoons[\substack{K_{aliphatic} < 10^4\ M^{-1} \\ aldehydes}]{K}$ $-\underset{SO_3^-}{\overset{OH}{\underset{|}{\overset{|}{C}}}}-$ 24

$$K_{D\text{-glucopyranose}} = 1.6\ M^{-1}$$

14.14   Menadione + HSO_3^- $\xrightleftharpoons{K}$ 25-27

$$K = 1 \times 10^6\ M^{-1} \quad pH\ 7.5,\ 25°C$$

14.15   Nicotinamide Adenine Dinucleotide NAD^+ + SO_3^{2-} $\xrightleftharpoons{K}$ 27-31

$$K = 36\ M^{-1} \quad pH\ 7.5,\ 25°C$$

Lactate Dehydrogenase + NAD^+ + SO_3^{2-} $\xrightleftharpoons[K \gg 36\ M^{-1}]{}$ $LDH \cdot NAD \cdot SO_3^-$

14.16   [structure] $+ HSO_3^- \rightleftharpoons$ [structure with SO_3^-]   32-35

K_{FAD} = 0.4   pH 7, 25°C
Flavin Adenine Dinucleotide

K_{FMN} = 0.53
Flavin Mononucleotide

D-Amino Acid $+ HSO_3^{2-} \rightleftharpoons$ D-Amino Acid $+ H^+$
Oxidase   Oxidase FAD · SO_3^-
     $K = 2.5 \times 10^2$ M^{-1} pH 8.5, 17°C

L-Amino Acid $+ HSO_3^{2-} \rightleftharpoons$ L-Amino Acid $+ H^+$
Oxidase FAD   Oxidase · FAD · SO_3^-
     $K = 4.1 \times 10^3$ M^{-1} pH 7.5, 17°C

14.17 a)   [structure] $+ HSO_3^- \rightleftharpoons$ [structure with SO_3^-]   36,37
       7-Hydroxypteridine

b)   [structure] $+ HSO_3^- \rightleftharpoons$ [structure with SO_3^-]
     Folate $K = 1.5$ M^{-1} pH 6.5, 31°C

c)   [structure] $+ HSO_3^- \rightleftharpoons$ [structure with SO_3^-]
     Dihydrofolate $K = 41$ M^{-1} pH 6.5, 31°C

Table 14.1, Continued

Reaction	Reference

14.18 Cytidine

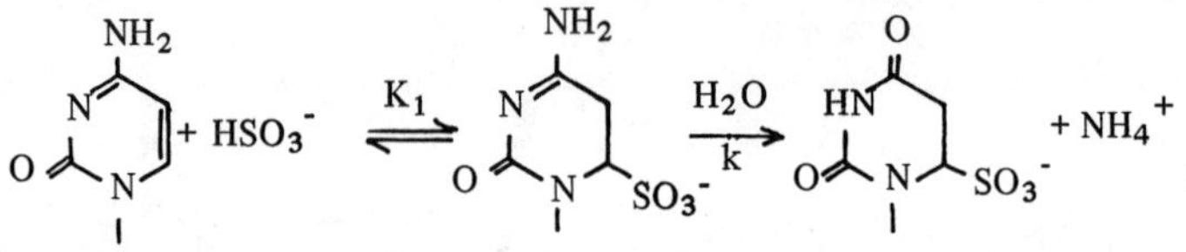

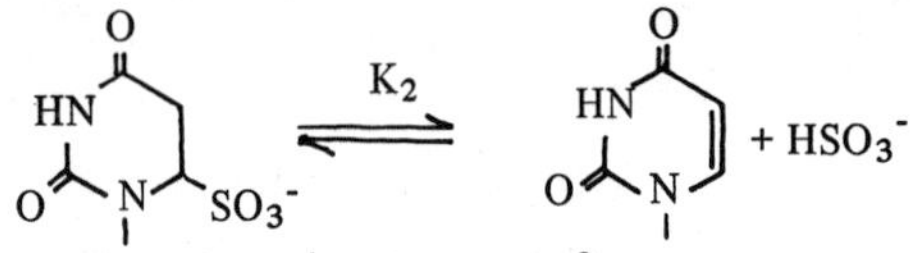

$$K_1 = 3.0 \text{ M}^{-1} \quad \text{pH } 7.0, \ 25°C$$
$$k = 1.8 \times 10^{-5} \text{ sec}^{-1} \quad \text{pH } 7.0, \ 37°C$$
$$K_2 \text{(uracil)} = 3.7 \times 10^{-3} \text{ M}^{-1} \quad \text{pH } 7.0, \ 24°C$$

38-42

14.19 Thiamine

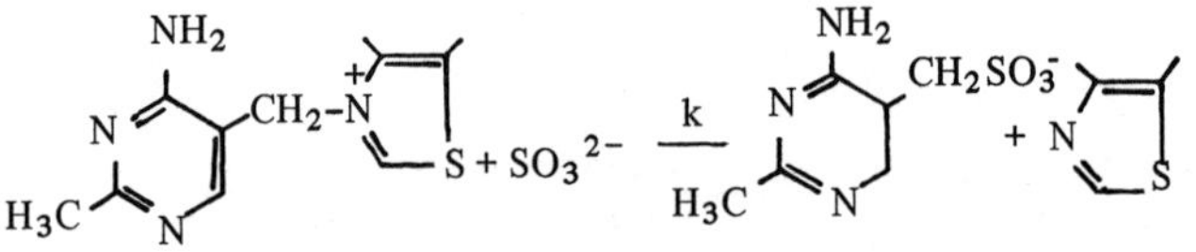

$$k = 50 \text{ M}^{-1} \text{ hr}^{-1} \quad \text{pH } 5.5\text{-}6.0, \ 25°C$$

43,44

14.20 Epinephrine

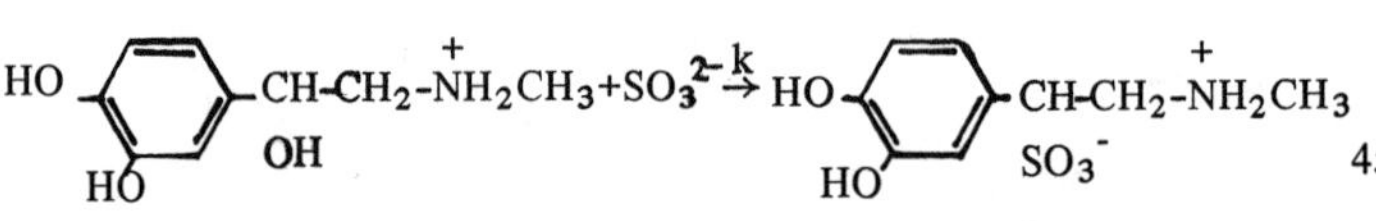

$$t_{1/2} = 74 \text{ hr} \quad \text{pH } 7.5, \ 25°C$$
$$[\text{EP}] = 0.082 \text{ M}$$
$$[\text{SO}_3{}^{2-}] = 0.96 \text{ M}$$

45-47

reversible reactions between HSO_3^- and various organic compounds, equilibrium constants for formation for the adducts are not large enough to assure stoichiometric interaction except in the presence of an excess of reactant (Equation 14.12-14.17). However, in the case of NAD^+ and the flavin FAD, the binding of these coenzymes to proteins such as lactate dehydrogenase, D-amino acid oxidase and L-amino acid oxidase markedly stabilizes the sulfonate adduct.[27,30-33] Hence, care must be taken in the interpretation of the thermodynamic data, for conditions within the cell may drastically alter these binding constants.

There are also examples here of irreversible reactions (Equations 14.18-14.20). In each reaction the rate constant for the irreversible step is small. It is so small for the reaction between sulfite and epinephrine that it can probably be discounted *in vivo* where both reactants are present at much lower concentration than those used in the determination of $t_{1/2}$.[47]

Some radical reactions of bisulfite of biochemical interest have also been observed (Table 14.2). In none of these cases is the precise nature of the reactive radical(s) known from among the several that arise during sulfite oxidation: HSO_3, SO_3, O_2^-, and OH (Equations 14.6-14.11). Several of the reactions in Table 14.1 are known to occur in biological systems. Recently it has been observed that $^{35}SO_2$ inhaled by animals reaches the circulatory system in significant amounts and is bound there as $RS^{35}SO_3^-$ according to Equation 14.12.[51-53] The large concentration of disulfides in blood plasma drives this reaction to completion so that no free bisulfite can be detected.

Table 14.2   Radical Reactions of Bisulfite

Equation		
14.22	DNA + SO_3^{2-} + O_2 $\xrightarrow{Mn^{2+}}$	Chain Cleavage
14.23	Unsaturated Lipid + SO_3^{2-} + O_2 $\rightarrow$	Oxidation of Double Bonds
14.24	$\underset{H_3\overset{+}{N}}{\overset{O_2C^-}{\diagup}}$ CHCH$_2$CH$_2$SCH$_3$ + SO_3^{2-} + O_2 $\xrightarrow{Mn^{2+}}$ $\underset{H_3\overset{+}{N}}{\overset{O_2C^-}{\diagup}}$ CHCH$_2$CH$_2\overset{O}{\overset{\|}{S}}CH_3$	
	Methionine	

It has long been known that foods preserved with SO_2 progressively lose thiamine content.[54] Now it is also evident that ingested bisulfite attacks thiamine *in vivo* to the extent that in experiments investigating the long-term adverse effects of bisulfite in foods, diets are fortified with thiamine to prevent the occurrence of thamine deficiency symptoms.[55]

The deamination of cytosine to uracil catalyzed by bisulfite is a highly specific method for generating G-C to A-T mutations in DNA.[39-42] In several test systems for mutagenic capability including bacteriophages and *E. coli* bacteria, bisulfite causes mutations and is classified as a moderately strong mutagen in the T-4 phage system.[56-58]

Besides these reactions, there is an enzyme that carries out the oxidation of sulfite to sulfate.[59]

$$SO_3^{2-} + 1/2\ O_2 \rightarrow SO_4^{2-} \tag{14.25}$$

This enzyme, sulfite oxidase, exists in the mitochondrion and may use cytochrome c as the proximate oxidizing agent, which then reduces oxygen via the electron transport chain.[60],[61] Sulfite oxidase contains molybdenum and cytochrome b_5 components. It serves the function of detoxifying bisulfite produced from the normal sulfur metabolism of the organism and is known to be crucial to the ability of organisms to withstand high levels of SO_2 exposure.[62-64]

Remarkably, only a few studies have been conducted on the effects of sulfur dioxide-bisulfite upon *in vitro* cell populations. Lymphocytes show reduced cell growth and DNA synthesis after exposure to 10^{-6} M bisulfite (calculation for 5 ml culture exposed once to 100 ml of 5.7 ppm SO_2).[65] At 10^{-5} M bisulfite HeLa cell survival is markedly reduced.[66] This effect is reversed by addition of vitamin E to the culture medium. Finally, at higher concentration, 10^{-3}-10^{-2} M, bisulfite inhibits normal aggregation of platelets.[67] These results warrant further investigation, for at 10^{-6} M one is working at a level of bisulfite that might accumulate from inhalation of ambient air.

It may now be asked what pattern of reactions of sulfur dioxide in biological systems are suggested by these results. Figure 14.1 summarizes one view of the available information.[68] Gaseous sulfur dioxide is converted to bisulfite at the surface of the lung. Although it may be possible for SO_2 to react directly at this surface, beyond this point HSO_3^- is expected to predominate. It has been claimed that sufficient sulfite oxidase exists in the lung to oxidize totally any reasonable ambient concentration of SO_2 to sulfate.[64] However, it is evident in rabbits and dogs that labeled sulfur of $^{35}SO_2$ reaches the blood plasma and is bound there as S-sulfocysteine compounds, $RS^{35}SO_3$.[51-53] Hence the presence of sulfite oxidase does not necessarily ensure detoxification. As a result, other reactions of bisulfite in lung cells may be expected to occur. Of concern are possible radical reactions perhaps initiated by O_2^-, the cleavage of thiamine, and the deamination of cytidine to uridine. Although the question has been raised whether SO_2 is a mutagen *in vivo*, one must also ask whether it has carcinogenic or cocarcinogenic properties in the lung. In fact, an epidemiological study of lung cancer in workers exposed to arsenic in the presence or absence of SO_2 and animal studies of the carcinogenicity of benz-(a)-pyrene as a function of the level of sulfur dioxide in the atmosphere both showed that cancer development was positively correlated with SO_2 exposure.[69],[70]

Once bisulfite has passed into the blood it is bound exclusively as $RSSO_3^-$, distributed among proteins and small molecules. In rabbits and

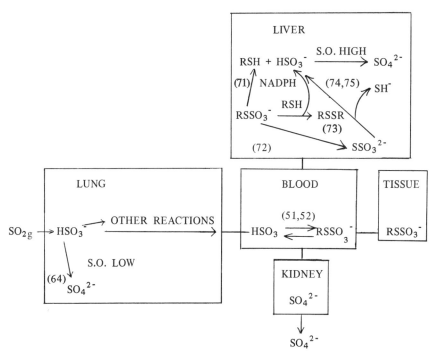

Figure 14.1 Metabolism of sulfur dioxide.

dogs subjected to 10-25 ppm SO_2, plasma S-sulfo compounds quickly rise to about 10^{-4} M.[51,53] It has not been determined whether the cleavage of disulfide bonds in plasma has significant detrimental effects upon constituent proteins.[68] Since there is no evidence of free HSO_3^- in plasma, the biochemistry of HSO_3^- becomes the biochemistry of $RSSO_3^-$ beyond the lung. Hence, unless free bisulfite is regenerated in germ cells by subsequent reaction of thiols with $RSSO_3^-$, it is unlikely that bisulfite acts as a mutagen in higher organisms.[27]

It is known that absorbed sulfur dioxide is ultimately converted to sulfate and excreted from the kidney. What has not been done, however, is a study, including material balance, of the kinetics of movement and the chemical forms of SO_2 that exist after its entrance into an organism until it leaves the biological system as sulfate. Yokoyama *et al.* have stated without details that inhaled $^{35}SO_2$ only slowly appears in the urine of dogs as $^{35}SO_4^{2-}$, that only a fraction is present in blood and that eventually most of the inhaled gas is metabolized to sulfate.[52] The implication is that most of the dose of SO_2 remains in the animal for long periods of time. Hence it is unclear what roles lung and liver sulfite oxidase play in detoxification of inhaled sulfur dioxide. Likewise, the metabolic fate and important S-sulfo compounds in the total interaction of sulfur dioxide with the organism is not known.

By using scattered reports in the literature, it may be hypothesized that S-sulfocysteinyl compounds that exist in blood plasma can react by various routes in the liver to regenerate bisulfite, which can then be oxidized efficiently to sulfate (Figure 14.1). It has also been shown recently that S-sulfo cysteine is a neurotoxic material that causes brain damage in rat pups after a single intravenous dose of 0.4 mmol/kg of the material.[77] Given the experience with lead in which increasingly sophisticated experiments are detecting brain abnormalities at progressively lower exposure levels of lead, this finding requires further study of the effects of S-sulfo compounds in $vivo$.[78]

It is clear that much remains to be done in the analysis of the interaction of sulfur dioxide with biological systems. It is also necessary now to undertake multivariable studies, as indicated at the outset. Figure 14.2 summarizes a view of the reaction of bisulfite with biomolecules, which can guide the development of such experiments. In simple terms

$$\text{Biosynthesis} \rightarrow X_n \rightarrow \text{Degradation}$$

$$X_1 \overset{K_{X1}}{\rightleftharpoons} X_1 \cdot SO_3^-$$

$$HSO_3^- + X_2 \rightleftharpoons X_2 \cdot SO_3^- \rightarrow \text{Degradation}$$

$$(C_{Total}$$

$$X_n \overset{k_1}{\underset{k_{-1}}{\rightleftharpoons}} X_n SO_3^-$$

$$\text{Intake} \rightarrow HSO_3^- + 1/2 \; O_2 \xrightarrow{\text{Sulfite Oxidase}} SO_4^{2-} \rightarrow \text{Excretion}$$

Toxicity
A. $X_n SO_3^-$ Depletion $[X_n]$ (Thiamine)
B. $X_n SO_3^-$ Direct Effect Independent of $[X_n]$
(Cytidine $\rightarrow$ Uridine; $RSSO_3^-$)

Figure 14.2   Reaction of bisulfite with biomolecules

bisulfite reacts with biomolecules $X_1 \ldots X_n$. Toxicity occurs when X_n is depleted by its conversion to $X_n \cdot SO_3^-$ or other products or when $X_n \cdot SO_3^-$ has a direct toxic effect. These effects are modulated by several general factors: (1) the concentration of bisulfite, which depends upon its rate of intake and transformation to other materials such as sulfate, (2) the concentration of X_n, which depends upon the relative rates of biosynthesis or incorporation into the organism of X_n and its degradation, and (3) the rate of degradation of $X_n \cdot SO_3^-$ or other product. In addition each reaction has its peculiar set of kinetic and thermodynamic parameters that govern the extent of the given reaction.

In terms of the reactions described here, Table 14.3 lists several parameters that might be varied in conjunction with exposure to sulfur dioxide in order to alter some of the dynamics of these biochemical reactions.

Table 14.3   Multivariable Experiments

	Reference

1. Reduction dietary thiamine
     To increase sensitivity of organism to thiamine depletion
       by bisulfite
	79

2. Reduction in Vitamin E
     To stress the antioxidant capacity of the organism in the
       face of the free radical forming capacity of bisulfite
	49

3. Reduction in dietary molybdenum To decrease the sulfite oxidase capability of the organism	64

4. Exposure to lead and/or presence of dietary iron deficiency
     To inhibit heme biosynthesis including cytochrome b_5 for
       sulfite oxidase
	80

5. Dietary copper deficiency
     To lower lung superoxide dismutase making radical reactions
       of bisulfite with O_2^- more favorable
	81

The emphasis upon diet as a fundamental variable in future experiments rests on the realization that a healthy nutritional status cannot be assumed for large numbers of the population, particularly among inner city dwellers who are exposed to sulfur dioxide and to many other pollutants as well.

REFERENCES

1. Reid, D. D. *Proc. Roy. Soc. Med.* 62:311 (1969).
2. National Air Pollution Control Administration. "Air Quality Criteria for Sulfur Oxides," Publication AP-50, pp. 72-87, 117-149 (1970).

3. McCarroll, J., E. J. Cassell, D. W. Walter, J. R. Mountain, J. R. Diammond and I. M. Mountain. *Arch. Environ. Health* 14:178 (1967).
4. French, J. G., G. Lowrimore, W. C. Nelson, J. F. Finklea, T. English and M. Hertz. *Arch. Environ. Health* 27:129 (1973).
5. Lewis, T. R., W. J. Moorman, W. F. Ludmann and K. I. Campbell. *Arch. Environ. Health* 26:16 (1973).
6. Alarie, Y., C. E. Ulrich, W. M. Busey, *et al. Arch. Environ. Health* 21:769 (1970).
7. Alarie, Y., C. E. Ulrich, W. M. Busey, A. A. Krumin and H. N. MacFarland. *Arch. Environ. Health* 24:115 (1972).
8. Alarie, Y., A. A. Krumin, W. M. Busey, C. E. Ulrich and R. J. Kantz, II. *Arch. Environ. Health* 30:254 (1975).
9. Johnson, H. D., E. M. Lincoln and R. E. Flatt. *Proc. Soc. Exp. Biol. Med.* 139:861 (1972).
10. Hirsch, J. A., E. W. Swenson and A. Wanner. *Arch. Environ. Health* 30:249 (1975).
11. Alarie, Y. *Arch. Environ. Health* 31:110 (1976).
12. Cassell, E. J., M. D. Lebowitz, D. W. Wolter and J. R. McCarroll. *Am. J. Public Health* 61:2348 (1971).
13. Ingle, D. J. *Persp. Biol. Med.* 14:410 (1971).
14. Giddens, W. E. and G. A. Fairchild. *Arch. Environ. Health* 25:166 (1972).
15. Fairchild, G. A., J. Roan and J. McCarroll. *Arch. Environ. Health* 25:174 (1972).
16. Zarkower, A. *Arch. Environ. Health* 25:45 (1972).
17. Eigen, M., Kusten and G. Maass. *Z. Phys. Chem.* 30:130 (1961).
18. Tartar, H. V. and H. H. Garetson. *J. Am. Chem. Soc.* 63:808 (1941).
19. Sillen, L. G. and A. E. Martell. *Stability Constants.* (Washington, D.C.: The Chemical Society, 1964), pp. 229-230.
20. Bourne, D. W. A., T. Higuchi and I. H. Pitman. *J. Pharm. Sci.* 63:865 (1974).
21. Abel, E. *Monatsh. Chem.* 82:815 (1951).
22. Yang, S. F. *Biochemistry* 9:5008 (1970).
23. Stricks, W. and I. M. Koltoff. *J. Amer. Chem. Soc.* 73:4569 (1951).
24. Schroeter, L. *Sulfur Dioxide.* (New York: Pergamon Press, 1966).
25. Carmack, M., M. E. Moore and M. E. Balis. *J. Amer. Chem. Soc.* 72:844 (1950).
26. Greenburg, F. H., K. K. Leung and M. Leung. *J. Chem. Ed.* 48:632 (1971).
27. Shih, N. T. and D. H. Petering. *Biochem. Biophys. Res. Commun.* 55:1319 (1973).
28. Colowick, S. P., N. O. Kaplan and M. M. Ciotti. *J. Biol. Chem.* 191:447 (1951).
29. Myerhof, O., P. Ohlmeyer and W. Mohler. *Biochem. Z.* 297:113 (1938).
30. Pfleiderer, G., D. Jeckel and T. Wieland. *Biochem. Z.* 328:187 (1956).
31. Holbrook, J. J. *Biochem. Z.* 344:141 (1966).

32. Massey, V., F. Müller, R. Feldberg, M. Schumann, P. A. Sullivan, L. G. Howell, S. G. Mayhew, R. G. Matthews and G. Foust. *J. Biol. Chem.* 244:3999 (1969).
33. Müller, F. and V. Massey. *J. Biol. Chem.* 244:4007 (1969).
34. Hevesi, L. and T. C. Bruice. *Biochemistry* 12:290 (1973).
35. Bruice, T. C., L. Hevesi and S. Shinkai. *Biochemistry* 12:2083 (1973).
36. Albert, A. and J. J. McCormack. *J. Chem. Soc.* 6930 (1965).
37. Vonderschmidt, D. J., K. S. Vitols, F. M. Huennekens and K. G. Scringeour. *Arch. Biochem. Biophys.* 122:488 (1967).
38. Notari, R. W. *J. Pharm. Sci.* 56:804 (1967).
39. Shapiro, R., R. E. Servis and M. Welcher. *J. Amer. Chem. Soc.* 92:422 (1970).
40. Hayatsu, H., Y. Wataya and K. Kai. *J. Amer. Chem. Soc.* 92:724 (1970).
41. Hayatsu, H., Y. Wataya, K. Kai and S. Iida. *Biochemistry* 9:2858 (1970).
42. Shapiro, R., V. Difate and M. Welcher. *J. Amer. Chem. Soc.* 96:906 (1974).
43. Williams, R. R., R. E. Waterman, J. C. Keresztesy and E. R. Buchman. *J. Amer. Chem. Soc.* 57:536 (1953).
44. Leichter, J. and M. A. Joslyn. *Biochem. J.* 113:611 (1969).
45. Higuchi, J. and L. C. Schroeter. *J. Amer. Chem. Soc.* 82:1904 (1960).
46. Riegelman, S. and E. Z. Fischer. *J. Pharm. Sci.* 51:206 (1962).
47. Hajratwala, B. R. *J. Pharm. Sci.* 64:45 (1975).
48. Hayatsu, H. and R. C. Miller, Jr. *Biochem. Biophys. Res. Commun.* 46:120 (1972).
49. Kaplan, D., C. McJilton and D. Luchtel. *Arch. Environ. Health* 30:507 (1975).
50. Yang, S. F. *Biochemistry* 9:5008 (1970).
51. Gunnison, A. F. and A. W. Benton. *Arch. Environ. Health* 22:381 (1971).
52. Yokoyama, E., R. E. Yoder and N. R. Frank. *Arch. Environ. Health* 22:389 (1971).
53. Gunnison, A. F. and E. D. Palmes. *Toxicol. Appl. Pharm.* 24:266 (1973).
54. Leichter, J. Ph.D. Dissertation, University Microfilms, Inc., 70-6153.
55. Til, H. P., V. J. Feron and A. P. DeGroot. *Fd. Cosmet. Toxicol.* 10:291 (1972).
56. Hayatsu, H. and A. Miura. *Biochem. Biophys. Res. Commun.* 39:156 (1970).
57. Mukai, F., I. Hawryluk and R. Shapiro. *Biochem. Biophys. Res. Commun.* 39:983 (1970).
58. Summers, G. A. and J. W. Drake. *Genetics* 68:603 (1971).
59. Cohen, H. J. and I. Fridovich. *J. Biol. Chem.* 246:359 (1971) and following articles.
60. Cohen, H. J., S. Betcher-Lange, D. L. Kessler and K. V. Rajagopalan. *J. Biol. Chem.* 247:7759 (1972).
61. Oshino, N. and B. Chance. *Arch. Biochem. Biophys.* 170:514 (1975).

62. Mudd, S. H., F. Irreverre and L. Laster. *Science* 156:1599 (1967).
63. Irreverre, F., S. H. Mudd, W. D. Heizer and L. Laster. *Biochem. Med.* 1:187 (1967).
64. Cohen, H. J., R. T. Drew, J. L. Johnson and K. V. Rajagopalan. *Proc. Nat. Acad. Sci. U.S.A.* 70:3655 (1973).
65. Schneider, L. K. and C. A. Calkins. *Environ. Res.* 3:473 (1970).
66. Kuroda, Y. *Exp. Cell Res.* 94:442 (1975).
67. Kikugawa, K. and I. Kazuhiro. *J. Pharm. Sci.* 61:1904 (1972).
68. Petering, D. H. and N. T. Shih. *Environ. Res.* 9:55 (1975).
69. Lee, A. M. and J. F. Fraumeni, Jr. *J. Nat. Cancer Inst.* 42:1045 (1969).
70. Kuschner, M. *Am. Rev. Res. Dis.* 98:573 (1968).
71. Erikson, B. and M. Rundfelt. *Acta Chem. Scand.* 22:562 (1968).
72. Sörbo, B. *Acta Chem. Scand.* 12:1990 (1958).
73. Winell, M. and B. Mannervik. *Biochim. Biophys. Acta* 184:374 (1969).
74. Villarejo, M. and J. Westley. *J. Biol. Chem.* 238:4016 (1963).
75. Sörbo, B. *Acta Chem. Scand.* 18:821 (1964).
76. Koj, A., J. Frendo and Z. Janek. *Biochem. J.* 103:791 (1967).
77. Olney, J. N., C. H. Misra and T. deGabareff. *J. Neuropath. Exp. Neurol.* 34:167 (1975).
78. Silbergeld, E. K. and J. J. Chisolm. *Science* 192:153 (1976).
79. Hoetzel, D. *Verhantl. Deut. Ges. Inn. Med.* 67:868 (1961).
80. Secchi, G. C., L. Erba and G. Cambiaghi. *Arch. Environ. Health* 28:130 (1974).
81. Petering, H. G. Personal communication.

CHAPTER 15

BIOLOGICAL ORIGIN AND METABOLISM OF SO$_2$

K. V. Rajagopalan and J. L. Johnson

Department of Biochemistry
Duke University Medical Center
Durham, North Carolina 27710

INTRODUCTION

In considering the biological effects of environmental SO$_2$ it is pertinent to inquire about the metabolic fate of the ingested molecule. The purpose of this chapter is to relate the environmental aspects of SO$_2$ to the overall pathways of sulfur metabolism in man. An appropriate experimental animal model is also discussed.

The discovery of the ability of animal tissues[1] and isolated rat liver mitochondria[2] to oxidize SO$_3^=$ to SO$_4^=$ led to successful attempts at purification of the enzyme sulfite oxidase from various sources.[3-6] The enzyme was characterized as a molybdohemoprotein[7,8] in all animals examined. Subsequently it was found that administration of tungstate to rats for several weeks resulted in a virtual state of sulfite oxidase deficiency in the animals.[9] This protocol has been of great usefulness in assessing the role of the enzyme in the detoxification of SO$_2$ and bisulfite and in providing an animal model for human sulfite oxidase deficiency first described by Mudd and co-workers in 1967.[10] The information gained from these studies will be discussed.

PATHWAYS OF SULFUR METABOLISM

The principal forms of dietary intake of sulfur are the amino acids methionine and cysteine. Under homeostatic conditions the absorbed sulfur is quantitatively excreted in the urine. The average daily excretion by an adult is about 25 milliatoms of sulfur, 60-90% of which is in the form of inorganic sulfate. Sulfate esters represent most of the remainder of excreted sulfur. The metabolic pathways by which the sulfur of methionine and cysteine is converted into sulfate are shown in Figure 15.1 and Figure 15.2. As shown in Figure 15.1, the metabolism of the sulfur moiety of methionine involves the initial formation of cysteine. Two

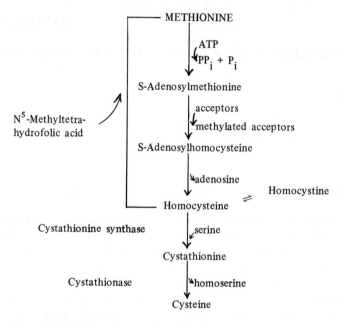

Figure 15.1 The pathway of methionine metabolism in higher vertebrates.

different pathways have been suggested for the further metabolism of cysteine sulfur to sulfate, as shown in Figure 15.2. While uncertainty exists regarding the enzymes and the intracellular site of the formation of sulfite from cysteine, it is now well established that the oxidation of $SO_3^=$ to $SO_4^=$, the terminal step in the pathway, is catalyzed by the mitochondrial enzyme sulfite oxidase. This molybdohemoprotein is localized in the intermembrane space of liver mitochondria[11-13] and, by utilizing cytochrome c as electron acceptor, serves to generate 1 ATP per molecule of $SO_3^=$ oxidized.[2,13,14] Liver and kidney contain the highest levels of sulfite oxidase in the rat, but activity is also present in other tissues such as intestine, lung and heart.[15]

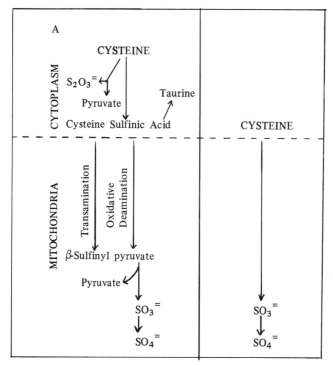

Figure 15.2 Metabolic pathways from cysteine to sulfate in higher vertebrates.

TOXICITY OF HSO₃⁻ AND SO₂ IN THE RAT

The functional presence of molybdenum in sulfite oxidase has made it possible to create sulfite oxidase deficiency in rats by feeding high levels of tungstate as a competitive inhibitor of molybdate uptake. Exposure of rats to higher than 100 ppm tungsten leads to a time-dependent decrease in tissue levels of sulfite oxidase, with a $t_{1/2}$ of about 4.7 days.[9] Adult rats with less than 1% residual tissue sulfite oxidase remain healthy indefinitely, indicating the absence of any stressful situation under normal conditions of laboratory maintenance.

The physiological importance of sulfite oxidase function in the rat has emerged from studies on the effects of acute doses of intraperitoneally injected HSO₃⁻ and respired SO₂ on normal and sulfite oxidase-deficient rats.[16] As shown in Table 15.1, the LD_{50} for injected bisulfite is three-fold higher for control rats than the level seen for deficient rats. In this experiment the fatalities invariably occurred within 10 min after injection

Table 15.1 LD_{50} for Intraperitoneal Bisulfite in Rats

Dose	Mortality	
(mg of $NaHSO_3$/kg)	Control	Tungsten-Treated
89	–	0/4
133	–	0/4
200	–	1/4
300	0/8	4/4
450	4/8	–
675	7/8	–
1012	8/8	–
LD_{50} (mg/kg)	475	181
95% Confidence range of LD_{50}	394-569	148-221

[a]Dashes, not tested.

of bisulfite. The effects of acute exposure of the two groups of rats to high levels of SO_2 are shown in Table 15.2. The design of this experiment was again to determine the effectiveness of sulfite oxidase as a detoxifying mechanism and thus entailed the use of very high levels of SO_2. Time of survival was used as the criterion since mortality was 100% in all groups. As expected, time of survival was inversely related to the dose of SO_2, and the two groups of animals were indistinguishable at the two high levels of SO_2. At the intermediate levels of SO_2 corresponding to 925 ppm and 2350 ppm control animals survived significantly longer than the sulfite oxidase-deficient animals. At 2350 ppm SO_2 and higher levels all animals in both groups showed symptoms of systemic toxicity similar to those seen in bisulfite-treated rats. At 925 ppm SO_2 the sulfite oxidase-deficient animals showed the same symptoms,

Table 15.2   Effect of Various Concentrations of Inhaled SO_2
on Survival Time of Rats

Concentration of SO_2	Survival Time (min ± SE)	
(ppm)	Control	Tungsten-Treated
590	1866 ± 210*	1542 ± 210*
925	750 ± 54	366 ± 36
2,350	176 ± 9	63 ± 3
50,000 (5%)	<10	<10
500,000 (50%)	<2	<2

but the control group of rats developed respiratory distress followed by exhaustion and death. Interestingly, at 590 ppm SO$_2$ both groups of rats showed respiratory toxicity, with less marked differences in survival time.

The experiments described above clearly demonstrate the ability of tissue sulfite oxidase to effect rapid detoxification, by oxidation, of large amounts of bisulfite either parenterally administered or derived from respired SO$_2$. As shown in Table 15.3, the total body content of rat sulfite oxidase should be capable of oxidizing 150 mmol of bisulfite to sulfate per day. The difference in the LD$_{50}$ for bisulfite between the

Table 15.3   Metabolism of SO$_2$ and Bisulfite in the Rat

	mmol/day
Total capacity for oxidation of HSO$_3^-$ in all tissues	150
Oxidation of HSO$_3^-$ in perfused liver	$>$ 40
Estimated from LD$_{50}$ studies on normal and sulfite oxidase-deficient rats	$>$ 100

control and sulfite oxidase-deficient groups, in conjunction with the fact that death occurred within 10 minutes after injection of bisulfite, clearly indicated that the rate of detoxification of bisulfite in the control rats was quite comparable to the maximum predicted capacity. In a direct study on the oxidation of SO$_3^=$ by perfused rat liver, Oshino and Chance[14] found that the rate of oxidation was at least 1.2 μmol/min/g liver, which is also in close agreement with the predicted maximum capacity. From a knowledge of the respiratory physiology of the rat and assuming 100% extraction of SO$_2$ during respiration, we have estimated that the capacity of rat tissue sulfite oxidase to oxidize SO$_3^=$ will be exceeded only at 5000 ppm SO$_2$ or higher levels. In conjunction with our observation that control rats exposed to 925 ppm SO$_2$ showed respiratory rather than systemic toxicity, these considerations justify the conclusion that at levels of SO$_2$ lower than 925 ppm there will not be any significant accumulation of bisulfite in the rat.

SULFITE OXIDASE IN MAN

The importance of sulfite oxidase in sulfur metabolism in humans was first underlined by Mudd and co-workers by the discovery in 1967 of a case of sulfite oxidase deficiency in a child.[10] The patient had dislocated ocular lenses, showed severe neurological aberrations and died at 30 months of age. The diagnosis of sulfite oxidase deficiency was made from the observation that the patient's urine contained the abnormal sulfur metabolites, sulfite, thiosulfate and S-sulfocysteine. The pathways of formation of thiosulfate and S-sulfocysteine from sulfite are shown in Figure 15.3. Since these compounds are not detectable in normal urine it is obvious that their formation is contingent on the accumulation of sulfite in the tissues. The correctness of the above diagnosis was revealed post-mortem by the total absence of sulfite oxidase in the tissues of the patient.

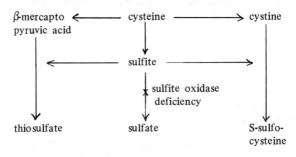

Figure 15.3   Formation of thiosulfate and S-sulfocysteine from sulfite.

From measurements of sulfite oxidase activity of autopsy samples of human liver and lung it has been possible to estimate the total capacity of adult human liver to detoxify bisulfite. From the data shown in Table 15.4 it can be seen that the daily endogenous production of bisulfite is but a minute fraction of the capacity of human liver sulfite oxidase. Further, even at 5 ppm SO_2 and assuming 100% extraction in the lung, the sulfite oxidase activity of human lung is fully capable of detoxifying the HSO_3^- formed. In short, it is extremely unlikely that detectable levels of HSO_3^- will accumulate in human tissues even in areas of prevalent high atmospheric SO_2 levels. Thus, it is our conclusion that the present day levels of atmospheric SO_2 do not constitute a genetic hazard, since the reactions that constitute the basis for the claims of genetic effects of HSO_3^- require extremely high concentrations of the compound.[17]

The average daily dietary intake of bisulfite in the form of food additives in the United States is less than 0.2 mmol per adult, with the maximum estimate being less than 2 mmol.[18] In studies with rats and mice, Gibson and Strong[18] found that prolonged dietary administration

Table 15.4   Metabolism of SO$_2$ and Bisulfite in Man

Organ	mmol/day
Liver	
Total capacity for oxidation of HSO$_3^-$	4,000-8,000
Average production of endogenous HSO$_3^-$	25
Average dietary intake of HSO$_3^-$ (USA)	0.2
Lung	
Total capacity for oxidation of SO$_2$	150
Maximum uptake of respired SO$_2$ at 5 ppm	1.3

of bisulfite to these animals even at doses 100-500 times the estimated average daily intake by man did not saturate their capacity for oxidation of bisulfite. No sulfite could be detected in the urine of the animals, indicating complete oxidation of the bisulfite. This is in contrast to the situation with patients with sulfite oxidase deficiency where sulfite, thio-sulfate and S-sulfocysteine are predominant urinary sulfur-containing constituents even at total excretion levels of 4-10 mmol/day. It is therefore apparent that, in the experiments of Gibson and Strong[18] tissue levels of HSO$_3$ were never large enough to cause the formation of abnormal sulfur metabolites. It may thus be concluded that levels of HSO$_3^-$ used as food additives are well below the oxidative capacity of tissue sulfite oxidase and do not constitute a genetic hazard. We would like to suggest that moni-toring urinary excretion of thiosulfate and S-sulfocysteine could very well be a useful method for detecting HSO$_3$-accumulation in the tissues, since these compounds appear to be formed even at low levels of accumulation of sulfite.

Since the immediate target of atmospheric SO$_2$ is the lung, careful studies are required to evaluate its possible deleterious effects on the epithelial tissue of the lung. The data presented above certainly do not rule out such a hazard. Hopefully future efforts of those concerned about the environmental effects of SO$_2$ will be directed towards answering this question.

REFERENCES

1. Heimberg, M., I. Fridovich and P. Handler. "The Enzymatic Oxi-dation of Sulfite," *J. Biol. Chem.* 204:913 (1953).
2. Hunter, F. E. and L. Ford. "Phosphorylation Coupled with Sulfite Oxidation in Liver Mitochondria," *Fed. Proc.* 13:234 (1954).
3. Cohen, H. J. and I. Fridovich. "Hepatic Sulfite Oxidase. Purifica-tion and Properties," *J. Biol. Chem.* 246:359 (1971).

4. Kessler, D. L. and K. V. Rajagopalan. "Purification and Properties of Sulfite Oxidase from Chicken Liver," *J. Biol. Chem.* 247:6566 (1972).
5. Kessler, D. L., J. L. Johnson, H. J. Cohen. and K. V. Rajagopalan. "Visualization of Hepatic Sulfite Oxidase in Crude Tissue Preparations by Electron Paramagnetic Resonance Spectroscopy," *Biochim. Biophys. Acta* 334:86 (1974).
6. Johnson, J. L. and K. V. Rajagopalan. "Purification and Properties of Sulfite Oxidase from Human Liver," *J. Clin. Invest.* 58:543 (1976).
7. Cohen, H. J. and I. Fridovish. "Hepatic Sulfite Oxidase. The Nature and Function of the Heme Prosthetic Groups," *J. Biol. Chem.* 246:367 (1971).
8. Cohen, H. J., I. Fridovich and K. V. Rajagopalan. "Hepatic Sulfite Oxidase. A Functional Role for Molybdenum," *J. Biol. Chem.* 246:374 (1971).
9. Johnson, J. L., H. J. Cohen and K. V. Rajagopalan. "Molecular Basis of the Biological Function of Molybdenum. Effect of Tungsten on Xanthine Oxidase and Sulfite Oxidase in the Rat," *J. Biol. Chem.* 249:859 (1974).
10. Irreverre, F., S. H. Mudd, W. D. Heizer and L. Laster. "Sulfite Oxidase Deficiency: Studies of a Patient with Mental Retardation, Dislocated Lenses, and Abnormal Urinary Excretion of S-Sulfo-L cysteine, Sulfite and Thiosulfate," *Biochem. Med.* 1:187 (1967).
11. Wattiaux-De Coninck, S. and R. Wattiaux. "Subcellular Distribution of Sulfite Cytochrome *c* Reductase in Rat Liver Tissue," *Eur. J. Biochem.* 19:552 (1971).
12. Ito, A. "Hepatic Sulfite Oxidase Identified as Cytochrome b_5-like Pigment Extractable from Mitochondria by Hypotonic Treatment," *J. Biochem.* 70:1061 (1971).
13. Cohen, H. J., S. Betcher-Lange, D. L. Kessler and K. V. Rajagopalan. "Hepatic Sulfite Oxidase. Congruency in Mitochondria of Prosthetic Groups and Activity," *J. Biol. Chem.* 247:7759 (1972).
14. Oshino, N. and B. Chance. "The Properties of Sulfite Oxidation in Perfused Rat Liver; Interaction of Sulfite Oxidase with the Mitochondrial Respiratory Chain," *Arch. Biochem. Biophys.* 170:514 (1975).
15. MacLeod, R. M., W. Farkas, I. Fridovich and K. V. Rajagopalan. "Purification and Properties of Hepatic Sulfite Oxidase," *J. Biol. Chem.* 236:1841 (1961).
16. Cohen, H. J., R. T. Drew, J. L. Johnson and K. V. Rajagopalan. "Molecular Basis of the Biological Function of Molybdenum. The Relationship between Sulfite Oxidase and the Acute Toxicity of Bisulfite and SO_2," *Proc. Natl. Acad. Sci., U.S.A.* 70:3655 (1973).
17. Hayatsu, H. and A. Muira. "The Mutagenic Action of Sodium Bisulfite," *Biochem. Biophys. Res. Commun.* 39:156 (1970).
18. Gibson, W. B. and F. M. Strong. "Metabolism and Elimination of Sulfite by Rats, Mice and Monkeys," *Food Cosmet. Toxicol.* 11: 185 (1973).

CHAPTER 16

CELLULAR MECHANISMS OF LUNG FIBROSIS

M. Chvapil

Department of Surgery
University of Arizona
Tucson, Arizona   85724

INTRODUCTION

For several years my co-workers and I have been studying various mechanisms of how to inhibit efficiently the various forms of fibrotic lesions in organisms. In our recent review on pharmacology of fibrosis[1,2] we arrived at the conclusion that with the exception of using lathyrogens, specifically β-aminopropionitrile, as a potential drug to control the physical characteristics of collagen, there is no method available now to specifically interfere with the deposition of collagen in the injured organ. However, fibrosis is the final stage of a dynamics of fibroproliferative inflammation, indicating that there are several other stages in the course of the inflammation that offer more promise of being affected by appropriate pharmacological treatment.

It seems that once the fibrogenic cell receives the message to produce more collagen it is already too late for any pharmacological interference. Thus our attention must be focused on the early stages of fibroproliferative inflammation, reflecting mainly the phase of cellular proliferation.
In this respect enough information has been accumulated to indicate that after any type of physical, chemical or biological injury to any tissue the cells follow a rather complex but stereotyped biological response. It was established that the proliferation or flux of different cells into the lesion is characteristic for every cell. Further, it was found that some cells communicate with each other while some cells do not. Polymorphonuclear

leucocytes that appear first in the lesion certainly communicate with macrophages but not with fibroblasts. The functional association of lymphocytes with macrophages has also been established. The high susceptability of mast cells to physical or chemical stimuli triggering the release of essential bioamines such as histamine or serotonin is well known. The participation of platelets, which are now recognized as an inflammatory cell, in the final outcome of the inflammatory lesion has been stressed recently by several authors.

This chapter will concentrate on the evidence showing that macrophages communicate with fibroblasts and that the functional state of the macrophage is essential for the type of message given to the fibroblast. Some data pointing to a method of how to interfere efficiently with the macrophage effect on fibroblast by using either divalent cations, specifically zinc, and specific anti-macrophage serum will also be presented.

ROLE OF MACROPHAGE FACTOR IN COLLAGEN FORMATION

One of the first reports indicating that silica-activated macrophages are producing a factor that enhances the synthesis of collagenous hydroxyproline by fibroblasts was presented by Heppleston and Styles.[3] Their results promoted several studies that had rather conflicting results. Some of them reproduced[4,5] and some of them failed to reproduce[6] the original observation. Presently, with more knowledge about this problem the reasons for the controversion are becoming better understood. For instance, it has been shown that only activated macrophages are stimulating-fibroblasts, and only fibroblasts (in the established culture) in logarithmic phase are susceptible to macrophage factor. Also, fibroblasts in the stationary phase are resistant and do not increase the activity after treatment with the extract from activated macrophages (Table 16.1).

Table 16.1   Effect of Extracts from Macrophages on GAG[a] Synthesis by 3T3 Fibroblast

Treatment of Fibroblast	Incorporated $^{35}SO_4$ (dpm/mg protein)	
	Log Phase	Stationary Phase
No extract, control	72.9 ± 1.7	614 ± 9
Macrophage–resting	87.8 ± 1.2 $\Big)$ P $<$ 0.001	742 ± 50
Activated by silica	125.3 ± 1.7	778 ± 40

[a]GAG–glycosaminoglycans

When viable peritoneal macrophages are injected intradermally and in the site of the injection, an incision wound is inflicted—the healing pattern of this wound is much faster when compared to the control, nontreated or just saline-treated wound (Table 16.2). In this case,

Table 16.2 Induction of Collagen Synthesis in Skin Wounds by Allogenic Macrophages

Treatment	Collagen Synthesis DPM ^{14}C Hyp/μmole	Breaking Strength g/0.5 cm
Macrophage	1726 ± 223[a]	215 ± 11[a]
Media Control	905 ± 105	127 ± 14
Control	792 ± 75	110 ± 19

[a]Greater than controls; $p < 0.001$ rat, 8-day-old skin wound (Casey, Peacock and Chvapil, unpublished results)

no activation of macrophages was needed because either the macrophages harvested from the peritoneal cavity have already been activated by the agent inducing the inflammation or the simple intradermal injection is stimulating the macrophage activity. As a result, the tensile strength as well as the rate of collagen synthesis in macrophage-treated wounds was significantly enhanced. This finding agrees with a similar one of Kilroe-Smith et al.[5] who demonstrated that a fibrogenic factor in alveolar macrophages of guinea pigs exposed to quartz dust produces granulomata when implanted subcutaneously into guinea pigs. Therefore there seems to be no doubt that macrophages activated either by silica or by any other activating agent are producing a factor that triggers the activity of fibroblasts to produce more collagen, eventually glycosaminoglycans, although the nature of this fibroblast-stimulating factor from macrophages has not been identified yet.

It is interesting to speculate on the possible nature of such a substance. It has been well-established that activated macrophages release the lysosomal enzymes. This is especially the case during the phagocytosis of the silica particles. In several studies[7,8] Allison demonstrated the enhancement of the release of lysosomal enzymes due to the lysis of lysosomal membrane. It may well be that modification of surface membrane of fibroblasts by lysosomal enzymes acting at a certain level of activity would trigger the fibroblast to higher activity. This seems to be supported by a recent finding by Dr. Rokosova (Portland, Oregon), who found an enhancement of fibroblast mitosis and activity at certain low concentrations of some lysosomal enzymes added to the cultivating medium (personal communication).

Another mechanism by which activated macrophages could stimulate the fibroblast activity may relate to increased synthesis of prostaglandins, especially PGE and PGE_2. During macrophage activation the oxidation of unsaturated fatty acids, specifically of arachidonic acid, is enhanced, resulting in the synthesis of prostaglandins.[9,10] Prostaglandins of the E and F type were found to stimulate adenyl cyclase activity in different fibroblasts' cultured cell lines, the most active being PGE_1. This suggests that prostaglandins synthesized by inflammatory cells like macrophage or platelet may regulate the synthesis and eventually the secretion of glyco-saminoglycans and of collagen by fibroblasts via cyclic AMP.[11] In our experiments the fibrogenic factor from macrophages was present in the extractable 15,000 x g supernate. In experiments by Kilroe-Smith et al.[5] the factor was found to be associated with the insoluble debris produced after sonic disintegration of the macrophages.

Another experiment indicates the fibroblast-promoting activity of ex-tract from the whole organ, in this case, from the lung of rats that were injected intratracheally with a suspension of quartz and sacrificed at dif-ferent time intervals from 3 to 24 days after the instillation of the dust. The lung was homogenized and extracted into the medium used for the cultivation of fibroblasts. Then the extract from various lungs was equilibrated to the same content of proteins. The same amount of ex-tract was added at two different concentrations to the established line of 3T3 fibroblasts. The function of fibroblasts was ascertained by mea-suring the synthesis of sulfated glycosaminoglycans. We found that within three days of the instillation of the silica particles the lung extract significantly enhanced the activity of fibroblasts (Table 16.3). Significant

Table 16.3   Effect of Extracts from Silicotic Lungs of Rats on GAG Synthesis by 3T3 Fibroblasts

Days After Silica Administration	GAG Synthesis—$^{35}SO_4$ in GAG (dpm/μg cell protein)
0	281 ± 24
3	625 ± 24
10	525 ± 45
17	293 ± 45
24	290 ± 27

Same lobe of the lungs at given times was extracted in MEM, protein content in 15,000 x g supernate of the extract was adjusted to the same protein content. Data (X ± SEM) refer to the effect of 10 μg protein of extracts added to 3T3 fibroblast culture in log phase. Cells were incubated for 36 hr, then $^{35}SO_4$ added (50 μCi/ flask) and incubated for another 24 hr. (Chvapil and Herring, unpublished results.)

activation was present on the tenth day. In later stages of silicotic fibro-proliferative inflammation the fibroblast-stimulating activity in the injured lung decreased and returned to the control values when a certain concentration of the extract was tested (10 μg protein).

Further experiments to characterize the chemical nature of this factor in the injured tissue are under way. So far we have learned that the factor is extractable in chloroform-ethanol and that it is unstable under storage. Therefore, we must work with fresh tissues and extracts.

REGULATION OF THE NUMBER AND ACTIVITY OF MACROPHAGES

In agreement with the concept that macrophage is essential for the formation of fibrosis is the well-established fact that in the silicotic fibrosis the damage of macrophages is of primary importance. Furthermore, the silicotic model is an excellent example of the erroneous reaction of macrophages which, while phagocytozing silica, undergo lysis of lysosomes with release of lysosomal enzymes and suicidal death of the cell. It may be assumed that during this process more fibroblast-activating substances are released. In addition the damaged macrophages attract more inflammatory cells to the lesion and a vicious circle is formed.

The participation of macrophages in the inflammatory lesion is certainly the essential feature of inflammation. I am suggesting, however, that the total number of macrophages entering the damaged area is often excessive, triggering too much fibroplasia. It seems that by limiting the amount as well as the function of macrophages to a certain extent less collagen might be deposited in the lesion. If this postulate is correct, then factors modifying macrophage reaction should also decrease collagen accumulation. In this context two approaches studied in my laboratories relate to the effect of zinc and the effect of antimacrophage serum.

Zinc

Recent evidence indicates that zinc ions administered either *in vitro* to incubated cells or eventually supplemented to animals *in vivo* inhibited various functions of cells like granulocytes, macrophages, platelets and mast cells.[12-14] For instance, disruption of mast cells induced by 48/80 substance is inhibited by 50% at 10 μM zinc concentration. Animals treated with zinc *in vivo* show less release of histamine from perfused rat lungs. Granulocytes *in vitro* showed less phagocytosis as measured by the oxygen consumption in the presence of zinc in the medium.

We showed recently that in rats kept on zinc-deficient or zinc-supplemented diet the amount of peritoneal inflammatory cells was indirectly proportional to zinc supplementation, *i.e.,* to the content of zinc in the serum (for review see Reference 13). We demonstrated that peritoneal macrophages isolated from animals fed high zinc diets, eventually supplemented parenterally with zinc, were rounded without any elongations and extrusions of the protoplasmatic membrane. This contrasted with multiple-shaped macrophages from control animals. Peratoneal macrophages from animals on high zinc diets did not migrate in an *in vitro* experiment that incubated macrophages and followed their migration from the capillary tube. Because of the decreased phagocytosis of these peritoneal macrophages isolated from animals treated with different doses of zinc, the lysis or the viability of macrophages exposed to 1-μ-size silica particles was significantly decreased in the presence of zinc.[15] This indicates that zinc ions are one of the factors controlling some functions of macrophages such as phagocytosis, chemotaxis, bacterial killing and function of hexosemonophosphate shunt.

We still do not know the actual mechanism of zinc effect on the cell, but a speculative scheme of proposed mechanisms is presented in Figure 16.1. It indicates that zinc acts either at the plasma membrane level,

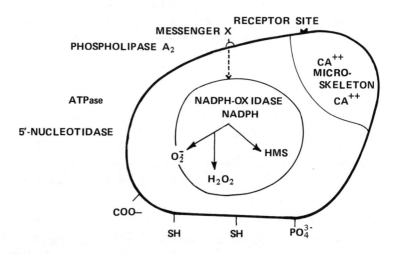

Figure 16.1 Proposed mechanisms of zinc effect on various cells.

affecting different reactive groups like sulfhydril, phosphate groups or carboxyl groups, or it interferes with some enzymes that control the function of the plasma membrane, such as 5'nucleotidase, ATPase or phospholipase A-2. Phospholipase A-2 and ATPase have been shown to be inhibited by zinc ions. Another mechanism postulates, however, that zinc is transported into the cell where it interacts with the calcium by displacing this cation from the microskeleton, thus modifying the function of microtubules or microfilaments.

Another mechanism relates to the now well-established effect of zinc on NADPH oxidation. Because this phenomenon seems to be of paramount biological importance, we studied the mechanism of Zn-NADPH interaction and found a competitive nature of the inhibition of NADPH oxidation by zinc. We are postulating that one NADPH molecule is linked with two zinc, which results in a piling of NADPH molecules that are becoming inactive. It is obvious that as a consequence of blocking NADPH oxidation NADPH-dependent lipid peroxidation and the NADPH oxidation-dependent function of mixed function oxidases will be inhibited as well. This actually was demonstrated in experiments *in vitro* using the liver microsomal mixed function oxidases system.[16,17]

How this would apply to the lung metabolism of xenobiotics through a similar metabolic pathway has not been studied yet. We believe that the protective effect of zinc supplementation against the hepatotoxicity of carbon tetrachloride to rats is related to the above-mentioned mechanism of blocking the oxidation of NADPH.[18] We found that after zinc supplementation the formation of malondialdehyde as an indicator of lipid peroxidation was significantly less. There was also less labilization of lysosomes, ascertained by measuring the free glucuronidase. But the most important finding was that parallel to the decrease of lipid peroxidation, and increased integrity of liver of lysosomes, there was significantly less collagen synthesized and deposited in the liver of animals treated with zinc. It will be of interest to see if a similar mechanism applies to the lung, which is exposed to some pollutants metabolized by mixed function oxidases.

If silicotic fibroplasia is primarily related to the damage of macrophages, then decrease of the number and eventually of the functional activity of the macrophages should decrease collagen deposition even in the presence of the same amount of silica. We tested this hypothesis, and the results, presented in Table 16.4, indicate that the rats supplemented parenterally with zinc and injected intratracheally with a suspension of silica showed significantly lower synthesis of collagen as well as total weight of the lung. As demonstrated by several authors, the fibrogenicity and degree of toxicity of silica particles correlates with the wet weight of the lung. It could be assumed that zinc significantly inhibited the fibroproliferative inflammation and the function of fibrogenic cells. These are, however, only preliminary results, which need to be expanded.

Table 16.4   Effect of Supplementation of Zinc on Lung Silicosis in Rats

Group	Lung w·wt (g)	Hyp/Lung (mg/lung)	Collagen Synthesis C^{14} HypDPN/μmole
Control	1.57 ± 0.07	$1.7 \pm$	474 ± 19
SiO_2	4.27 ± 0.59	2.6 ± 0.44	1572 ± 31
SiO_2 + Zn	3.57 ± 0.51	1.3 ± 0.16	872 ± 79

$X \pm SEM$ $^a p < 0.05$ $^b p < 0.001$

Male, 250-g rats, treated with single intratracheal 50 mg SiO_2.
Zinc administered as zinc sulfate 1 mg/100 g/day, i.m. or i.p. for a total of 6 weeks.
(Chvapil, unpublished results.)

Antimacrophage Serum

The second method of eliminating a certain cell from participation in the chain of reaction leading to the activation of fibroblasts is to prepare a specific antiserum against a certain cell, thus either inactivating or lysing the cell. This has already been done with antilymphocyte serum or anti-granulocyte serum. There have also been some studies performed with antimacrophage serum, which indicated that less collagen was deposited in treated skin wounds of rats treated with specific antimacrophage serum.[19]

In our studies we used antimacrophage serum against rat peritoneal macrophages. After 8 days of administration of antimacrophage serum to rats implanted subcutaneously with Ivalon sponges, we found significantly less collagen and significantly lower activity of prolyl hydroxylase in the reactive granuloma tissue as compared with controls treated either with saline or normal serum and eventually with antithymocyte serum. All three groups served as controls. This indicates that at certain time periods of inflammation antimacrophage serum administered in adequate concentrations to the animal may eliminate the macrophage stimulus for fibroblasts. We also produced the specific antiserum against fibroblasts in order to modify the function of collagen-synthesizing cells. We found EM evidence on disruption of fibroblasts and collagen with lower activity of prolyl hydroxylase in those sponges of animals treated with antifibroblast serum. Here again, these experiments are rather preliminary, but they indicate a potential method of how to interfere, at least on the experimental level, with participation of a certain inflammatory cell in the kinetics of fibroproliferative inflammation.

ACKNOWLEDGMENTS

The experiments reported in this chapter were performed by my co-workers Dr. Ronald Misiorowski, Dr. Karen Steinbronn, Dr. Del Steinbronn, Dr. Linda Karl, Dr. William Casey, Janet Ludwig and Craig Herring. Their skilled assistance is highly appreciated.

These research projects were supported in part by NIH grants #HL 19633 and #AM 16489.

REFERENCES

1. Chvapil, M. "Pharmacology of Fibrosis: Definitions, Limits, and Perspectives," *Life Sci.* 16:1345 (1975).
2. Chvapil, M. "Pharmacology of Fibrosis and Tissue Injury," *Environ. Health Persp.* 9:283 (1974).
3. Heppleston, A. G. and J. A. Styles. "Activity of a Macrophage Factor in Collagen Formation by Silica," *Nature* 214:521 (1967).
4. Richards, R. J. and F. S. Wusteman. "The Effects of Silica Dust and Alveolar Macrophages on Lung Fibroblasts Grown *In Vitro*," *Life Sci.* 14:355 (1974).
5. Kilroe-Smith, T. A., I. Webster, M. V. Drimmelen and L. Marasas. "An Insoluble Fibrogenic Factor in Macrophages from Guinea Pigs Exposed to Silica," *Environ. Res.* 6:298 (1973).
6. Harington, J. S., M. Ritchie, P. C. King and K. Miller. "The *In Vitro* Effects of Silica-Treated Hamster Macrophages on Collagen Production by Hamster Fibroblasts," *J. Pathol.* 109:21 (1973).
7. Allison, A. C., J. S. Harington and M. Birbeck. "An Examination of the Cytotoxic Effects of Silica on Macrophages," *J. Exp. Med.* 124:141 (1966).
8. Harington, J. S. and A. C. Allison. "Lysosomal Enzymes in Relation to the Toxicity of Silica," *Medna. Law* 56:471 (1965).
9. Tan, W. C., R. Cortesi and O. S. Privett. "Lipid Peroxide and Lung Prostaglandins," *Arch. Environ. Health* 28:82 (1974).
10. Stossel, T. P., R. J. Mason and A. L. Smith. "Lipid Peroxidation by Human Blood Phagocytes," *J. Clin. Invest.* 54:638 (1974).
11. Peters, H. D., K. Karzel, D. Padberg, P. S. Schonhofer and V. Dinnendahl. "Influence of Prostaglandin E_1 on Cyclic 3', 5'-AMP Levels and Glycosaminoglycan Secretion of Fibroblasts Cultured *In Vitro*," *Pol. J. Pharmacol. Pharm.* 26:41 (1974).
12. Chvapil, M. "New Aspects in the Biological Role of Zinc: A Stabilizer of Macromolecules and Biological Membranes," *Life Sci.* 13:1041 (1973).
13. Chvapil, M. "Effect of Zinc on Cells and Biomembranes," *Med. Clinics North Amer.* 60(4) (June 1976).
14. Chvapil, M., L. Stankova, C. F. Zukoski, and C. F. Zukoski. "Inhibition of Some Functions of Polymorphonuclear Leucocytes by *In Vitro* Zinc," *J. Lab. Clin. Med.* (accepted for publication).

15. Karl, L., M. Chvapil and C. F. Zukoski. "Effect of Zinc on the Viability and Phagocytic Capacity of Peritoneal Macrophages," *Proc. Soc. Exp. Biol. Med.* 142:1123 (1973).
16. Chvapil, M., I. G. Sipes, J. C. Ludwig and S. C. Halladay. "Inhibition of NADPH Oxidation and Oxidative Metabolism of Drugs in Liver Microsomes by Zinc," *Biochem. Pharmacol.* 24:917 (1975).
17. Chvapil, M., J. C. Ludwig, I. G. Sipes and R. L. Misiorowski. "Inhibition of NADPH Oxidation and Related Drug Oxidation in Liver Microsomes by Zinc," *Biochem. Pharmacol.* 25:1787 (1976).
18. Chvapil, M., J. N. Ryan, S. L. Elias and Y. M. Peng. "Protective Effect of Zinc on Carbon Tetrachloride-Induced Liver Injury in Rats," *Exp. Mol. Pathol.* 19:186 (1973).
19. Leibovich, S. J. and R. Ross. "The Role of the Macrophage in Wound Repair," *Amer. J. Pathol.* 78:73 (1975).

CHAPTER 17

LUNG ELASTIC TISSUE

Judith Ann Foster and Carl Franzblau

Boston University
School of Medicine
80 East Concord Street
Boston, Massachusetts 02118

INTRODUCTION

Elastic recoil or compliance is of paramount importance in lung function as well as lung structure. Physiologists have, for many years, been studying lung compliance through measurements of pressure-flow relationships. In recent years biochemists have begun to examine the tissue elements responsible for lung elasticity. Much of the impetus for these studies originated from the observation that elastic tissue was intimately involved in several chronic obstructive lung diseases such as emphysema.[1,2]

The following discussion is aimed at describing the major structural protein of lung elastic tissue, namely elastin. Particular emphasis will be given to recent advances in the understanding of elastin biosynthesis as a foundation for future insight in elastic fiber pathogenesis.

BACKGROUND

The elastic fibers of lung have been studied by many investigators since the turn of the century. The pleura, blood vessels, bronchi and respiratory units of the lung all contain elastic tissue by three months of human fetal life.

Before one discusses the synthesis of elastic fibers in detail, the chemical nature of these fibers must be defined. Ross and his collaborators[3,4] have noted that elastic fibers are composed of two distinct entities, an

325

amorphous elastin component and a microfibrillar component. The latter component has been described as a glycoprotein or a family of glycoproteins. It is proposed that these glycoprotein moieties serve as a matrix for the formation of the insoluble elastin component of elastic fibers. The microfibrillar component is purported to be present in high concentration early in the development of elastic fibers, and as the fiber develops, its synthesis decreases to a low or nonexistent level. When compared to the amorphous elastin component, the microfibrillar component will be present in relatively high concentration early in the development of the fiber and, as the tissue develops, it will become diluted with increasing amounts of the amorphous elastin component. Studies on the chemistry of the microfibrillar component have truly just begun and suffice it to say that it is a glycoprotein(s) which contains significant quantities of cysteine in its structure.[3,5]

The chemistry of the amorphous elastin component requires some background description as well. Elastin is usually defined as that protein material which remains after all other connective tissue components have been removed by chemical procedures. When isolated in relatively pure form, fibers of elastin behave as true rubberlike elastomers.[6] This means that they are capable of stretching to several times their length under tension and, when released, rapidly return to their original size and shape.

The protein is usually purified by removal of other biological materials which can be solubilized under conditions in which elastin itself appears to be inert. In the case of the elastin from *ligamentum nuchae,* one is required to autoclave the previously milled and saline-extracted material for successive periods of 1 hr until no further protein appears in the supernatant.[7] This treatment, although harsh, yields a preparation of elastin with an amino acid composition which remains constant upon further treatment in the autoclave. Preparations of elastin from aorta require the use of 0.1 N sodium hydroxide for 45 min at 98°C.[8] It has been suggested that this treatment is required to remove from elastin, a closely associated glycoprotein which is present in aortic tissue but not in *ligamentum nuchae.*[9] Recent studies suggest that this unusual glycoprotein is also present in skin and lung.[10,11] This component may well be the microfibrillar protein described above.

Milder treatments are presently being examined for the purification of elastin. Specifically, Hospelhorn and Fitzpatrick[11], Richmond[12], Ross and Bornstein[3], and others[13,14] have utilized enzymatic procedures coupled with the use of denaturing agents to purify lung elastin. Regardless of the method of preparation, the amino acid composition of purified elastin is unique. As in collagen, one-third of the amino acid residues in elastin are glycine and one-ninth of the residues are proline. In contrast to collagen, elastin contains very little hydroxyproline (approximately one percent), no hydroxylysine, and a preponderance of the nonpolar amino acids alanine, valine, leucine, and isoleucine. There are very few residues of aspartic acid, glutamic acid, lysine, or arginine. As shown in Table 17.1, the amino acid composition of elastin from aorta, *ligamentum nuchae,* and lung are similar to one another but considerably different from calf skin collagen.

Table 17.1. Amino Acid Composition of Elastin From Various Sources[a]

	Collagen	Elastin		
Amino Acid	Calf Skin	Aorta	Ligamentum Nuchae	Lung
Hydroxyproline	85.1	15.3	7.1	14.5
Aspartic Acid	44.9	3.1	7.3	3.2
Threonine	17.8	9.9	10.1	10.1
Serine	37.4	11.71	9.0	13.2
Glutamic Acid	71.6	16.7	17.4	15.6
Proline	135.5	119.2	125.4	109.4
Glycine	326.4	344.6	316.2	337.3
Alanine	111.7	243.3	213.3	242.6
Valine	22.5	98.6	134.0	106.9
Methionine	6.4	0	0	0
Isoleucine	10.9	20.9	26.6	22.8
Leucine	24.6	54.0	64.7	59.3
Tyrosine	3.0	23.2	6.1	29.4
Phenylalanine	13.4	19.1	33.6	20.8
Hydroxylysine	7.3	0	0	0
Lysine	26.5	5.2	3.6	5.0
Histidine	5.1	0.5	0.5	0.5
Arginine	50.1	5.8	6.6	6.8
Isodesmosine	0	0.7	1.1	0.9
Desmosine	0	1.1	1.4	1.2
Lysinonorleucine	0	0.6	0.9	0.4

[a]Residues/1000 Residues.

Electron micrographs of elastic fibers from a variety of sources reveal no ordered structure.[15] There is no recognizable periodicity such as the 640 Å spacing one observes with native collagen fibrils. Because of the insoluble nature of elastin, no information concerning the size or shape of its molecule is available. Wide angle X-ray diffraction data reveal no axial periodicity and, at present, elastin is thought to be a three-dimensional network of polypeptide chains joined by covalent cross-links.[16]

Since it has been suggested by Hoeve and Flory[6] that elastic fibers behave as rubber-like elastomers, certain key cross-links should be present between the various polypeptide chains that make up the elastic fiber. These cross-links, as Baumann[17] points out, impart a necessary restriction on the elastic fiber such that, upon stretching, the individual chains are constrained so that they will not slip past one another. Release of the tension will allow the individual chains to snap back to their original conformation. In the manufacturing of rubber, one introduces the process of vulcanization to create a cross-linking between chains. The cross-links in elastin are unique and the origin of their structure was initially described by Partridge and his collaborators[18] as two unusual amino acids from strong acid hydrolysates of purified elastin. Both were found to be polyfunctional amino acids containing a pyridine nucleus and alkylated in four positions including the ring nitrogen. These two compounds were found to be geometric isomers differing only in position of ring substitution. The structures of these amino acids are shown in Figure 17.1 and have been designated by Thomas et al.[19] as desmosine and isodesmosine, respectively.

Franzblau et al.[20] found, in addition to desmosine and isodesmosine, another unusual compound. Isolation and chemical characterization led to the identification of still another amino acid which was assigned the trivial name of lysinonorleucine. The structure of lysinonorleucine, shown in Figure 17.2, suggests that it, too, probably serves a cross-linking function in elastin.[20]

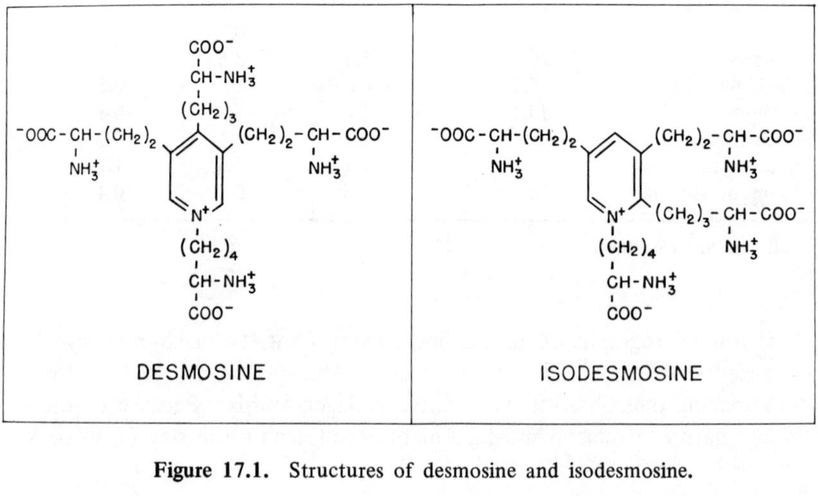

Figure 17.1. Structures of desmosine and isodesmosine.

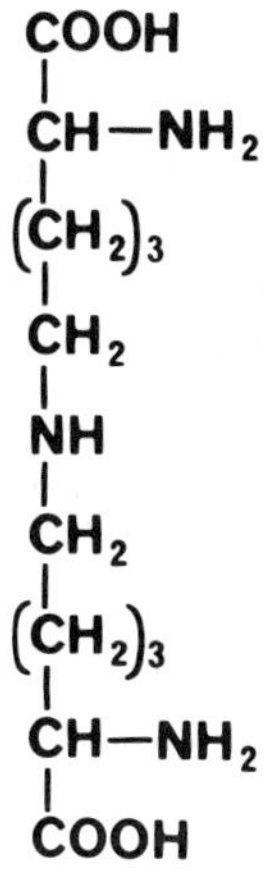

COOH
|
CH—NH₂
|
(CH₂)₃
|
CH₂
|
NH
|
CH₂
|
(CH₂)₃
|
CH—NH₂
|
COOH

Figure 17.2. Structure of lynsinonorleucine.

The discovery of these newly described amino acids provide true chemical markers for elastin, just as hydroxylysine and hydroxyproline are labels for collagen. Studies by Miller et al.[21] on chick embryo aorta, and Partridge et al.[22] on rat aorta, suggested that lysine is the precursor of both desmosine and isodesmosine. That lysine is also the precursor of lysinonorleucine as well as the desmosines was proposed by Franzblau et al.[23] Repeating the studies of Miller et al.[21] on developing chick embryos, it was found that the concentration of lysinonorleucine in aortic elastin increased at the same rate as the desmosines.

Knowing that lysine is the precursor of these unusual amino acids, one may then ask how they may be synthesized or incorporated into the structure of elastic fibers. Recent studies have yielded some insights into the cell or cell type responsible for the biosynthesis of elastin. One group of investigators believes that muscle cells are chiefly responsible and another group implicates the fibroblast.

Recent studies by Ross, Wissler and their collaborators[24,26] and Franzblau and his collaborators[27] have clearly shown that elastin is synthesized by smooth muscle cells grown in tissue culture. The sources of these latter cells is from medial portions of thoracic aortae of several animal species. To our knowledge, no chemical data have been presented which suggests that elastin is synthesized by fibroblasts.

No matter which cell or cell types are responsible for the synthesis of elastic fibers, the first step in the biosynthesis of elastin requires formation of a soluble "pro-elastin," which should be recognizable by its amino acid composition. Compared to mature elastin, "pro-elastin" should contain little or no desmosine, isodesmosine, or lysinonorleucine residues, but relatively more lysine.

Soluble Elastin

A major advance in elastin research came with the isolation of an elastin-like, soluble component from the aortae of copper-deficient swine.[28] Further purification and characterization of this soluble protein have led to the proposal that it is indeed the precursor to insoluble elastin and, accordingly, it has been designated tropoelastin.[28]

Soluble elastin, as well as the mature insoluble elastin, is rich in glycine (33%) and the nonpolar amino acids alanine, valine, and proline. It differs from the insoluble protein in its high content of lysine residues and lack of any cross-links.

Recently, Sandberg et al.[29] have reported on a strong clustering of alanine and lysine residues in the soluble protein, as evidenced by the structures of small tryptic peptides and of the carboxy-terminal fragments of the large tryptic peptides. This clustering of alanine near the lysine residues of the molecule is in agreement with the isolation of alanine-enriched, cross-linked peptides from mature elastin. Through the characterization of large tryptic peptides, Foster et al.[30] have recently been able to sequence over 400 residues which correspond to approximately half of the residues present in the tropoelastin molecule.

To date, the sequences obtained reveal a tropoelastin primary structure quite distinct from that of tropocollagen. Tropoelastin possesses repeat units of a tetrapeptide, Gly-Gly-Val-Pro, a pentapeptide, Pro-Gly-Val-Gly-Val and a hexapeptide, Pro-Gly-Val-Gly-Val-Ala. In addition, alanine residues are close to the lysyl residues of elastin. Several of the peptides contain a partial substitution of hydroxyproline for proline, especially in the sequences Gly-Leu-Pro-Gly and Gly-Ile-Pro-Gly. Since the sequences of these peptides resemble those of other tropoelastin peptides and also lack glycine in every third position (contrary to collagen), we feel that this is definitive evidence for the existence of hydroxyproline in elastin. The combined data of the sequences from the soluble elastin have led to a model of elastin which resembles a huge extension of coiled springs with the desmosines located in alanine-rich areas.[31]

Recently, we have isolated tropoelastin from lung tissue. Because of the mild procedures utilized in the isolation,[32] the data obtained provide a direct comparison of different tissue tropoelastins. We were particularly interested in exploring the possibility that elastin may exhibit tissue differences analogous to the existence of various types of collagen. However, as can be seen from the amino acid analyses of the aortic and lung tropoelastins (see Table 17.2), the two tissue elastins appear very similar if not identical in amino acid composition, molecular weight and immunoreactivity. Immunodiffusion of the purified tropoelastins is given in

Table 17.2. Amino Acid Compositions of Lung and Aortic Elastins[a]

| | Chick | | | |
| | Tropoelastin | | Insoluble Elastin[b] | |
Amino Acid	Lung	Aorta	Lung	Aorta
Lys	46	39	15	13
His	3	—	3	—
Arg	8	8	3	6
Hyp	10	10	22	18
Asp	7	4	13	3
Thr	13	11	11	8
Ser	11	7	8	5
Glu	16	14	23	13
Pro	125	124	115	141
Gly	310	338	338	340
Ala	177	178	172	168
Val	170	175	142	166
Ile	18	17	25	21
Leu	55	54	67	54
Tyr	11	12	10	13
Phe	19	20	26	21

[a]Residues per 1000.
[b]Isolated from lathyritic tissue by the hot alkalai procedure.

Figure 17.3. The double diffusion technique demonstrates that the lung tropoelastin is antigenic toward the aortic antibody and shows identity to the aortic tropoelastin.

Proelastin

Since the isolation of a soluble form of elastin,[29] it has been generally accepted that this molecular species is the precursor to insoluble elastin. Hence, soluble elastin possessing a molecular weight of approximately 72,000 is referred to as tropoelastin, analogous to the nomenclature first described for the tropocollagen to collagen transition.[29] With the recent discovery of a pro-form of collagen, the finding of a larger molecular weight species of soluble elastin would not be surprising.

Our laboratory has been concerned for the last several years with the isolation of soluble elastin from a variety of animal tissues. It has become apparent to us as well as to others that a major problem in dealing with soluble elastin is the presence of proteolytic enzymes in the various preparations which readily attack tropoelastin. As reported earlier, we have

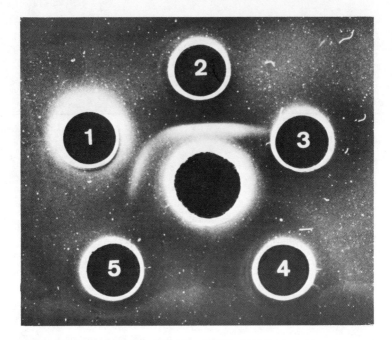

Figure 17.3. Immunodiffusion plate showing reaction of: 1) chick aortic tropoelastin; 2) chick lung tropoelastin; 3) pig tropoelastin; 4) chick skin collagen; 5) whole chick sera.

isolated an enzyme which is closely associated with tropoelastin and is carried along with tropoelastin throughout various purification steps.[33] With this knowledge we have tried to minimize proteolytic degradation of soluble elastin by increasing the concentrations of those inhibitors known to inactivate the enzyme(s) associated with tropoelastin, *i.e.*, N-ethylmaleimide and N-ε-aminocaproic acid. Eight-day-old chicks were raised on a diet supplemented with β-aminopropionitrile (BAPN) and their aortae and lungs extracted as previously described.[32]

The final product from the neutral salt extract was a homogeneous protein of approximately 130,000 daltons as determined by sodium dodecyl sulfate (SDS) polyacrylamide electrophoresis. The amino acid composition of this high-molecular-weight protein together with chick tropoelastin is given in Table 17.3. As can be seen from the analyses, the higher-molecular-weight protein resembles tropoelastin in that it has an elevated glycine, alanine and valine content. More importantly, it differs from tropoelastin by possessing increased amounts of hydroxyl and acidic amino acid and in possessing histidine, cystine and methionine residues. It is also of interest that the higher-molecular-weight protein contains more hydroxyproline than tropoelastin.

Table 17.3. Amino Acid Compositions of Soluble Elastins[a]

Amino Acid	Tropoelastin	Proelastin	C-Terminal Extension
Lysine	39	48	52
Histidine	—	16	32
Arginine	8	26	40
Hydroxyproline	10	28	52
Aspartic	4	40	68
Threonine	11	28	43
Serine	7	40	74
Glutamic	14	57	100
Proline	124	88	65
Glycine	338	250	158
Alanine	178	137	101
½ Cysteine	—	4	8
Valine	175	116	64
Methionine	—	4	7
Isoleucine	17	3	29
Leucine	54	59	64
Tyrosine	12	19	25
Phenylalanine	29	27	34

[a]Residues/1000 residues.

The high-molecular-weight protein was tested for immunoreactivity against antisera developed against chick tropoelastin.[34] Double diffusion revealed that the protein was antigenic and displayed identity to tropoelastin. Immunoelectrophoresis[35] of the high-molecular protein revealed a single precipitin electrophoretic arc positioned differently from the precipitin arc resulting from tropoelastin. When both tropoelastin and the high-molecular-weight protein were run together (see Figure 17.4), the

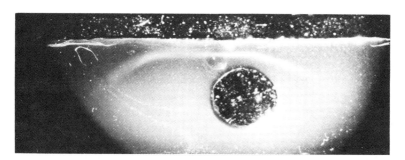

Figure 17.4. Immunoelectrophoretic pattern of a mixture of tropoelastin and proelastin.

pattern revealed two components electrophoretically distinct yet immuno-chemically related or identical with arcs joining in a continuous reaction. As a control, chick tropoelastin was incubated in phosphate buffer to insure activation of a closely associated enzyme.[33] This degraded sample (evidenced by SDS-polyacrylamide electrophoresis) was also examined by immunoelectrophoresis. There was no precipitin arc in the position of the high-molecular-weight protein nor was there any evidence, that more than one antigenic component was present.

One of the first clues to the identification of the high-molecular-weight protein as a pro-form of elastin was the finding that the high-molecular-weight species does break down to fragments including tropo-elastin and its characteristic degradation products[33] and also a more acidic component (see Figure 17.5). This observation points to the fact that proelastin as well as tropoelastin contains a closely associated enzyme which is carried along during the isolation procedures. We do not know as yet if the same enzyme(s) or enzyme system is responsible for cleavage of both forms of soluble elastin.

Ion exchange chromatography of a partially degraded DEAE-cellulose sample of proelastin has resulted in the isolation of an acidic component possessing a molecular weight of 65,000. The amino acid composition of this protein is included in Table 17.3. The acidic protein was found in approximately equimolar amounts to the tropoelastin and its degrada-tion products.

Automated sequence analysis of the high-molecular-weight soluble elastin revealed that the prominent N-terminal sequence was identical to that reported for tropoelastin.[32] These data suggest that the 65,000-MW acidic component is attached onto the C-terminus of the tropoelastin molecule. These data have prompted us to develop a model for elastin fibrogenesis based on the higher-molecular-weight soluble material (pro-elastin) being the primary precursor to insoluble elastin. This model is illustrated schematically in Figure 17.6. The model allows for the initial assembly and alignment of proelastin molecules via disulfide bonds either between individual molecules or on a specific template in the extra-cellular matrix such as the microfibril. This association via disulfide bond would serve to "fix" the precursor molecules thereby presenting an insoluble substrate to the enzyme lysyl oxidase for lysine-derived cross-link formation. The next step in elastin maturation may be the cleavage of the nonpolar portion of the proelastin molecule by an enzyme(s) analogous to procollagen peptidases. It is also possible that this cleavage is not significant *in vivo* and may represent a con-trol mechanism for degrading proelastin molecules which do not become cross-linked. This would be the case in situations where the enzyme lysyl oxidase is inhibited.

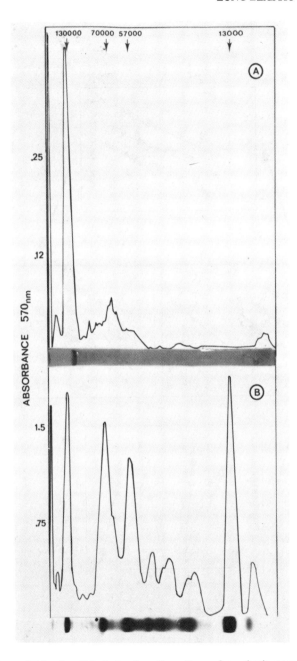

Figure 17.5: A. Gel electrophoretic pattern of proelastin together with a densitometer tracing. B. Gel electrophoretic pattern of proelastin after storage.

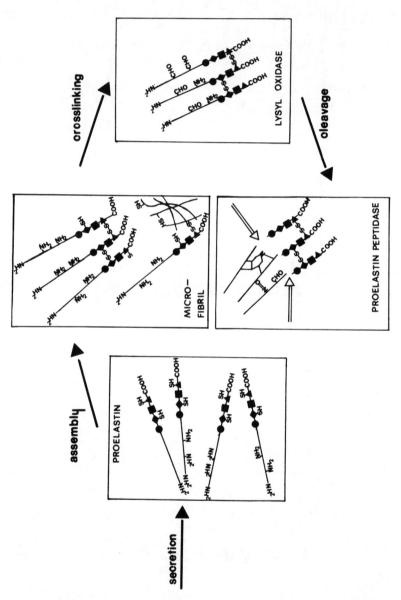

Figure 17.6 Model for elastin fibrogenesis.

REFERENCES

1. Loeven, W. A. "Elastolytic Enzymes and Lung Elastic Tissue," In: *Pulmonary Emphysema and Proteolysis,* C. Mittman, Ed. (New York: Academic Press, 1972), pp. 275-280.

2. Janoff, A. "Elastase-Like Proteases of Human Granulocytes and Alveolar Macrophages," In: *Pulmonary Emphysema and Proteolysis,* C. Mittman, Ed. (New York: Academic Press, 1972), pp. 205-224.

3. Ross, R. and P. Bornstein. "The Elastic Fiber. I. The Separating and Partial Characterization of Its Macromolecular Components," *J. Cell Biol.* 40:366-381 (1969).

4. Ross, R. and S. Klebanoff. "The Smooth Muscle Cell. I. *In Vivo* Synthesis of Connective Tissue Proteins," *J. Cell Biol.* 50:159-171 (1971).

5. Serafini-Fracassini, A., J. M. Field and C. Armitt. "Characterization of the Microfibrillar Component of Bovine *Ligamentum Nuchae,*" *Biochem. Biophys. Res. Commun.* 65:1146-1152 (1975).

6. Hoeve, C. A. and P. J. Flory. "The Elastic Properties of Elastin," *Biopolymers,* 13:677-686 (1974).

7. Partridge, S. M., H. F. Davis and G. S. Adair. "The Chemistry of Connective Tissues. 2. Soluble Proteins Derived from Partial Hydrolysis of Elastin," *Biochem. J.* 61:11-21 (1955).

8. Lansing, A. I., T. B. Rosenthal, M. Alex and E. W. Dempsey. "The Structure and Chemical Characterization of Elastic Fibers as Revealed by Elastase and by Electron Microscopy," *Anat. Rec.* 114:555-575 (1952).

9. Gotte, L., V. Meneghelli and A. Castellani. "Electron Microscope Observations and Chemical Analyses of Human Elastin," In: *Structure and Function of Connective and Skeletal Tissues,* S. Fitton Jackson, R. D. Harkness, S. M. Partirdge and G. R. Tristram, Eds. (London: Butterworth, 1965), pp. 93-100.

10. Varadi, D. P. and D. A. Hall. "Cutaneous Elastin in Ehlers-Danlos Syndrome," *Nature* (London) 208:1224-1225 (1965).

11. Hospelhorn, V. D. and M. J. Fitzpatrick. "The Isolation of Elastic Tissue from Lung," *Biochem. Biophys. Res. Commun.* 6:191-195 (1961).

12. Richmond, V. "Lung Parenchymal Elastin Isolated by Non-Degradative Means," *Biochem. Biophys. Acta,* 351:173-177 (1974).

13. Miller, E. J. and H. M. Fullmer. "Elastin: Diminished Reactivity with Aldehyde Reagents in Copper Deficiency and Lathyrism," *J. Exp. Med.* 123:1097-1106 (1966).

14. Gallop, P. M. and M. A. Paz (Unpublished observations).

15. Grant, R. A. "Preparation of Elastin-Like Material from Collagen by Cross-Linking Followed by Heat Treatment," *Biochem. J.* 97:5c-7c (1965).

16. Franzblau, C. "Elastin," *Comp. Biochem.* 26C:659-712 (1971).

17. Baumann, P. "The Present State of Our Knowledge in the Field of Elastomeres," *Chem. and Indust.* 48:1498-1504 (1959).

18. Partridge, S. M., D. F. Elsden and J. Thomas. "Constitution of the Cross-Linkages in Elastin," *Nature* (London) 197:1297-1298 (1963).

19. Thomas, J. D. F. Elsden and S. M. Partridge. "Degradation Products from Elastin," *Nature* (London) 200:651-652 (1963).
20. Franzblau, C., B. Faris and R. Papaioannou. "Lysinonorleucine. A New Amino Acid from Hydrolysates of Elastin," *Biochemistry* 8: 2833-2837 (1969).
21. Miller, E. J., G. R. Martin and K. A. Piez. "The Utilization of Lysine in the Biosynthesis of Elastin Cross-Links," *Biochem. Biophys. Res. Commun.* 17:248-253 (1964).
22. Partridge, S. M., D. F. Elsden, J. Thomas, A. Dorfman, A. Telser, and P. L. Ho. "Incorporation of Labelled Lysine into the Desmosine Cross-Bridges in Elastin," *Nature* (London) 209:399-400 (1966).
23. Franzblau, C., F. M. Sinex, B. Faris and R. Lampidis. "Identification of a New Crosslinking Amino Acid in Elastin," *Biochem. Biophys. Res. Commun.* 21:575-581 (1965).
24. Ross, R. and J. A. Glomset. "Atherosclerosis and the Arterial Smooth Muscle Cell. Proliferation of Smooth Muscle is a Key Event in the Genesis of the Lesions of Atherosclerosis," *Science* 180:1332-1339 (1973).
25. Fisher-Dzoga, K., R. Chen and R. W. Wissler. "Effects of Serum Lipoproteins on the Morphology, Growth and Metabolism of Arterial Smooth Muscle Cells," In: *Arterial Mesenchyme and Atherosclerosis,* W. D. Wagner and T. B. Clarkson, Eds. *Adv. In Exp. Med. and Biol.* 43:299-311 (1974).
26. Ross, R. "The Smooth Muscle Cell. II. Growth of Smooth Muscle in Culture and Formation of Elastic Fibers," *J. Cell Biol.* 50:172-186 (1971).
27. Faris, B., L. L. Salcedo, V. Cook, L. Johnson, J. A. Foster and C. Franzblau. "The Synthesis of Connective Tissue Protein in Smooth Muscle Cells," *Biochim. Biophys. Acta* 418:93-103 (1976).
28. Sandberg, L. B., N. Weissman and D. W. Smith. "The Purification and Partial Characterization of a Soluble Elastin-Like Protein from Copper-Deficient Porcine Aorta," *Biochemistry* 8:2940-2945 (1969).
29. Sandberg, L. B., N. Weissman and W. R. Gray. "Structural Features of Tropoelastin Related to the Sites of Crosslinks in Aortic Elastin," *Biochemistry* 10:52-56 (1971).
30. Foster, J. A., E. Bruenger, W. R. Gray and L. B. Sandberg. "Isolation and Amino Acid Sequences of Tropoelastin Peptides," *J. Biol. Chem.* 248:2876-2879 (1973).
31. Gray, W. R., L. B. Sandberg and J. A. Foster. "Molecular Model for Elastin Structure and Function," *Nature* (London) 246:461-466 (1973).
32. Foster, J. A., R. Shapiro, P. Voynow, B. Faris, G. Crombie and C. Franzblau. "Isolation of Soluble Elastin from Lathyritic Chicks. Comparison to Tropoelastin from Copper-Deficient Pigs," *Biochem.* 14:5343-5346 (1975).
33. Mecham, R., J. A. Foster and C. Franzblau. "Intrinsic Enzyme Activity Associated with Tropoelastin," *Biochim. Biophys. Acta* (1976) in press.
34. Foster, J. A., D. Knaack, B. Faris, R. Moscaritolo, L. Salcedo, M. Skinner and C. Franzblau. "Development of a Specific Immunological

Assay for Tropoelastin and Its Application to Tissue Culture Studies,"
Biochim. Biophys. Acta (1976) in press.

35. Foster, J. A., R. Mecham and C. Franzblau. "Isolation of a High
Molecular Weight Species of Soluble Elastin," *Biochem. Biophys.
Res. Commun.* (1976) in press.

CHAPTER 18

BIOCHEMICAL MECHANISMS OF INTERACTION OF ENVIRONMENTAL METAL CONTAMINANTS WITH LUNG CONNECTIVE TISSUE

M. Zamirul Hussain, Rajendra S. Bhatnagar

Laboratory of Connective Tissue Biochemistry
School of Dentistry 630 Sciences
University of California, San Francisco
San Francisco, California 94143

and S. D. Lee

U.S. Environmental Protection Agency
Health Effects Research Laboratory
Cincinnati, Ohio 45268

INTRODUCTION

Heavy metals are becoming increasingly significant as a potential hazard in the environment, and the ions of these metals are implicated in causing a wide variety of biological effects. For example, Cd^{2+} decreases glucose metabolism[1] and adversely affects the respiration of pulmonary macrophages by uncoupling oxidative phosphorylation and inhibiting mitochondrial oxygen uptake.[2] Also Cd^{2+} and Hg^{2+} interact with a large number of enzymes through —SH groups[3,4] and destabilize lysosomal membranes, resulting in the release of lysosomal hydrolases.[5] They also have been shown to impair ion transport through membranes.[6] Pd^{2+} also binds to protein —SH groups[7] and is thereby expected to interfere with biological systems. Recent studies in our laboratory have shown that Cd^{2+}, Hg^{2+} and Pd^{2+} ions inhibit prolyl hydroxylase, a critical enzyme in the synthesis of collagen.[8] These effects directly contribute to biochemical injury in the lung, which presumably evokes a repair response culminating in fibrosis. Chronic exposures of cadmium compounds[9,10] and mercury vapors[11,12] have been reported to cause fibrotic lesions in the lung *in vivo*.

Biochemical study of pulmonary injury-repair process has been difficult. This difficulty arises from the large number of heterogeneous lung cell types, their interactions and the constant presumed effects exerted by blood-borne agents. Use of lung organ culture avoids some of these complexities and provides a convenient system to study lung cellular mechanisms involved in adaptive response to tissue environmental changes. We have utilized lung organ cultures from neonatal rats to investigate the effects of Cd^{2+}, Hg^{2+} and Pd^{2+} on lung collagen synthesis and have compared the effects of these metals with the effects of hydralazine, a drug known to induce pulmonary fibrosis *in vivo*.

MATERIALS AND METHODS

Lung Organ Cultures

The lungs were removed from newborn rats (timed-bred, Long Evans from Simonsen Laboratories, Gilroy, California) and washed in a medium consisting of Dulbecco's Vogt MEM with Earle Salts Solution (Grand Island Biological Co., Sunnyvale, California), 90 μg/ml ascorbate, 2 mM glutamine, 50 μg/ml each of streptomycin and penicillin under sterile conditions. They were split lengthwise into 2.0-mm strips (devoid of major airways and vasculatures) and placed on Millipore filter discs (SSWP 3μ) floated over 1 ml of the medium supplemented with 10% fetal calf serum in a disposable, 35 x 10-mm plastic organ culture dish (Falcon plastics, Oxnard, California). Each culture contained two lung sections. The surrounding chamber of the dish was saturated with sterilized distilled water. The dishes were placed in a gas-tight Lucite chamber (38 x 16 x 8 cm) lined with water-saturated filter paper. The chamber was then placed inside a tissue culture incubator maintained at 37°C and high humidity. A constant flow (0.3 ml/min) of a filtered humidified gas mixture containing 5% CO_2 in air was passed through the chamber. This allowed the lung cultures to grow at the gas-liquid interface in a humid atmosphere. The medium was changed every other day.

Analysis of Collagen Synthesis

At the appropriate times, the cultures were pulse-labeled with 5 μC of ^{14}C-proline (uniformly labeled ^{14}C-proline, 254 mC/m mol, from New England Nuclear) for 3 hr. The incorporation was stopped by harvesting the cultures in chilled hypotonic buffer (0.01 M Tris-HCl, pH 7.5 and 0.9% NaCl). The incorporation of ^{14}C-proline into the collagen sequence was examined using a highly purified protease-free preparation of clostridial collagenase (Advance Biofactures Corp., Lynbrook, New York). The tissues were excised into small pieces and dialyzed at first against water to remove unbound radioactivity and then against collagenase buffer (0.1 M Tris-HCl, pH 7.5, 0.1 mM CaCl$_2$) for 20 hr at 4°C. They were homogenized (10 strokes in a glass homogenizer) in 1-2 ml of the same buffer and placed in a dialysis bag with the appropriate amount of collagenase.

The collagenase treatment was performed according to a previously described method.[13] The dialyzed peptides were further analyzed for ^{14}C-hydroxyproline. Samples were concentrated to a small volume (2-4 ml) and hydrolyzed with 6 N HCl for 20 hr at 120°C, and ^{14}C-hydroxyproline was determined according to the method of Juva and Prockop.[14] Total amino acid content was measured by ninhydrin using leucine as standard.[15] Total ninhydrin material in the hydrolysate was taken as an index of protein content. The radioactive incorporation has been related to the total protein content and is expressed as specific activity (DPM/ μmol leucine equivalent).

RESULTS AND DISCUSSION

We have examined the effect of two known fibrogenic metals, Cd^{2+} and Hg^{2+}, and the fibrogenic drug hydralazine on collagen synthesis. We have also examined the effect of Pd^{2+}, a component of catalytic convertor devices used in automobiles, on collagen synthesis in lung organ cultures. The synthesis of collagen was determined by measuring the incorporation of ^{14}C-proline into collagenase-susceptible polypeptides. This is a highly specific assay for collagen polypeptide synthesis. For reasons to be discussed below, hydroxyproline synthesis, the usual criterion for collagen synthesis, was not a good index in these studies.

Neonatal rat lungs in our organ culture system exhibited a constant rate of "growth" for over 6 days. Specific activity of proteins by the incorporation of radioactive proline was used as the index of growth. The total protein content of the lung cultures also increased during the period. Collagen synthesis proceeded at a constant rate during the 5-6 day growth period, and therefore in all experiments the effects of various agents on the lung cultures were followed over a period of 5 days. The three metals as well as hydralazine stimulated the incorporation of ^{14}C-proline into collage-related polypeptides. ^{14}C-hydroxyproline synthesis was also stimulated, but the increase in hydroxyproline did not parallel the increase in ^{14}C-proline incorporation into collagenase-susceptible polypeptides. This discrepancy is explained by our previous observations that Cd^{2+}, Hg^{2+}, Pd^{2+} and hydralazine are all potent inhibitors of prolyl hydroxylase.[13,16-19]

As seen in Figure 18.1A, 24 hr after the initial exposure to 0.1 μM Cd^{2+} incorporation of ^{14}C-proline into collagen sequence was comparable to the control. A significant increase in collagen synthesis at this concentration of Cd^{2+} was not apparent until 120 hr after the initial exposure. However, after 120 hr the cultures incorporated 30% more radioactivity into collagen. Cd^{2+} in concentrations of 1.0 and 10.0 μM caused an initial decline in the synthesis of collagenous polypeptides, followed by a 30-40% stimulation after 72 hr exposure and over 50% stimulation after 120 hr exposure. Similar increases were observed in the synthesis of ^{14}C-hydroxyproline (Figure 18.1B). Maximal ^{14}C-hydroxyproline synthesis was obtained after 72 hr of exposure to 10 μM Cd^{2+}.

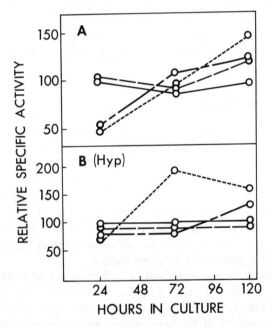

Figure 18.1 Incorporation of ^{14}C-proline and synthesis of ^{14}C-hydroxyproline into collagenase-susceptible protein in the presence of Cd^{2+}. Lung cultures were grown in the presence of various concentrations of $CdCl_2$ as shown below. At each indicated time, cultures were incubated for 3 hr with 5 μC of ^{14}C-proline, and dialyzed homogenates of the labeled tissues were analyzed for (A) ^{14}C-proline incorporation and (B) ^{14}C-hydroxyproline synthesized as described in the Methods Section.

———— Control medium; – – – 0.1 μM;
– – – – 1.0 μM; and · · · · · 10 μM $CdCl_2$.

Exposure of the cultures to Hg^{2+} resulted in similar patterns of stimulation of ^{14}C-proline incorporation into collagenase-susceptible material and ^{14}C-hydroxyproline synthesis (Figures 18.2A and 18.2B). After an initial decline in the incorporation and hydroxyproline synthesis, maximal stimulation was observed at 72 hr after 24 hr of exposure. This was followed by a decreased incorporation as well as decreased hydroxyproline synthesis.

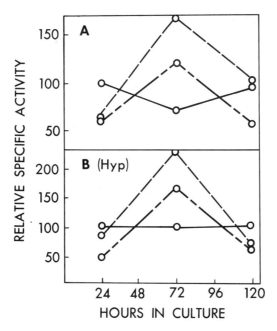

Figure 18.2 Incorporation of ^{14}C-proline and synthesis of ^{14}C-hydroxyproline into collagenase-susceptible protein in the presence of Hg^{2+}. Lung cultures were grown in the medium containing various concentrations of $HgCl_2$ as indicated below. The rest of the procedure was the same as described in Figure 18.1.

———— Control medium; – – – – 0.1 μM and – - – - 1.0 μM $HgCl_2$

A somewhat different temporal pattern of stimulation of ^{14}C-proline incorporation was observed in the presence of Pd^{2+} (Figure 18.3A). The maximal incorporation of proline into collagenase-susceptible polypeptides was observed after 24-hr exposure to 0.1-10.0 μM Pd^{2+}. Incorporation was reduced after 72-hr exposure and was somewhat lower than control levels after 120 hr. Synthesis of ^{14}C-hydroxyproline followed the same pattern (Figure 18.3B).

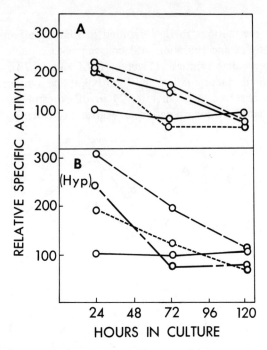

Figure 18.3 Incorporation of ^{14}C-proline and synthesis of ^{14}C-hydroxyproline into collagenase-susceptible protein in the presence of Pd^{2+}. Lung cultures were grown in the medium containing various concentrations of PdCl$_2$ as indicated below. The rest of the procedure was the same as described in Figure 18.1.

——— Control medium; – – – – 0.1 μM;
– - – - – 1.0 μM; and - - - - 10 μM PdCl$_2$

Data presented above suggested that metal toxins known to induce fibrosis *in vivo* stimulated the synthesis of collagen in lung organ cultures. Other fibrogenic agents were examined to see if they would have similar effects on these cultures. Hydralazine (1-hydrazine phthalazine), a hypertensive drug, is known to cause pulmonary fibrosis.[20-22] When lung organ cultures were exposed to hydralazine (10.0-100 μM), increased collagen synthesis was observed (Figure 18.4). The stimulation was dependent both on the concentration and the length of exposure. Thus, at 10.0 and 100 μM hydralazine, maximal ^{14}C-proline incorporation was seen after a 72-hr exposure (Figure 18.4A). The maximal stimulation by hydralazine was greater at the higher concentration. As in the case of the metal toxins, incorporation of ^{14}C-proline declined after the maximal rate had been attained. Synthesis of ^{14}C-hydroxyproline was maximal at 48 hr in the case of 10 μM hydralazine and at 72 hr in the presence of 100 μM hydralazine. The increases in ^{14}C-hydroxyproline synthesis

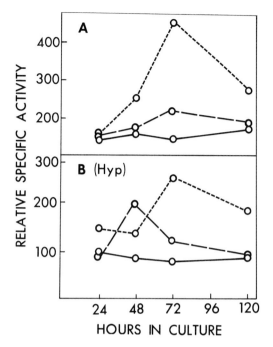

Figure 18.4 Incorporation of ^{14}C-proline and synthesis of ^{14}C-hydroxyproline into collagenase-susceptible protein in the presence of hydralazine. Lung cultures were grown in the presence of different concentrations of hydralazine as shown below. Cultures were pulse-labeled and processed as described in Figure 18.1.

——— Control medium; – – – – 10 μM and - - - - - 100 μM hydralizine.

did not parallel the increase in incorporation of ^{14}C-proline into the collagen sequence.

Studies on the regulation of collagen synthesis, in our laboratory, have shown that hydralazine, Cd^{2+}, Hg^{2+} and Pd^{2+} inhibit the reaction of purified prolyl hydroxylase.[16-19] As seen in Table 18.1, the Ki_{app}s for these agents are very similar in magnitude. A common feature of these inhibitory processes involves Fe^{2+}, the prosthetic metal of prolyl hydroxylase. Hydralazine is an excellent chelating agent and competes with the enzyme for Fe^{2+} and also binds to enzyme-bound Fe^{2+}.[16] Pd^{2+}, Hg^{2+} and Cd^{2+} also compete for the Fe^{2+} binding site.[13,17,18] The similarity in the *in vivo* and *in vitro* effects of hydralazine, Cd^{2+}, Hg^{2+} and Pd^{2+} suggests that these unrelated agents may elicit a fibrogenic response through some common mechanism, for instance by causing a transient inhibition of prolyl hydroxylase. This transitory inhibition of collagen synthesis and secretion may interfere with regulatory processes controlling tissue growth and elicit connective tissue proliferation.

Table 18.1   Some Fibrogenic Agents and Their Ki_{app} for Prolyl Hydroxylase[a]

Hydralazine	0.03 mM
Hg^{2+}	0.025 mM
Cd^{2+}	0.01 mM
Pd^{2+}	0.02 mM

[a]Values have been taken from References 13 and 16-18.

As far as we are aware, this is the first report suggesting that organ cultures of lungs may mimic some of the pulmonary disease processes when exposed to etiologic agents. Our organ culture system provides a promising tool for studying environmental interactions. Among its practical applications, one may envisage its use as a screening procedure for examining pulmonary toxicity of any agent that can be presented to the cultures in solution or in the gaseous phase. Our studies suggest that the primary response to an airborne toxin may be elicited directly in pulmonary tissues and that this response may in itself be sufficient to precipitate a fibrotic reaction. Any systemic involvement such as immunological phenomena and other reactions mediated or carried by the circulatory system may in effect exacerbate the initial response of lungs, the primary target of environmental injury stimulus.

Although Hg, Cd and hydralazine are recognized fibrogenic agents, little is known about the toxicity of Pd. The use of Pd in catalytic converter devices in the exhaust systems of many new automobiles is likely to introduce significant amounts of this metal in various forms into the environment. Previous studies in our laboratory have shown the potent effects of this metal on connective tissues.[13] Data presented here suggest that inhalation of Pd^{2+} may lead to pulmonary fibrosis and suggest caution in the use of this metal.

ACKNOWLEDGMENTS

The expert technical support of Ms. Maximita Tolentino and the secretarial assistance of Ms. Sandra Hodess are greatly appreciated. This study was supported by EPA Research Contract #68-03-2005 and NIH Grants DE-03861 and HL-19668.

REFERENCES

1.   Ithakissios, D. S., T. Ghafgazi, J. H. Mennear and W. V. Kessler. "Effect of Multiple Doses of Cadmium on Glucose Metabolism and Insulin Secretion in the Rat," *Toxicol. Appl. Pharmacol.* 31:143 (1975).

2. Mustafa, M. G. and C. E. Cross. "Pulmonary Alveolar Macrophage: Oxidative Metabolism of Isolated Cells and Mitochondria and Effects of Cadmium Ion on Electron and Energy Transfer Reactions," *Biochem.* 10:4176 (1971).
3. Brenner, I. "Heavy Metal Toxicities," *Quar. Rev. Biophys.* 7:75 (1974).
4. Hughes, W. L., Jr. "Protein Mercaptides," Cold Spring Harbor *Symp. Quant. Biol.* 14:79 (1950).
5. Taylor, N. S. "Histochemical Studies of Nephrotoxicity with Sublethal Doses of Mercury in Rats," *Amer. J. Pathol.* 46:1 (1965).
6. Fleisher, L. N., T. Yorio and P. J. Bentley. "Effect of Cadmium on Epithelial Membrane," *Toxicol. Appl. Pharmacol.* 33:384 (1975).
7. Akerfeldt, S. and G. Lovgren. "Spectrophotometric Determination of Disulfides, Sulfinic Acids, Thiol Ethers and Thiols with the Palladium (11) Ion," *Anal. Biochem.* 8:223 (1964).
8. Bornstein, P. "The Biosynthesis of Collagen," *Ann. Rev. Biochem.* 43:567 (1974).
9. Hayes, J. A., G. L. Snider and K. C. Palmer. "The Evolution of Biochemical Damage in the Rat Lung after Acute Cadmium Exposure," *Amer. Rev. Resp. Dis.* 113:121 (1976).
10. Carrington, C. B. "Organizing Interstitial Pneumonia: Definition of the Lesion and Attempts to Devise an Experimental Model," *Yale J. Biol. Med.* 40:352 (1968).
11. Trakhtenberg, I. M. "Chronic Effects of Mercury on Organisms," DHEW Publication #NIH 74-473 (1974).
12. Tennant, R., H. J. Johnson and J. B. Wells. "Acute Bilateral Pneumonitis Associated with the Inhalation of Mercury Vapor," *Conn. Med.* 25:106 (1961).
13. Rapaka, R. S., K. R. Sorensen, S. D. Lee and R. S. Bhatnagar. "Inhibition of Hydroxyproline Synthesis by Palladium Ions," *Biochim. Biophys. Acta* 429:63 (1976).
14. Juva, K. and D. J. Prockop. "Modified Procedure for the Assay of ^{3}H- or ^{14}C-Labeled Hydroxyproline," *Anal. Biochem.* 15:77 (1966).
15. Rosen, H. "A Modified Ninhydrin Colorimetric Analysis for Amino Acid," *Arch. Biochem. Biophys.* 67:10 (1957).
16. Bhatnagar, R. S., R. S. Rapaka, T. Z. Liu and S. M. Wolf. "Hydralazine-Induced Disturbances in Collagen Biosynthesis," *Biochim. Biophys. Acta* 271:125 (1972).
17. Rapaka, R. S., A. M. Vare and R. S. Bhatnagar. "Biochemical Mechanism of Cleft Palate Induction by Cadmium," *J. Dent. Res.* 53:91 (1974).
18. Kagawa, K. and R. S. Bhatnagar. "Mechanism of Mercury Toxicity: Inhibition of Prolyl Hydroxylase by Mercuric Ions," *J. Dent. Res.* 55:240B (1976).
19. Bhatnagar, R. S., T. Z. Liu, R. S. Rapaka, M. Z. Hussain, K. Kagawa, K. R. Sorensen and F. von Dohlen. "Allosteric Properties of Prolyl Hydroxylase," 10th International Congress of Biochemistry (Hamburg) (1976), p. 370.
20. Perry, H. M. and H. A. Schroeder. "Syndrome Stimulating Collagen Disease Caused by Hydralazine," *J. Amer. Med. Assoc.* 154:670 (1954).

21. Reinhardt, D. J. and J. M. Waldron. "Lupus Erythematosus-Like Syndrome Complicating Hydralazine Therapy," *J. Amer. Med. Assoc.* 155:1492 (1954).

22. Dustan, H. P., D. Taylor and A. C. Corcoran. "Rheumatic and Febrile Syndrome During Prolonged Hydralazine Treatment," *J. Amer. Med. Assoc.* 154:23 (1954).

CHAPTER 19

LEAD, ZINC AND δ-AMINOLEVULINATE DEHYDRATASE

V.N. Finelli
> Kettering Laboratory
> Department of Environmental Health
> College of Medicine
> University of Cincinnati
> 3223 Eden Avenue
> Cincinnati, Ohio 45267

For several years the hematological effects of lead have been principal targets of many investigators due to the facts that a) hematological disturbances are important aspects of saturnism and b) the specificity and sensitivity by which lead inhibits certain enzymes involved in the pathway of heme synthesis yielded valuable tools in the diagnostic procedures for lead exposure. Lead at very low concentrations inhibits δ-aminolevulinic acid dehydratase (ALA-D) which catalyzes the formation of porphobilinogen (PBG), a precursor of heme. At least one more enzyme of the heme synthesis pathway is inhibited by lead, that is ferrochelatase (heme synthetase) which catalyzes the insertion of iron in protoporphyrin IX to form heme (Figure 19.1). Due to the lead inhibition of these enzymes, heme precursors are elevated in body fluids (urine and blood) of lead exposed individuals.

There are many indices utilized for the assessment of lead absorption, such as ALA-D, blood lead, urinary lead with and without administration of chelators, urinary δ-aminolevulinic acid (ALA) and porphyrins, free erythrocyte porphyrins (FEP), and zinc protoporphyrin (ZPP). Among these, erythrocyte ALA-D activity is the method of choice for assessing low levels of exposure since its inhibition by lead is highly specific and sensitive.

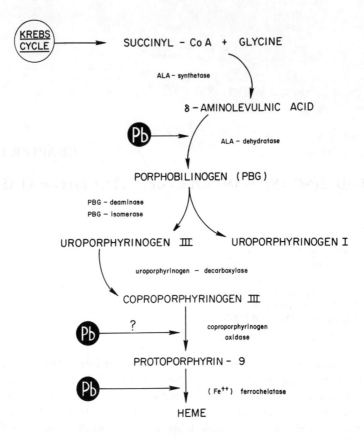

Figure 19.1. Interference of lead on heme synthesis.

The biological significance of ALA-D inhibition by lead is still uncertain. ALA-D is not a rate limiting enzyme in the synthesis of heme. Therefore, extensive inhibition of this enzyme does not affect the synthesis of hemoglobin and it can be tolerated by the exposed organisms. We have not observed anemia in rats or humans when as much as 80% of red blood cell ALA-D activity was inhibited by lead. However, when the extent of ALA-D inhibition is such as to produce great elevation of ALA in tissues and body fluids it is evident that porphyrinogenesis has been impaired and, furthermore, abnormal concentration of ALA in tissues may possess a toxicity of its own.

Until recently there have been numerous contrasting reports on the metal requirement of ALA-D. In the last few years zinc has been shown both *in vitro*[1-6] and *in vivo*[4,6,7] to be the metal required for the activity of ALA-D. In our laboratory we have also shown *in vivo* and *in vitro* the antagonistic effect of zinc on ALA-D inhibition by lead.[6] Other investigators have since confirmed our findings.[8,9]

Zielhuis[10] in a recent article has reviewed literature data and discussed the relationship between blood lead levels and various effects on hematological and biochemical parameters. He, like Pietrovski,[11] subdivides the total body burden of lead into 3 separate pools, essentially: a) rapid exchange lead in blood and soft tissue, b) intermediate exchange lead in skin and muscles and c) intermediate and slow exchange lead in bone marrow and dense bones, respectively. The idea of various pools of lead is widely accepted and is substantiated by a large volume of data generated in animal and human experiments. However, one could hypothesize the existence of numerous small pools since there may be a variety of Pb-binding sites in organs and tissues of the body. The rates of exchange between these pools depend on the stability of the Pb complexes, the abundance of binding sites, the concentration of competing cations and affinity of these cations for the same binding sites. This concept is also valid in elucidating the interaction of lead and zinc on ALA-D. This enzyme which is activated by Zn^{++} and inhibited by Pb^{++} is rich in sulfhydryl groups, there being 56 SH groups per molecule. A great portion of blood lead must be strongly bound to this enzyme since it takes minute concentrations of lead to substantially inhibit its activity. In our studies, rats with blood lead levels of approximately 50 μg/100 ml showed more than 80% ALA-D inhibition. Addition of $ZnCl_2$ to the lead-inhibited ALA-D preparation fully restored its enzymatic activity. Figure 19.2 shows the activation of ALA-D in the blood of a lead-exposed rat (50 μg Pb/100 ml blood) by the *in vitro* addition of $ZnCl_2$. It seems that Zn^{++} and Pb^{++} compete for the same binding sites; therefore the amount of erythrocyte lead bound to ALA-D may depend not only on the blood lead level, but also on the concentration and availability of Zn^{++} in the red blood cell. The reversal of the lead inhibition by addition of Zn^{++} also suggests the involvement of zinc at the active site.[6] It is not surprising that zinc may be involved in the catalytic site of this enzyme, since it is known to be one of the possible catalysts in enzymatic and nonenzymatic dehydration and aldol condensation reactions. A possible mechanism of PBG synthesis involving zinc and $-NH_2$ groups at the active site is reported in Figure 19.3.

Other heavy metals such as Hg^{++}, CH_3Hg^+, Cu^{++} and Cd^{++}, with affinity for -SH group higher than or similar to Pb^{++} show much less ALA-D inhibition. The preferential affinity of Pb^{++} to ALA-D may be due to the steric configuration of the protein molecule at the active site and/or to the presence of other ligands in the system with higher binding capacity

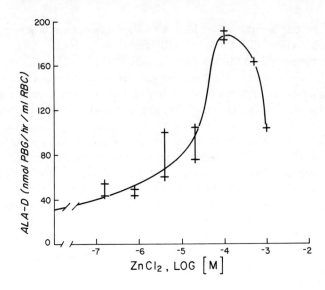

Figure 19.2. Activation of ALA-D by addition of $ZnCl_2$ in blood of Pb-exposed rat with blood lead concentration of 50 μg/100 ml.

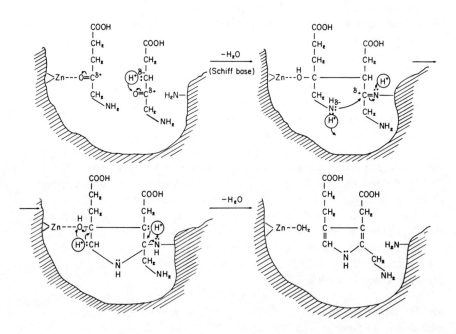

Figure 19.3. Proposed mechanism of ALA-D catalyzed synthesis of PBG involving an amino group and a zinc atom at the enzymatic active site.

for the other metals. Another possibility is that some of the heavy metal ions may also replace zinc at the active site without any appreciable loss of enzymatic activity, *e.g.*, Cd^{++} and Fe^{++} have been reported to enhance the activity of purified ALA-D.[5]

DOSE-EFFECT RELATIONSHIP

The question has arisen whether the blood lead level may be considered a good indicator of biologically effective body burden of lead. The Health Protection Commission of the European Communities (HPCEC) have produced certain guidelines for assessing the problem of lead exposures based both on blood lead levels and on δ-aminolevulinic acid dehydratase activity.[12]

It is our opinion and that of other investigators[13,14] that while blood lead may be a good indicator of lead exposure it may not be correlated to biological effects. Certain criteria for dose-effect relationship, abstracted from available scientific data, have been proposed to and reported by the HPCEC[12] and, for convenience of the reader, it is worthwhile restating them:

- Blood lead levels higher than 80 μg/100 ml may produce effects on the central nervous system in adults.
- Effects on central nervous system in children (hyperactivity and mental retardation) do not appear at blood levels lower than 50-60 μg/100 ml.
- Effects on peripheral nervous system begin to show at blood levels over 40-50 μg/100ml.

The document also states that the above effects are of pathological nature and therefore should not be considered in establishing exposure standards.

The above clinical symptoms may be manifest only in a certain percentage of exposed population. Blood lead levels which can cause disturbances in some individuals may therefore be tolerated by others. The dose-effect relationship may vary significantly from individual to individual due to age, sex, nutritional state and probably many other variables encountered in the exposed population.

Even though a negative correlation between blood lead and ALA-D activity has been observed by many investigators,[15,16] often there is an enormous scattering of ALA-D values especially at higher levels of blood lead. This scattering may sometimes be explained by the nutritional state of the individual with regard to zinc, or by other factors which may also affect erythrocyte ALA-D. In our laboratory we have shown that nutritional levels of zinc affect ALA-D. Table 19.1 shows the effects of dietary zinc and copper on rat erythrocyte ALA-D.[7]

Table 19.1. Effect of Dietary Zinc and Copper on Red Blood Cells
ALA-Dehydratase Activity

Group	Metals in Drinking H_2O (μg/ml)		Enzyme Activity (nmols PBG/hr/ml RBC±S.E.M.)
	Cu	Zn	
1	0	2.5	83.2 ± 15.3
2	2	2.5	119.7 ± 5.8
3	2	20	169.4 ± 4.4
4	2	40	212.4 ± 13.9
5	0	40	213.2 ± 14.6

In this experiment male Sprague-Dawley rats were kept for 30 days under
controlled environmental conditions and fed a semipurified diet low in
copper and zinc. Various levels of these metals were added to the drinking water, as reported in Table 19.1. It is evident from these data that
ALA-D depends on the dietary levels of zinc and is independent of
dietary copper. These effects were also evident in liver ALA-D..
  Alteration of hormonal balance in rats through surgical manipulations,
gonadectomy and/or adrenalectomy, affects ALA-D. It is evident from
the data reported in Table 19.2 that both castration and adrenalectomy
reduced erythrocyte ALA-D. However, in the rats where both operations
were performed ALA-D activity became almost twice the control value.
We do not yet know whether the alteration of ALA-D is a consequence
of the hormonal effects on trace metal metabolism or on erythropoiesis.

Table 19.2. Effects of Gonadectomy and Adrenalectomy
on Erythrocyte ALA-D Activity

Experimental Groups	ALA-D Activity (nmols PBG/hr/ml RBC ± S.E.M.)
Control	165 ± 11
Gonadectomy	33 ± 4
Adrenalectomy	129 ± 3
Gonadectomy and Adrenalectomy	320 ± 4

Exposure of rats to carbon monoxide (200 ppm) or to automobile
exhaust emissions with similar concentration of CO produced more than
20% elevation in red blood cell ALA-D (Table 19.3). Hematocrit and

Table 19.3. Erythrocyte ALA-D in Rats Exposed to Carbon Monoxide or Auto Exhaust Emissions

Group	CO (ppm)	Hct. % ± S.E.M.	Serum Zinc (μg/ml ± S.E.M.)	ALA-D (nmols PBG/hr/ml RBC ± S.E.M.)
CA Control	0	46.9 ± 1.2	1.61 ± 0.05	289 ± 17
CO Control	230	54.1 ± 0.7[a]	2.01 ± 0.10[c]	347 ± 20[b]
AEE NI	228	53.2 ± 1.3[a]	1.97 ± 0.09[c]	359 ± 10[b]
AEE I	210	52.0 ± 1.7[a]	1.85 ± 0.05[c]	372 ± 24[b]

Significantly different from control: [a] $p < 0.001$, [b] $p < 0.005$, [c] $p < 0.01$

Four groups of 15 male rats were fed a semipurified diet containing controlled levels of micro and macro nutrients (NRC requirements). Dietary zinc and copper levels were 40 and 4 ppm, respectively. All animals were exposed 23 hrs/day for 28 days to the following: a) clean air control (CA); b) carbon monoxide control—average concentration 230 ppm—(CO); c) non-irradiated auto exhaust emissions (AEE NI); d) irradiated auto exhaust emissions (AEE I). The exhaust emissions were diluted with air (1:10 ratio). Other experimental procedures were similar to those previously reported.[27]

serum zinc were also elevated in the exposed animals. The increment in ALA-D may therefore, be explained either by a possible increase in immature red blood cells due to CO induced erythrocytosis or by increased availability of zinc for enzyme synthesis and activation.

These are studies done on laboratory animals and may or may not have clinical importance. On the other hand we have shown in few clinical cases that total red blood cell ALA-D levels, that is the enzyme reactivated with 10^{-4} M $ZnCl_2$, may differ substantially from control values. In such instances the susceptibility to lead exposure may depend on the total amount of blood and tissue ALA-D.

Depressed ALA-D activity was observed in a 14-year old girl affected by tyrosinemia (a genetic impairment of tyrosine metabolism) even though her blood lead level was less than 10 μg/100 ml (Table 19.4).[17] Addition of $ZnCl_2$ to the enzyme preparation did not activate ALA-D to normal levels (Figure 19.4) indicating that either the enzyme synthesis is impaired or that an abnormality in the enzyme molecule affects its activity.

Table 19.4.   ALA-D Activity in Tyrosinemic Patient

Date		ALA-D Activity (nmols PBG/hr/ml RBC ± S.D.)	% of Control
—	Control (n=13)	1085 ± 255	100
1/7/75	C.B. (patient)	173	16
6/11/75	C.B. (patient)	143	13
3/25/75	C.B. (patient)	88	8

Activation of Pb-inhibited ALA-D by *in vitro* addition of $ZnCl_2$ to the incubation mixture can be seen in Figure 19.4). The enzymatic activity in a control group composed of male and female human adults (n=13) averaged 1085 ± 255 units (nmols PBG/hr/ml RBC). Activation of ALA-D in the control group ranged between 30 to 40% of initial activity when the concentrations of $ZnCl_2$ were between 10^{-4} and 5 x 10^{-4} M.

In the same figure are also reported ALA-D activation curves in the blood of two occupation Pb-exposed workers. Patient A[18] at the time of the admission to the hospital had extremely high blood lead levels (260 μg/100 ml) and unexpectedly mild symptoms. At the time of this assay, that is, 2 months post admission including 5 days of parenteral therapy with 500 mg $CaNa_2$ EDTA daily, his blood lead level dropped to 70 μg/100 ml and ALA-D activity was 310 units without added Zn^{++} and 2139 with 10^{-4} M Zn^{++}. Patient B[19] at the time of admission showed

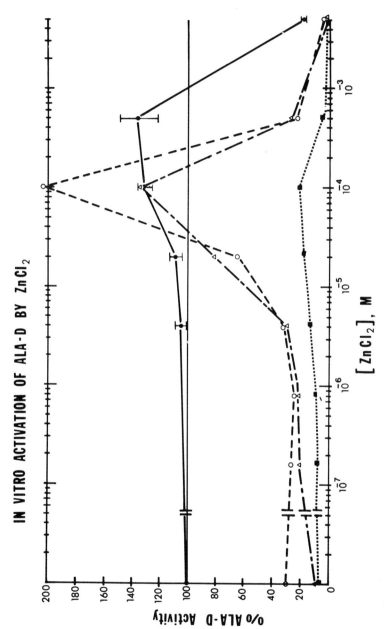

Figure 19.4. *In vitro* activation of blood ALA-D by addition of ZnCl₂: Control group (– • — • –); Occupational Pb-exposed patient A (- - ○ - - ○ - -); Occupational Pb-exposed patient B (- △ - — - · △ -); Tyrosinemic patient (• • • • ■ • • • •). The mean unactivated ALA-D value for the control group was 1085 ± 255 nmols PBG/hr/ml RBC (set as 100%).

severe symptoms of lead poisoning, had a blood lead level of 89.5 μg/100 ml and ALA-D activity of 93 nmols PBG/hr/ml RBC. After one week, his blood lead level was 80.7 μg/100 ml and ALA-D activity was 134 units without zinc and 1468 with 10^{-4}M Zn^{++}. At that time this patient had not yet received chelation therapy. The higher level of ALA-D activity with 10^{-4}M Zn^{++} in patient A remains unexplainable since Zn^{++}-activated ALA-D in patient B and in experimental Pb-exposed animals reached, but did not surpass, control values.

These reported observations are only examples of factors which may affect ALA-D activity. Nevertheless, ALA-D still remains a sensitive indicator of lead exposure and may also be an indicator of the biologically significant body burden since, when its activity is below 30% of control value, there is a detectable increase of urinary ALA[20] which indicates a metabolic disturbance of porphyrinogenesis. Nakao et al.[21] reported that only 2 of 12 symptomatic lead-exposed patients, with blood lead levels ranging between 39.5 and 165 μg/100 ml, showed ALA-D activity higher than 30% of the activity found in a control group with blood lead average of 22.9 ± 8.2 μg/100 ml.

Another zinc-dependent enzyme which seems susceptible to lead exposure is carbonic anhydrase-B. Taniguchi et al.[22] reported a significant decrease in carbonic anhydrase isoenzyme B in lead-exposed workers with blood lead levels above 30 μg/100 ml. This parameter, however, was not as sensitive to blood lead as the inhibition of ALA-D. In this case lead seems to inhibit the synthesis of the isoenzyme B and, with the assay procedure used, it is impossible to assess any direct effect of lead on the enzymatic activity.

EFFECTS OF CHELATION THERAPY

It is a common procedure to administer chelating agents, usually calcium disodium ethylenediaminetetracetate (EDTA), to lead-exposed adults and children for diagnostic and therapeutic purposes. The principle of this treatment is that EDTA, which is not metabolized by the human organism, increases the urinary excretion of lead, consequently lowering the total body burden. The problem arises from the fact that EDTA is not selective in binding lead but complexes a variety of other metals many of which are essential trace metals. The same can be said for other chelating agents used in the therapy of heavy metal poisoning. The stability constants of EDTA with Pb^{++} and with some of the essential trace metals, such as Zn^{++}, Fe^{++}, Fe^{+++}, and Cu^{++} lie in the range of 10^{14} to 10^{25},[23] with increasing affinity for $Fe^{++} < Zn^{++} < Pb^{++} < Cu^{++} < Fe^{+++}$. Intraperitoneal administration of $CaNa_2$EDTA to lead-exposed rats increased the urinary excretion of zinc, lead, iron and copper 11, 4.5, 3 and 1.2 times the normally excreted levels, respectively.[24] The discrepancy between the stability constants and the excretion rates is due to the fact that Cu^+ and Fe^{+++} are strongly bound to serum proteins, ceruloplasmin and transferrin, respectively. The competition between EDTA and the metal-binding protein therefore favors the latter and the excretion of iron and copper remains relatively low. A different story can be told for zinc which in serum is bound mainly to albumin and globulins with relatively low stability and consequently its excretion with EDTA therapy is highly increased.

Farina et al.[25] reported abnormally high urinary excretion of zinc from lead-exposed adults treated with EDTA. The excreted levels of zinc were such that in prolonged EDTA therapy the zinc balance could very well have been negative with severe depletion resulting therefrom. In one isolated case[18] we have observed that in 5 days of treatment with 500 mg/day parenteral dose of $CaNa_2EDTA$ the total excretion of zinc was 27.3 mg which may have been much greater than the zinc absorbed from dietary sources. During the EDTA treatment the Zn/Pb molar ratio in urine increased from 7.5 (pretreatment) to 17.2 (5th day treatment) and erythrocyte ALA-D activity, in nmols PBG/hr/ml RBC, decreased from 204.4 (pretreatment) to 130.7 (4th day treatment).

From many reports and experiments it is obvious that chelation therapy significantly alters the metabolism of trace metals. From our results zinc seems more susceptible to EDTA therapy than iron or copper. It is therefore possible that, zinc-dependent enzyme systems other than ALA-D may also be deleteriously altered. Furthermore, zinc seems to be a direct antagonist of lead, at the absorption site[26] and at enzymatic levels.[7,26]

From these considerations it would seem that nutritional or therapeutic supplementation of zinc may be beneficial in treating and preventing lead toxicity.

ACKNOWLEDGMENTS

The author acknowledges the kindness of Dr. S. Brooks, Dr. R. El-Gazzar and their coworkers for releasing unpublished data. He also wishes to thank R. Danner and W.B. Peirano for their valuable assistance.

REFERENCES

1. Gurba, P. E., R. E. Sennett and R. D. Kobes. "Studies on the Mechanism of Action of δ-Aminolevulinate Dehydratase from Bovine and Rat Liver," Arch. Biochem. Biophys. 150:130 (1972).

2. Cheh, A. and J. B. Neilands. "Zinc, an Essential Metal Ion for Beef Liver δ-Aminolevulinate Dehydratase," *Biochem. Biophys. Res. Comm.* 55:1060 (1973).

3. Border, E. A., A. C. Cantrell and T. A. Kilroe-Smith. "The *in vitro* Effect of Zinc and Other Metal Ions on the Activity of Human Erythrocyte Aminolevulinic Acid Dehydratase," *Environ. Res.* 11:319 (1976).

4. Abdulla, M. and B. Haeger-Aronsen. "ALA-Dehydratase Activation by Zinc," *Enzyme* 12:708 (1971).

5. Komai, H. and J. B. Neilands. "Effect of Zinc Ions on δ-Aminolevulinate Dehydratase in Ustilago Sphaerogena," *Arch. Biochem. Biophys.* 124:456 (1968).

6. Finelli, V. N., D. S. Klauder, M. A. Karaffa and H. G. Petering. "Interaction of Zinc and Lead on δ-Aminolevulinate Dehydratase," *Biochem. Biophys. Res. Comm.* 65:303 (1975).

7. Finelli, V. N., L. M. Murthy, W. B. Peirano and H. G. Petering. "δ-Aminolevulinate Dehydratase, a Zinc Dependent Enzyme," *Biochem. Biophys. Res. Comm.* 60:1418 (1974).

8. Haeger-Aronsen, B., A. Schutz and M. Abdulla. "Antagonistic Effect *in vivo* of Zinc on Inhibition of δ-Aminolevulinic Acid Dehydratase by Lead," *Arch. Environ. Health* 31:215 (1976).

9. Border, E. A., A. C. Cantrell and T. A. Kilroe-Smith. "The *in vitro* Effect of Zinc on the Inhibition of Human δ-Aminolevulinic Acid Dehydratase by Lead," *Brit. J. Ind. Med.* 33:85 (1976).

10. Zielhuis, R. L. "Dose-Response Relationship for Inorganic Lead," *Int. Arch. Occup. Hlth.* 35:1 (1975).

11. Pietrovsky, J. K. "Kinetic Behaviour of Lead," Congr. Chem. Poll. and Human Ecology, Prague (1970).

12. "The Health Protection Directorate, European Community Draft Directives Regarding the Environmental Health Aspects of Lead," *Int. Arch. Occup. Environ. Hlth.* 35:189 (1975).

13. Chisolm, J. J., Jr., M. B. Barrett and H. V. Harrison. "Indicators of Internal Dose of Lead in Relation to Derangement in Heme Synthesis," *The JohnsHopkins Med. J.* 137:6 (1975).

14. Chisolm, J. J., Jr., M. B. Barrett and E. D. Mellits. "Dose-Effect and Dose-Response Relationship for Lead in Children," *J. Ped.* 87:1152 (1975).

15. Haeger-Aronsen, B., M. Abdulla and B. I. Fristedt. "Effect of Lead on δ-Aminolevulinic Acid Dehydratase Activity in Red Blood Cells," *Arch. Environ. Health* 29:150 (1974).

16. Granick, J. L., S. Sassa, S. Cyranick, R. D. Levere and A. Kappas. "Studies in Lead Poisoning," *Biochem. Med.* 8:149 (1973).

17. Strife, F. C., E. L. Zuroweste, V. N. Finelli, E. A. Emmett, H. G. Petering and H. K. Berry. "Tyrosinemia with Acute Intermittent Porphyria: Aminolevulinic Acid Dehydratase Deficiency Related to Elevated Urinary Aminolevulinic Acid Levels," *J. Ped.* (1977) in press.

18. Thomasino, J. A., E. L. Zuroweste, S. M. Brooks, H. G. Petering, S. I. Lerner and V. N. Finelli. "Relationship of Lead, Zinc and Erythrocyte ALA-D in Lead Toxicity," *Arch. Environ. Health* (1977) in press.

19. Brooks, S. *et al.*, Dept. Environ. Health, Univ. of Cincinnati, College of Medicine, Cincinnati, Ohio 45267 (personal communication).

20. Lauwerys, R., J. P. Buchet, H. A. Roels and D. Materne. "Relationship Between Urinary δ-Aminolevulinic Acid Excretion and the Inhibition of Red Cell δ-Aminolevulinate Dehydratase by Lead," *Clin. Toxicol.* 7:383 (1974).

21. Nakao, K., O. Wada and Y. Yano. "δ-Aminolevulinic Acid Dehydratase Activity in Erythrocytes for the Evaluation of Lead Poisoning," *Clin. Chim. Acta* 19:319 (1968).

22. Taniguchi, N., T. Sato, T. Kondo, H. Tamachi, K. Saito and E. Takakuwa. "Carbonic Anhydrase Isozymes, Hemoglobin-F and Glutathione Levels in Lead Exposed Workers," *Clin. Chim. Acta* 59:29 (1975).

23. Sillen, L. G. and A. E. Martell. *Stability Constants of Metal-Ion Complexes,* Special Publ. No. 17, The Chemical Society (London: Burlington House, W1, 1964).

24. El-Gazzar, R. *et al.* (unpublished results), Dept. Environ. Health, Univ. of Cincinnati, College of Medicine, Cincinnati, Ohio 45267.

25. Farina, G., A. M. Griffini and R. Grisler. "Eliminazione Orinaria dello Zinco in Corso di Trattamento con Versenato," *Med. Lavoro* 61:372 (1970).

26. Cerklewski, F. L. and R. M. Forbes. "Influence of Dietary Zinc on Lead Toxicity in the Rat," *J. Nutr.* 106:689 (1976).

27. Lee, S. D., M. Malanchuk and V. N. Finelli. "Biological Effects of Auto Emissions. I. Exhaust from Engine with and without Catalytic Converter," *J. Toxicol. Environ. Health* 1:705 (1976).

CHAPTER 20

ROLE OF NUTRITION IN HEAVY METAL TOXICITY

H. G. Petering, L. Murthy and F. L. Cerklewski

Kettering Laboratory
Department of Environmental Health
College of Medicine
University of Cincinnati
Cincinnati, Ohio 45267

INTRODUCTION

The role of nutrition in heavy metal toxicity is really only one aspect of the more general topic of the role of nutrition in toxicology in its broadest sense. In this regard we are *rediscovering* the importance of nutrition to human health in a special way, one which suggests that scientists themselves must make certain changes in their viewpoints. Nutritional science is being recognized as having new and special roles in surgery, as evidenced by the interest in hyperalimentation of surgical patients and the relationship of nutrition to wound healing and host resistance to infection.

In toxicology vitamin A and some analogs have been found to prevent chemical carcinogenesis, and some chemical carcinogens are less potent in experimental animals if adequate or excessive dietary intakes of copper, zinc, or riboflavin are used.[1] Vitamin E has been reported to reduce the toxic effects of the atmospheric oxidant gases NO_x and O_3.[2] Therefore, the role of nutrition in heavy metal toxicity for this aspect of toxicology must be discussed because it is one that is always with us in our modern urban civilization, and it is one that may be worsened by the increased use of coal as a source of energy.

We have selected for this discussion the role of nutrition in the toxicity of lead and cadmium, since our group has been active in this area for a number of years and since these studies illustrate the concept of a protective role for optimal nutrition in heavy metal toxicity.

The Effect of Dietary Variations on Lead Toxicity

A review of the literature shows that the nutritional status of the animal model greatly alters absorption, retention, and toxic effects of oral ingestion of lead. A summary of the most striking interrelationship of dietary constituents with oral toxicity of lead is given in Table 20.1.

Table 20.1 Relationships Between Lead and Essential Nutrients

| Nutrient | Dietary Intake of Individual Nutrients[a] | | | |
	Normal[b]	Deficiency[c]	Excess[d]	Reference[e]
Protein	+	+	+	A
Calcium	+	+	±	B
Phosphorus	±	+	−	C
Vitamin D	0	−	−	D
Vitamin E	0	+	0	E
Ascorbic acid	0	0	+	F
Niacin	?	0	?	G
Pyridoxine	?	0	?	F
Iron	+	+	+	H
Zinc	+	+	±	I
Selenium	+	+	±	I
Copper	+	±	±	J

[a]+ = Yes, - = No, 0 = undefined, ? = not established in all species tested.
[b]Lead affects the metabolism of the nutrient
[c]Deficiency of the nutrient increases the severity of lead toxicity
[d]An excess of the nutrient decreases the toxicity of lead

[e](A) Baernstein, H. D. and J. A. Grand. *J. Pharm. Exp. Ther.* 74:18 (1942).
(B) Six, K. M. and R. A. Goyer. *J. Lab. Clin. Med.* 76:933 (1970).
(C) Shields, J. B. and H. H. Mitchell. *J. Nutr.* 21:541 (1940).
(D) Sobel, A. E., H. Yuska, D. D. Peter and B. Kramer. *J. Biol. Chem.* 132:239 (1940).
(E) Levander, O. A., V. C. Morris, D. J. Higgs and R. J. Ferretti. *J. Nutr.* 105:1481 (1975).
(F) Kao, R. L. C. and R. M. Forbes. *Arch. Env. Health* 27:31 (1973).
(G) deBruin, A. *Arch. Env. Health* 23:249 (1971).
(H) Six, K. M. and R. A. Goyer. *J. Lab. Clin. Med.* 79:128 (1972).
(I) Cerklewski, F. L. and R. M. Forbes. *J. Nutr.* 106:689 and 778 (1976).
(J) Klauder, D. S., L. Murthy and H. G. Petering. *Trace Substances in Env. Health* (University of Missouri), VI, 131 (1973).

We see that there are many nutritional elements that affect the fate of orally ingested lead, ranging from amounts of protein, through the mineral contents of the diets to the vitamin intakes of the animals. In order to limit this discussion and to illustrate the importance of the dietary relationships involved we have focused our attention on the effects of dietary zinc, copper and iron.

Zinc vs. Lead

In a recent publication Cerklewski and Forbes[3] reported that an inverse relationship existed between the absorption of orally ingested lead (200 ppm in the diet) and the log concentration of zinc in the semipurified diet fed to rats. They also found that the lead concentration of tibia from the same rats (a measure of lead retention) was inversely related to dietary zinc, as was the excretion of urinary δ-aminolevulinic acid, which is a measure of the metabolic effect of lead on the heme synthetic pathway. A summary of some of their data is given in Table 20.2. These data indicate the important role that dietary zinc can play in altering absorption, retention, and metabolic effects of oral lead ingestion.

Table 20.2   The Influence of Dietary Zinc and Lead on Tibia Lead Concentration and on the Excretion of Urinary Delta-Aminolevulinic Acid (ALA)[a]

ppm Pb	0			50			200		
ppm Zn	8	35	200	8	35	200	8	35	200
Tibia Pb μg/g Ash Mean ± SEM		10		118^{A*} ±25	83^{B*} ±15	37^{A*B*} ±10	191^C ±11	204^D ±29	91^{CD} ±12
μg ALA/mg Creatinine % of Control Mean ± SEM		100		175^E ±15	125^E ±9	138 ±12	361^F ±24	318^G ±30	183^{FG} ±12

[a]Data taken from Cerklewski and Forbes.[3]

[b]Matching superscripts along a horizontal line denote statistical difference at $P < 0.05*$ and at $P < 0.01$.

Copper, Iron vs. Lead

Because of the intimate metabolic relationship of copper and iron, we shall consider together the effects of dietary copper and iron on oral lead toxicity. In 1972, Klauder et al.[4] reported that reducing the copper levels below the optimal in a semipurified diet based on 20% egg white,

63% corn starch and 10% corn oil caused an increase in lead absorption and toxicity in male rats. About the same time Six and Goyer[5] also reported that reducing the iron level in a different semipurified diet below the optimal level also caused exacerbation of some of the toxic effect of orally ingested lead. Since then Klauder and Petering[6] and Klauder[7] have elaborated on these findings, showing that copper and iron are interrelated in many ways in altering oral lead toxicity. Some of their data are presented here to illustrate again the effect of nutritional status on lead toxicity.

Tables 20.3 and 20.4 present data taken from the work of Klauder and Petering,[6] showing the effects of iron and copper on lead toxicity.

Table 20.3   The Effect of Iron and Copper on Erythrocyte Lead in Rats[a]

| Dietary Levels | | Erythrocyte Lead (μg/100 g Wet Weight)[b] |
Iron ppm	Copper ppm	(Lead in Diet 500 ppm)
6	0.5	355^A
6	8.5	412^B
40	0.5	155^A
40	8.5	125^B

[a]Data taken from Klauder and Petering.[6]

[b]Geometric means given: matched superscript letters indicate significant differences ($P < 0.01$):

Table 20.4   The Influence of Iron, Copper, and Lead on Hematopoiesis in Rats[a]

| Dietary Levels | | Hematocrit % Volume Lead | | Hemoglobin g/100 ml Blood Lead | |
Iron ppm	Copper ppm	0 ppm	500 ppm	0 ppm	500 ppm
6	0.5	$22.4^{A,I}$	$14.6^{C,I}$	$5.2^{E,L}$	$3.1^{G,L}$
6	8.5	$33.7^{A,J}$	$26.7^{C,J}$	$8.2^{E,M}$	$6.5^{G,M}$
40	0.5	43.3^{B*K}	$34.7^{D,K}$	$12.3^{F,N}$	$8.8^{H,N}$
40	8.5	47.3^{B*}	46.9^{D}	13.9^{F*}	13.1^{H}

[a]Data taken from Klauder and Petering.[6]

[b]Arithmetic means given. Matched letters indicate significance at $P < 0.01$. Asterisk indicates $P < 0.05$.

Table 20.3 shows that iron has a marked effect on erythrocyte lead, the most reliable measure of current lead absorption. When iron is suboptimal (6 ppm), the lead content of erythrocytes is three times that found in rats receiving the optimal level (40 ppm). In this experiment copper had only a minor effect on erythrocyte lead levels and then only when iron was optimal. The data in Table 20.4 shows that the severity of the anemia produced by lead ingestion in rats is reduced by both iron and copper, but that copper appears to be the more important element, as indicated by both hemoglobin and hematocrit values.

Other data obtained by Klauder[7] revealed that body weight gain was suppressed or reduced by lead. This effect was minimized by iron (40 ppm *vs.* 6 ppm) or copper (8.5 ppm *vs.* 0.5 ppm), but it was only when both copper and iron were optimal that this effect of lead was completely eliminated. In related data given in Table 20.5, we see that lead causes an enlargement of the liver or heart when copper is low, but it does not have this effect when copper is optimal. Iron does not seem to be influential in this regard.

Table 20.5 The Effect of Dietary Iron and Copper on Lead-Induced Hypertrophy of Liver and Heart of Rats[a]

Dietary Levels		Specific Organ Weight			
Iron ppm	Copper ppm	Liver g/100 g Body Weight		Heart g/100 g Body Weight	
		Pb=0 ppm	Pb=500 ppm	Pb=0 ppm	Pb=500 ppm
6	0.5	$2.7^{A,D}$	$3.6^{B,D}$	$0.54^{F,I}$	$0.78^{G,I}$
6	8.5	2.3^{A}	2.7^{B}	0.35^{F}	0.38^{G}
40	0.5	2.6^{E}	$3.2^{C,E}$	0.35	0.42^{H*}
40	8.5	2.4	2.5^{C}	0.32	0.30^{H*}

[a]Data taken from Klauder.[7]

[b]Arithmetic means given. Matched letters indicate significant at $P < 0.01$, * $P < 0.05$.

In a related observation it was found that lead reduces plasma zinc levels significantly when copper is low but not when it is optimal. This effect is more pronounced when iron and copper are low than when only copper is low. So here again we see that lead has an important effect on zinc metabolism if dietary copper and iron are suboptimal.

These results are just a few of those found that indicate that decreased dietary intakes of zinc, copper and iron may greatly enhance the toxicity of a given level of lead exposure. They also indicate that optimal and supraoptimal dietary levels of these nutrients may be protective of the effects of lead exposure of rats.

The Effect of Dietary Variations on Cadmium Toxicity

Turning now to the role that nutrition plays in cadmium toxicity we find also that the literature strongly supports the concept that the level and type of dietary component can greatly alter the biologic response of an animal to cadmium exposure in a variety of forms. The scope of nutritional interaction with cadmium toxicity is shown in Table 20.6.

Table 20.6   Relationships Between Cadmium and Essential Nutrients[a]

Nutrient	Dietary Intake of Individual Nutrients		
	Normal[b]	Deficiency[c]	Excess[d]
Zinc	+	+	+
Iron	+	+	+ (Fe^{2+})
Manganese	+	?	?
Copper	+	+	+
Selenium	+	?	+
Calcium	+	+	?
Ascorbic acid	?	?	+
Vitamin D	?	+	?
Protein	?	+	+

[a]Data taken from Fox.[8]
[b]+ = cadmium affects metabolism and/or function of the nutrient;
 ? = no relationship has been established.
[c]+ = a deficiency of the nutrient increases the severity of cadmium toxicity
[d]+ = an excess of the nutrient decreases the toxicity of cadmium.

This summary, taken from a review by Fox[8] shows that as with the case of lead toxicity, so here: the spectrum of interrelationships of nutrients is very broad. Because Fox has indicated the breadth of the effect of dietary components of cadmium toxicity, we shall again emphasize only the relationships of dietary levels of zinc and copper and relate these to parameters of zinc, copper and iron metabolism.

Zinc–Cadmium

Nutritional science not only is a basic science for understanding the growth and function of complex organisms, but also is of primary importance in the physiology of cells *per se* whether prokaryates or eukaryates. Thus Christian *et al.*[9] showed that dose-related cadmium toxicity could be shown in a mammalian cell culture system and that this effect was prevented by additions of zinc to the medium in a fashion that appeared to be governed by the molar ratio of zinc/cadmium in the medium.

In a more complex experiment with rats fed a semipurified diet in which zinc was absent, Petering *et al.*[10] showed that the growth inhibitory effect of orally administered cadmium could be prevented by ingestion of additional zinc. This effect also appeared to be governed by an antagonism that depended on the molar ratio of zinc/cadmium in the diet.[11]

Zinc—Copper vs. Cadmium

Since dietary zinc and copper appear to have an antagonistic interaction in the physiological range of intake, which is reflected in metabolic variations, we have usually carried out our experiments on cadmium toxicity under conditions which varied dietary levels of both zinc and copper in a block design. These normal nutritional interactions of zinc and copper have been described in detail by Murthy *et al.*[12] and by Murthy and Petering[13] in recent publications. The biochemical and physiologic parameters that are affected by zinc and/or copper are growth, serum and tissue levels of zinc and copper, hemoglobin, hematocrit, and serum values of uric acid, GOT and cholesterol.

In 1974 Petering[14] reviewed some of the work carried out by his group and showed that when dietary copper was varied from the suboptimal level of 0.5 ppm to 4.0 ppm (an optimal level) and dietary zinc from 2.5 ppm (suboptimal) to 40 ppm (superoptimal), oral ingestion of cadmium could be shown to lower serum zinc and serum copper, depending on the ration of zinc/cadmium or copper/cadmium. The inhibition of serum zinc by cadmium was small but definite, and greater when copper was low than when it was optimal. The effects of cadmium on serum copper levels were reduced by both increased dietary copper and zinc, showing the metabolic relationship of zinc and copper.

Whanger and Weswig[15] found that dietary cadmium at 100 ppm had a depressive effect on serum ceruloplasmin levels of rats, and in 1973 Whanger[16] reported that dietary cadmium reduced liver iron on a dose-related basis up to 50 ppm.

Murthy and Petering[17] investigated the effect of cadmium on zinc, copper and iron metabolism in male rats when copper was varied; some of their data are given in Tables 20.7 and 20.8. In Table 20.7 we see

Table 20.7 Influence of Dietary Copper on Toxicity of Cadmium-Blood Parameters[a,b]

Dietary Copper	– Cadmium		+ Cadmium[d]	
	0.5 ppm[a]	7.5 μg/ml[d]	0.5 ppm[a]	7.5 μg/ml[d]
Serum zinc (μg%)	139.1(10.4)	121.6(12.2)	178.0(7.1)	129.1(10.3)
Serum copper (μg%)	92.9(17.3)	109.1(4.8)	10.1(2.0)	102.9(2.9)
Ceruloplasmin (mg%)	26.1(4.5)	31.3(3.9)	0.64(0.63)	32.9(4.0)
Serum iron (μg%)	134.2(19.3)	244.6(84.3)	87.0(36.0)	140.7(22.0)
Hemoglobin (g%)	13.4(0.25)	14.1(0.24)	10.9(1.1)	11.7(0.87)
Hematocrit (% vol.)	42.2(1.1)	43.7(0.9)	37.0(2.6)	38.7(2.5)

[a]The diet was a semipurified one based on 20% egg white, 63% corn starch, 10% corn oil, adequate vitamins, and Bernhard-Tomarelli salt mix without copper, which provided NRC requirement of minerals, except copper, for the rat—e.g., 20 ppm Zn, 40 ppm Fe, 55 ppm Mn, and 0.5 ppm Cu. Numbers in parentheses indicate SEM.

[b]Unpublished data of Murthy and Petering.[17]

[c]Cadmium (as chloride) given in drinking water at 34.4 μg/ml.

[d]Copper (as sulfate) given in drinking water.

Table 20.8 Influence of Dietary Copper on Toxicity of Cadmium-Liver and Kidney Metal Values[a,b]

Dietary Copper	– Cadmium		+ Cadmium (17.2 μg/ml)[c]	
	0.5 ppm	7.5 mg/ml[d]	0.5 Cu	7.5 μg/ml[d]
A. Liver				
Zinc μg/g (dry wt)	110.4(6.3)	114.1(2.4)	159.7(9.8)	149.1(6.8)
Copper μg/g (dry wt)	15.0(1.1)	22.9(10.3)	6.2(1.3)	18.5(1.1)
Iron μg/g (dry wt)	531.8(114.4)	385.5(43.2)	335.3(32.0)	190.2(78.4)
Cadmium μg/g (dry wt)	0	0	78.5(5.5)	96.2(12.6)
B. Kidney				
Zinc μg/g (dry wt)	109.4(3.2)	110.4(2.3)	145.3(7.9)	134.3(5.9)
Copper μg/g (dry wt)	24.9(4.3)	49.9(5.2)	14.8(0.3)	66.5(1.5)
Iron μg/g (dry wt)	302.4(28.9)	258.9(12.1)	159.7(10.3)	166.0(17.6)
Cadmium μg/g (dry wt)	0	0	103.1(12.2)	104.3(12.5)

[a]The diet was a semipurified one, described in Table 20.7. Numbers in parentheses indicate SEM.

[b]Unpublished data of Murthy and Petering.

[c]Cadmium (as chloride) given in the drinking water at 34.4 μg/ml levels.

[d]Copper (as sulfate) given in drinking water.

that serum zinc is elevated by cadmium when dietary copper is low, while serum copper and ceruloplasmin levels are markedly lowered under the same condition. Of particular interest is the finding that cadmium lowers serum iron at both levels of dietary copper, although the higher level of copper is somewhat protective. This effect occurs even though dietary iron was at 40 ppm, considered to be an optimal level, which indicates that higher levels of iron may be needed to prevent this effect of cadmium. The reduced serum iron and copper may also be related to the reduction in hemoglobin and hematocrit values that cadmium induces.

In the same experiment they examined total tissue concentration of zinc, copper and iron in liver and kidney as these were affected by oral ingestion of cadmium. These results, given in Table 20.8, show the following variations, which we believe are significant and indicative of nutritional interactions with cadmium. Liver zinc was elevated by cadmium, while liver copper was reduced, the latter being less pronounced when dietary copper was elevated. Liver iron, which normally is high when dietary copper is low, was reduced at both levels of copper.

Kidney zinc was also elevated by cadmium ingestion, and kidney copper was only diminished when dietary copper was low. Again in the case of kidney iron, cadmium caused a significant lowering of this parameter; thus the data of this experiment point to a definite perturbation of zinc, copper and iron metabolism by oral cadmium, a perturbation prevented by extra dietary copper. The data with respect to iron in liver complement those reported by Whanger;[16] in fact they show that much lower levels of cadmium are effective and that the action of cadmium on iron metabolism in the liver is prevented to some extent by copper.

In a recent investigation of the effect on the development of fetuses of cadmium given to rat mothers, Choudhury et al.[18] found that whole body iron and copper levels of rat neonates were seriously depressed by administration of a low level of oral cadmium prior to and during gestation. These same neonates grew normally during the lactation period, during which the mothers received no cadmium, and in the postweaning period, but they were found to have spontaneous activity deficits in the postweaning period. Some of the data obtained in this experiment are given in Table 20.9.

DISCUSSION

The concept that heavy metal toxicity in experimental animals and human beings may be greatly modified and indeed modulated by the

Table 20.9   Effect on Neonates of Cadmium Given to Rat Mothers[a]

Neonatal Parameter	Group Control[b]	Cadmium Treated[c]
Litter Size	16 (1)	23 (0)
Male/Female	8/8	11/12
Avg. Wt. of Neonate	6.06 g	6.32 g
Avg. Body Weight at Weaning	55.9 g	45.7 g
Whole Body Cd (μg/g)	15.2	22.1
Whole Body Zn (μg/g)	120	100
Whole Body Cu (μg/g)	10.9	7.6
Whole Body Fe (μg/g)	301	237

[a]Unpublished data of Choudhury et al.[18]

[b]Control mothers received rat chow and deionized water throughout the experiment.

[c]Cadmium treated mothers received chow throughout the experiment and 17.2 μg cadmium (chloride)/ml of drinking water for 180 days prior to conception and during the gestational period. No cadmium was given to mothers during the lactation period.

nutritional status of the animal or person is firmly rooted in a great number of reports, some of which are of long standing. In this chapter we have emphasized the effects of varying dietary zinc, copper and iron on the toxic manifestations of exposure to lead or cadmium and have only indicated in passing that other nutritional elements also have an important role in this regard. This chapter could also have been expanded to consider the role of nutritional status in the toxicology of mercury, silver, cobalt and other heavy metals.

Most of our illustrations relate to oral exposure to lead and cadmium and other studies need to include absorption by the respiratory route; however, one study, namely that of Lal,[11] certainly indicates that nutritional status is also a factor in the toxicity of cadmium oxide given by inhalation.

The whole thrust of this effort has been to point out (1) that toxicity of heavy metals cannot be assessed adequately without definitive control of dietary intake and nutritional status of either the experimental animal or the human subject, (2) that extrapolation of results of animal experiment to human problems of heavy metal toxicity may be much more reliable and more satisfactory if attention were paid to comparing similar nutritional conditions as well as environmental exposures, and finally (3) that nutritional status and dietary intake should be viewed as one of the most important preventive measures available to public health officials to reduce the consequences of environmental or occupational exposure to lead or cadmium.

The concept of nutritional modulation of chemical toxicity is an important one and one which should be exploited to its fullest. A recent review[19] emphasized the resurgence of interest in the relationship of nutritional status to chemical toxicity or drug action. In the specific cases of the toxicity of lead or cadmium we believe that much can be done to minimize the health effects of the widespread dissipation of these toxic elements by paying attention to the diets of those in danger of ingesting these elements.

ACKNOWLEDGMENT

The authors wish to acknowledge the generous support for this work furnished to them under UL-EPA Contract 68-03-2011 USPHS Grant ESH-00159.

REFERENCES

1. Falk, H. L. *Anticarcinogenesis—An Alternative in Progress in Experimental Tumor Research,* vol. 14, F. Homburger, Ed. (Basel, New York: S. Karger, 1971), p. 105.
2. Menzel, D. B., J. N. Roehm and S. D. Lee. "Vitamin E: The Biological and Environmental Antioxidant," *J. Agric. Food Chem.* 20:481 (1972).
3. Cerklewski, F. L. and R. M. Forbes. "Influence of Dietary Zinc on Lead Toxicity in the Rat," *J. Nutr.* 106:689 (1976).
4. Klauder, D. S., L. Murthy and H. G. Petering. "Effect of Dietary Intake of Lead Acetate on Copper Metabolism in Male Rats," In: *Trace Substances in Environmental Health,* VI, D. D. Hemphill, Ed. (Columbia, Missouri: University of Missouri, 1972), p. 131.
5. Six, K. M. and R. A. Goyer. "The Influence of Iron Deficiency on Tissue Content and Toxicity of Ingested Lead in the Rat," *J. Lab. Clin. Med.* 79:128 (1972).
6. Klauder, D. S. and H. G. Petering. "Protective Value of Dietary Copper and Iron Against Some Toxic Effects of Lead in Rats," *Environ. Health Persp.* 12:77 (1975).
7. Klauder, D. S. "The Effects of Dietary Copper, Iron and Zinc on the Toxicity of Lead in Male Rats," Ph.D. Dissertation, University of Cincinnati (1975).
8. Fox, M. R. S. "Effect of Essential Minerals on Cadmium Toxicity, A Review," *J. Food Sci.* 39:321 (1974).
9. Christian, R. T., T. E. Cody, C. S. Clark, R. Lingg and E. J. Cleary. "Development of a Biological Chemical Test for the Potability of Water," *Water—1973,* Amer. Inst. Chem. Eng. Symp. Series, 70(136): 15 (1974).

10. Petering, H. G., M. A. Johnson and K. L. Stemmer. "Studies of Zinc Metabolism in the Rat," *Arch. Environ. Health* 23:93 (1971).
11. Lal, J. B. "The Effects of Low and High Levels of Dietary Zinc on Pathology in Rats Exposed to Cadmium," Ph.D. Dissertation, University of Cincinnati (1976).
12. Murthy, L., L. M. Klevay and H. G. Petering. "Interrelationships of Zinc and Copper Nutriture in the Rat," *J. Nutr.* 104:1458 (1974).
13. Murthy, L. and H. G. Petering. "The Effect of Dietary Zinc and Copper Interrelationships on Blood Parameters of the Rat," *J. Agr. Food Chem.* 24:808 (1976).
14. Petering, H. G. "The Effect of Cadmium and Lead on Copper and Zinc Metabolism," In: *Trace Elements in Animals,* 2nd ed. W. G. Hoekstra, J. W. Suttie, H. E. Ganther and W. Mertz, Eds. (Baltimore: University Park Press, 1974), p. 311.
15. Whanger, P. D. and P. H. Weswig. "Effect of Some Copper Antagonists on Induction of Ceruloplasmin in the Rat," *J. Nutr.* 100:341 (1970).
16. Whanger, P. D. "Effect of Dietary Cadmium on Intracellular Distribution of Hepatic Iron in Rats," *Res. Comm. Chem. Pathol. Pharm.* 5:733 (1973).
17. Murthy, L. and H. G. Petering. Unpublished (1976).
18. Choudhury, H., L. Hastings, H. G. Petering and G. P. Cooper. "Dietary Cadmium: Embryotoxicity and Behavioral Effects in Rats," In *Annual Report of Center for the Study of the Human Environment* (Cincinnati, Ohio: University of Cincinnati, Department of Environmental Health, 1976), p. 111.
19. Hathcock, J. N. "Nutrition: Toxicology and Pharmacology," *Nutr. Rev.* 34:65 (1976).

CHAPTER 21

METABOLIC INTERACTIONS OF SELENIUM WITH HEAVY METALS

R. A. Rimerman, D. R. Buhler and P. D. Whanger

Department of Agricultural Chemistry and
Environmental Health Sciences Center
Oregon State University
Corvallis, Oregon 97331

INTRODUCTION

Selenium (Se) appears to be a natural protective agent against heavy metal toxicity to biological systems. Most of the available information on Se interactions with metals relate only to its effect on toxicity or to its influence on tissue or subcellular distribution of metals. The known roles of Se in biological processes are quite limited,[1-4] consequently, there are only a few enzymatic or other interactions possible between Se and heavy metals. Possible mechanisms for Se protection against heavy metal toxicity discussed in this paper include: 1) Se-metal binding; (2) Se-metal or Se-metal-protein aggregation, (3) enhancement of immune response by Se, (4) tissue and/or subcellular redistribution of metal by Se; (5) Se induced shift of metals among soluble cytosol proteins; (6) Se requirement for metal excretion; and (7) enhanced or reduced metabolism of metal, for example, in the demethylation of $MeHg^+$.

RESULTS AND DISCUSSION

Effect on Toxicity

Protection by Se against heavy metal toxicity was first shown by Kar and co-workers[5] in 1960 who observed that Se prevented Cd-induced testicular damage. Protection against the toxicity of other metals including

Cd^{+2}, Hg^{+2}, Ag^+ and Tl^+ have been subsequently observed by other researchers.[1,6] Se is effective against both Hg^{+2} and the environmentally important $MeHg^+$ form of the metal.[1,6,7] Ganther and co-workers[8,9] found that dried tuna fish in the diet protected rats against $MeHg^+$. The agent in tuna responsible for reduced toxicity of $MeHg^+$ was Se. The same group[8] also observed that the levels of Hg and Se in tuna increased in a 1:1 molar ratio. These observations point out the difficulty in assigning maximum allowable limits based only on the levels of metal present in foods and suggest that a more realistic guideline for the metal may involve actual measurement of the relative toxicities of foods containing the metal.

Conversely, metals such as Cd^{+2}, Hg^{+2} and Cu^{+3} protect against the toxicity of Se compounds. In addition, Ag^+ in the rat[7] and $MeHg^+$ in the pig[11] have been reported to induce Se deficiency. $MeHg^+$, however, failed to elicit such a response in the rat.[7]

The chemical forms of the Se and the metal, the dosages and ratio of Se to metal employed, the route of administration, and the sequence of timing of treatment all can influence metal toxicity. Thus Stillings $et\ al.$[12] observed that selenite (SeO_3^{-2}) was more effective than selenomethionine in overcoming $MeHg^+$ toxicity. A 1:1 molar ratio of Se:metal gives maximum protection against Hg^{+2} toxicity.[13] If Cd^{+2} or Hg^{+2} are given first, the animals are protected against the heavy metals by subsequent treatment with selenite.[6] If Hg^{+2} is given after selenite administration, however, toxicities of the relatively harmless excretory products dimethylselenide and trimethylselenonium are greatly enhanced (about 10^4 times). This effect was observed only in male rats. In contrast, Cd^{+2} does not appear to alter Se toxicity.

Other factors such as vitamin E,[14-17] sulfur compounds[12,18,19] and arsenite[18,19] also have been shown to have an effect on relieving toxicity of $MeHg^+$ and Ag^+. A combination of these chemicals with Se was more protective against $MeHg^+$ than were the compounds alone: $i.e.$, arsenite + methionine + selenite > arsenite + selenite > arsenite. Te did not protect against $MeHg^+$ toxicity;[16] however, tellurate or tellurate plus selenate (SeO_4^{-2}) was more protective than selenate alone against Hg^{+2}-induced kidney nephritis.[13] A balance between Br, Hg and Se levels has been noted in the livers of California sea lions that had normal pups, but not in those that had premature pups.[20] This suggests that Br may have a role in protection against the toxicity of $MeHg^+$ or Hg^{+2}, although Br^- ion did not protect rats against $MeHg^+$.[21]

Macromolecular Binding

Fang and Fallin[22] have shown that the binding of Hg to various plasma and red blood cell proteins *in vitro* depended on whether the metal was present as Hg^{+2} or $MeHg^+$. Hg^{+2} firmly bound to both serum albumin and hemoglobin, whereas $MeHg^+$ interacted strongly only with hemoglobin. Fang et al.[23] also have shown that orally administered Se increased the affinity of Hg^{+2} for plasma with a 0.5 ppm Se diet, and appeared to decrease the number of available binding sites at dietary levels of 5.0 ppm. Similar results were obtained with $MeHg^+$. Changes in binding affinities or binding sites could account for the Se-induced redistribution of metals among tissues, subcellular fractions, and cytosol components.

Burk and co-workers[24] have found that simultaneous administration of Hg^{+2} and selenite at various Hg:Se ratios resulted in 1:1 binding of a large proportion of the dose to a single plasma protein. Se appeared to be bound to a protein sulfhydryl group in which Hg was subsequently bound to Se. Administration of Hg^{+2} or selenite alone, however, resulted in binding to different plasma components.

The low molecular weight, high cysteine protein metallothionein has been thought to protect against Cd^{+2} and Hg^{+2} intoxification.[25,26] Day et al.[27] have reported that Cu salts cause induction of a similar but distinct protein, chelatin, to which Cu is bound. Metallothionein is induced in response to Cd^{+2}, Hg^{+2},[25,26] or Zn^{+2} and may protect against tissue injury until its metal binding capacity is saturated. Recently Bryan and co-workers[28,29] have established a correlation between the disappearance of injected Cd^{+2} from nuclei or nonspecific cytosol macromolecules and the uptake of Cd^{+2} by newly synthesized metallothionein. Injected selenite diverts similarly administered Cd^{+2} or Hg^{+2} from metallothionein into high molecular weight proteins.[30-32] Fang,[33] however, has shown that oral administration of Hg^{+2} and selenite did not reduce the metal content of metallothionein and Whanger[21] obtained similar results for dietary Cd^{+2} and selenite. These results suggest that metallothionein may still play a role in the detoxification and metabolism of metals.

Tissue Distribution

Ecologically significant correlations of Se with heavy metals have been found by Koeman et al.[34,35] in the brains and livers of marine mammals, which contain Hg and Se in a 1:1 molar ratio (2.5:1 weight ratio). The highest Hg and Se concentrations in the tissues of marine mammals were found in the liver, and values as high as 765 ppm Hg were observed in specimens of the common seal.[34] Liver Hg values in apparently healthy marine mammals as high as 172 ppm have been noted in Northern fur seals by Anas,[36] and up to 120 ppm in California sea lions by Buhler *et al.*[37] These findings emphasize that metal levels in tissue, blood, or excretory products by themselves can be deceiving as a measure of metal intoxication.

Buhler *et al.*[37] had shown that sea lion liver contains much more Hg than the kidney and that in many sea lion tissues, especially liver, a large percentage of the metal is Hg^{+2} rather than $MeHg^+$. The main dietary source of the metal for these animals, however, is $MeHg^+$ in fish or other marine organisms that also contain considerable Se. A considerable portion of orally administered $^{14}CH_3^{203}Hg^+$ was found to be demethylated over a period of 105 hr by sea lions.[38] Hg and Se are present in a 1:1 molar ratio in sea lion liver[39] and in the liver of other marine mammals[34,35] which, along with the tissue distribution data, suggests that Se plays a major role in protecting sea lions against Hg toxicity.

There have been many reports that treatment of animals with Se can alter the tissue distribution of heavy metals. In addition to affecting tissue concentrations of Cd^{+2}, Hg^{+2}, and $MeHg^+$, Se can alter levels of other metals such as Ag^+,[40] Tl^+,[1,41] or Zn^{+2}, Cu^{+2}, Mg^{+2}, and Ca^{+2} in animals.[42] There is some disagreement, however, as to whether the Cd or Hg content of tissues are increased or decreased by Se compounds. The lack of agreement appears to be related to differences in the metal or Se dose, metal to Se ratios, route, and time sequence of administration, as well as a failure to correct for the metal content of blood retained in tissues. In addition, the level of Se in the control diet may be significant (>0.02-0.05 ppm Se) and/or other uncontrolled dietary factors may play a role. As an example, Chen *et al.*[43] found that 0.5 ppm Se as selenite in the diet decreased the Hg content of liver and kidney when 2 ppm Hg as dietary $MeHg^+$ was fed but caused increases when 10 ppm Hg as $MeHg^+$ was used. A 1:1 molar ratio of Se:metal has been shown to produce maximum modification in the tissue distribution of Hg^{+2} by selenite when both elements were administered by injection.[44]

Chen and co-workers also showed that injection of 0.8 mg/kg body weight Se as ^{75}Se-selenite 30 min prior to injection with 1 ppm $^{109}Cd^{+2}$/ kg body weight increased the uptake of Cd in testis of rat at both 30 min[30] and 1 hr[31] after treatment. They also showed that Se greatly increased blood and plasma Cd but lowered liver and kidney Cd levels. In most of these studies, however, metal and Se levels were not corrected for retained blood in tissues.

Johnson and Pond[45] observed that 3 ppm Se as selenite in the diet increased the metal content of liver when 320 ppm Hg^{+2} was fed to rats for 4 weeks. Dietary Hg^{+2} increased Se levels in kidney, had no effect on the brain, but decreased levels in liver and muscle. Potter and Matrone[46] found similar results in liver and small increases of Hg in spleen and testis due to Se when 40 or 400 ppm Hg^{+2} and 5 ppm Se as selenite were fed to rats for 3 weeks. Hg in kidney was decreased by Se at dietary levels of 40 ppm Hg^{+2} and 5 ppm Se as selenite were fed to rats for 3 weeks. Hg in kidney was decreased by Se at dietary levels of 40 ppm Hg^{+2} and increased at 400 ppm Hg^{+2}. Chen et al.[32] found that injection of 0.8 mg Se/kg as ^{75}Se-selenite 30 min before injection of 2 mg [203]Hg^{+2}/body weight in rat caused large increases in blood and plasma Hg, and increase in testis, a slight increase in liver, and a large decrease in kidney at 1 hr. Groth[13,47] showed that administration of 50 ppm Hg^{+2} and 5-15 ppm Se as selenate in the drinking water of rats over 20 months caused an increase in the Hg and Se content of lymph nodes and, contrary to the findings of short-term experiments, also in kidney. This increase was associated with the formation of black particles containing Hg and Se.

Fang[33] observed that oral administration by intubation of 0.6-2 mg[203] Hg^{+2}/kg and 0.1-0.3 mg Se/kg body weight as[75] Se-selenite caused increases in the Hg contents of blood, liver, spleen, pancreas, heart, lung, muscle, brain, reproductive organ and a large decrease in kidney of rats over a 96 hr period. The order of effectiveness in inducing these changes was selenomethionine > selenocystine > selenate > selenite.

Moffitt and Clary[44] carried out a long-term study on Se-Hg interactions in rats fed a standard laboratory diet containing 0.2-0.3 ppm Se. Levels of Se and Hg in tissues were corrected for retained blood. Simultaneous injection of 1 mg [203]Hg^{+2} and 1 mg Se/kg body weight as selenite caused a large decrease in kidney Hg and an increase in blood Hg at 1 day relative to the results obtained in the absence of Se treatment (Table 21.1). When Hg^{+2} alone was given to the animals, Hg was eliminated from all tissues after one day, but significant metal was retained by kidney at 28 days. Including selenite in the diet caused all tissues, except kidney, to retain more Hg at 28 days than in those rats not receiving selenite. Between 4 and 28 days, there was a delayed buildup of Hg in liver, spleen, and kidney in the selenite fed animals, with the liver accumulating the largest portion of the dose. The delayed buildup in Hg may be related to the formation of black bodies containing Hg and Se as seen by Groth[13,47] in these tissues.

We have also studied the influence of Se on the tissue and subcellular distribution of Hg in two separate studies with rats.[48,49] Two weeks prior to dosing with Se and Hg, animals were placed on a torula yeast Se-deficient diet containing 0.02 ppm Se. In the first experiment,[48] doses of 0.5 mg [203]Hg^{+2}/kg and 0.5 mg Se/body weight as ^{75}Se-selenite

Table 21.1 Distribution and Excretion of ^{203}Hg in Rats at Various Times After Administration of ^{203}HgCl$_2$ or ^{203}HgCl$_2$ and Sodium Selenite[a]

Day	Group	Percent of Administered Dose ^{203}Hg/Tissue or Fraction[b]					
		Blood	Liver	Kidney	Lung	Spleen	Urine and Feces (cumulative)[d]
1	Hg	4.0 (10.3)	9.2 (6.8)	33.5 (29.9)	0.3 (0.1)	0.4 (0.3)	20.6
	Hg+Se	21.1 (27.2)	16.6 (12.0)	2.0 (1.8)	1.2 (0.61)	1.6 (1.3)	1.7
4	Hg	1.0 (5.3)	2.6 (1.9)	27.5 (24.0)	0.1 (<0.1)	0.1 (<0.1)	53.8
	Hg+Se	9.2 (15.7)	18.1 (13.2)	3.1 (2.7)	1.1 (0.4)	2.4 (2.0)	3.5
14	Hg	<0.1 (2.2)	0.3 (0.2)	15.9 (13.9)	<0.1 (<0.1)	<0.1 (<0.1)	61.8
	Hg+Se	3.7 (16.6)	40.3 (29.4)	6.1 (5.3)	0.9 (0.4)	4.1 (3.4)	7.7
28	Hg	<0.1 (1.5)	0.2 (0.2)	10.2 (8.9)	<0.1 (<0.1)	<0.1 (<0.1)	64.5
	Hg+Se	1.3 (17.6)	51.7 (37.7)	8.8 (7.7)	0.7 (0.3)	4.5 (3.7)	12.3

[a]Data from Moffitt and Clary.[44]

[b]Values in parentheses represent data corrected for retained blood in the tissues.

[c]For estimation of % administered dose ^{203}Hg/total blood, it was assumed that the blood represents 5.5% of the total body weight.

[d]Urine and feces data represent cumulative percentage excretion.

were simultaneously injected. At day 1 the distribution of Se and Hg in tissues resembled that found by Moffitt and Clary[44] but differed significantly at later times (Tables 21.2 and 21.3). We observed no delayed

Table 21.2 Distribution of Mercury in Rats Receiving Inorganic Mercury

Day	Group	Blood	Liver	Kidney	Brain	Muscle
1	Hg	1.96	10.1	48.6	0.01	2.06
	Hg+Se	17.3	20.7	2.41	<0.01	0.60
8	Hg	0.10	2.00	52.6	0.02	0.73
	Hg+Se	9.66	19.0	7.16	0.02	2.20
29	Hg	0.02	0.50	23.6	< .01	0.21
	Hg+Se	1.89	10.6	11.5	0.02	0.94
85	Hg	< 0.01	0.05	3.03	<0.01	0.07
	Hg+Se	0.05	8.59	4.67	0.01	1.69

Percent of Administered Mercury[a]

[a]Mean of two adult male Wistar rats, corrected for retained blood. Animals received a simultaneous intraperitoneal dose of 0.5 mg $^{203}Hg^{+2}$/kg and 0.5 mg Se/kg body weight as ^{75}Se-selenite. [48]

Table 21.3 Distribution of Selenium in Rats Receiving Inorganic or Methyl Mercury

Percent of Administered Selenium[a]

Day	Group	Blood	Liver	Kidney	Brain	Muscle
1	Hg+Se	12.02	21.1	3.29	0.07	2.30
8	Hg+Se	5.14	15.7	1.27	0.07	4.18
29	Hg+Se	3.49	7.04	2.16	0.11	4.31
85	Hg+Se	1.52	4.62	0.30	0.04	3.61
1	MeHg+Se	6.00	17.8	4.23	0.14	3.88
8	MeHg+Se	2.99	3.75	1.29	0.06	3.06
29	MeHg+Se	5.93	3.95	2.72	0.22	9.16
85	MeHg+Se	0.66	0.21	0.10	0.02	1.89

[a]Mean of two adult male Wistar rats, corrected for retained blood. Animals received a simultaneous intraperitoneal dose of 0.5 mg Hg/kg as $^{203}Hg^{+2}$ or Me$^{203}Hg^{+}$ and 0.5 mg Se/kg body weight as ^{75}Se-selenite. [48,49]

buildup of Hg in the liver (Figure 21.1) and spleen. The findings of Groth[13,47] and the observation that Se stimulates the immune response[50] suggested that the absence of a delayed accumulation of Hg in liver and

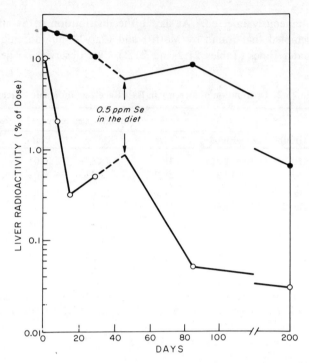

Figure 21.1 Percent of radioactivity administered as ^{203}HgCl$_2$ recovered in rat liver with respect to time and dietary Se content. ○ ^{203}HgCl$_2$ alone; ● ^{203}HgCl$_2$ plus Na$_2$^{75}SeO$_3$.[48]

spleen may be due to the depletion of Se in the animals. Nevertheless, liver contained much more Hg when Se was injected than without initial Se treatment (Figure 21.1), whereas accumulation of Hg in kidney (Table 21.2) was delayed by Se. By day 85, more Hg accumulated in liver than in kidney due to initial Se treatment, as found in the case of sea lions.[37,51] At day 200, however, the distribution was reversed and kidney contained more Hg than liver. Even at this time, blood and all tissues of Se treated animals contained more Hg than those not dosed with Se (Table 21.2). Similar molar quantities of Se and Hg were present in most of the tissues. Addition of 0.5 ppm Se as selenite to the diet at day 46 did not affect elimination of Hg from liver (Figure 21.1) or other tissues (Table 21.2), except possibly in the kidney.

Chen et al.[43] found that dietary selenite (0.5 ppm Se) decreased Hg levels in liver and kidney in rats fed a diet containing 2 ppm Hg as MeHg$^+$, but increased Hg concentrations in these organs when 10 ppm Hg as MeHg$^+$ was included in the diet. Johnson and Pond[45] fed 25 ppm Hg as MeHg$^+$ and 3 ppm Se as selenite to rats for 4 weeks. High dietary Se generally increased the levels of Se in most tissues, except brain and also caused an accumulation of Hg in liver. In animals fed high concentrations of Se in the diet, dietary MeHg$^+$ increased the level of Se in kidney, slightly increased Se in muscle, had no effect on Se in liver, but markedly increased the content of the brain. This latter effect could be involved in Se protection of the central nervous system against MeHg$^+$ toxicity. Potter and Matrone[46] showed that dietary selenite (5 ppm Se) did not significantly increase Hg accumulation in kidney from dietary MeHg$^+$ (10-40 ppm Hg) yet prevented MeHg$^+$ induced reduction in kidney size. This was undboutedly due to the increase in kidney Se noted by Johnson and Pond.[45] Potter and Matrone[46] noted that the selenite-induced differences between rats actually increased when MeHg$^+$ dosing was stopped, yet the Se-induced differences in Hg content in liver and kidney disappeared. Chen et al.[52] found that pretreatment of rats with 0.8 ppm Se as selenite by injection followed by injection of 2 mg Hg/kg body weight as MeHg$^+$ resulted in a high Hg accumulation in brain; small increases in the Hg content of blood, spleen, and testis; no change in Hg concentration of liver or heart; and decreases in plasma and kidney Hg. The large increase in brain Hg found by Chen et al.[52] is accompanied by a similar increase in Se.[45]

Iwata et al.[53] analyzed the MeHg$^+$ content of tissues in rats injected with 0.5 mg Se/kg as selenite and dosed orally with 10 mg Hg/kg body weight as MeHg$^+$ for 8-10 days. Selenite treatment caused an increase in the MeHg$^+$ concentration in brain and little change in heart, liver, kidney, or blood at day 1, but greatly decreased MeHg$^+$ levels in all organs after 7 days over those observed in rats receiving MeHg$^+$ alone. Stillings et al.[12] found that 0.6 ppm Se as selenite or 17% fish protein concentrate and 25 ppm Hg as MeHg$^+$ in the diet decreased total Hg levels in rat liver, kidney and brain after 6 weeks, but caused an increase in muscle and blood Hg. Dietary selenite decreased both urinary and fecal excretion of Hg. Fish protein concentrate also decreased urinary Hg excretion but increased fecal excretion moderately, suggesting that factors other than Se may be important.

Froseth et al.[11] fed a low Se diet (0.03-0.05 ppm Se) alone or supplemented with 0.1 or 5.0 ppm Se as selenite for up to 7 weeks to swine which were given 7 mg Hg/kg body weight as MeHg$^+$ orally at 5 weeks into the experiment. Se produced a decrease in total Hg levels of bicep muscle, cerebrum, heart, liver, kidney and blood.

We also conducted a second 200-day rat experiment[49] identical to that described for Hg^{+2},[48] except that 0.5 mg Hg/kg body weight as Me^{203}Hg$^+$ was injected into the animals. At day 1, Hg levels in blood, liver, kidney and spleen were much lower in selenite-treated animals than in those not given selenite but caused large increases in Hg concentration of brain and muscle (Table 21.4). In fact, 56% of the dose of

Table 21.4 Distribution of Mercury in Rats Receiving Methylmercury

Day	Group	Blood	Liver	Kidney	Brain	Muscle
			Percent of Administered Mercury[a]			
1	MeHg	43.6	2.47	4.14	0.06	15.9
	MeHg+Se	21.2	1.72	1.00	0.84	56.4
8	MeHg	24.2	0.87	4.30	0.17	25.3
	MeHg+Se	27.3	1.14	3.77	0.30	31.5
29	MeHg	14.5	1.90	8.64	0.15	21.2
	MeHg+Se	10.9	1.83	7.23	0.17	15.7
85	MeHg	0.25	0.03	0.83	0.01	0.62
	MeHg+Se	0.28	0.08	0.87	0.01	0.44

[a]Mean of two adult male Wistar rats corrected for retained blood. Animals received a simultaneous intraperitoneal dose of 0.5 mg Hg/kg $Me^{203}Hg^+$ and 0.5 mg Se/kg body weight as ^{75}Se-selenite. [49]

$MeHg^+$ accumulated in the muscle of selenite injected rats (Figure 21.2). While the molar amounts of ^{75}Se in other tissues were comparable to the ^{203}Hg present, the ^{75}Se content of skeletal muscle was considerably lower than that of ^{203}Hg (Table 21.3). This suggests that Se may divert $MeHg^+$ into muscle. It is known that selenomethionine is deposited in muscle to a greater extent than selenocysteine or selenite.[54] This may account in part for the protective effect of Se against $MeHg^+$ toxicity.

In the absence of continuing Se treatment, the Hg content in tissues and blood became similar to values found in those animals that received no Se injection (Table 21.4). The total amount of Hg and Se in various tissues and blood remained almost constant, however, through day 29. When 0.5 ppm Se as selenite was added to the diet at day 46 there was a drastic reduction in Hg levels in all tissues and blood (Table 21.4) as shown for muscle in Figure 21.2. The apparent half-life of ^{203}Hg on the basis of two data points was about 7 days for all tissues. Since the data are limited, however, the actual half-life of $MeHg^+$ may be less initially in some tissues. The biological half-life of $MeHg^+$ in the rat has been reported to be approximately 16 days.[55] This suggests that Se may be required for elimination of $MeHg^+$ from tissues and blood and provides another mechanism for Se protection against $MeHg^+$ toxicity.

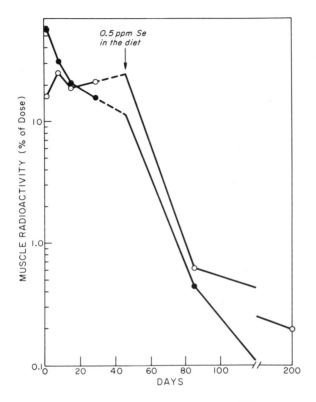

Figure 21.2 Percent of radioactivity administered as [203]Hg-methylmercury recovered in rat muscle with respect to time and dietary Se content. ○ [203]Hg-methylmercury alone; ● [203]Hg-methylmercury plus Na_2[75]SeO_3.[49]

Subcellular Distribution

There is little information on the influence of Se on the subcellular distribution of heavy metals in animal tissues. Chen et al.[30] found that administration of ^{75}Se-selenite to rats 30 min before [109]Cd^{+2} administration, increased the percentage of [109]Cd in the cell cytosol fraction of testis while decreasing the metal content of the crude nuclear fraction. Chen et al.[31] showed selenite treatment resulted in a decrease in the percentage of [109]Cd in the crude nuclear fractions of these tissues. The changes in the cell cytosol seemed to reflect decreases in [109]Cd levels of liver and kidney and an increase in that of testis. Chen and co-workers extended their studies[32,52] to Hg^{+2} and $MeHg^+$. Selenite pretreatment of rats dosed with [203]Hg^{+2} produced changes in the Hg content of subcellular fractions similar to those observed previously with Cd. In this case, the ^{203}Hg content of liver was slightly increased over non-Se-treated animals, due to ^{203}Hg in retained blood, but the percentage of ^{203}Hg in the cell cytosol decreased as with Cd. With MeHg$^+$, no selenite induced change in the subcellular distribution of ^{203}Hg was noted with brain, liver, kidney or spleen.

We have determined the subcellular distribution of Hg and Se in the tissues of rats simultaneously injected with 0.5 ppm Hg as ^{203}Hg^{+2},[48] or Me^{203}Hg$^+$,[49] and 0.5 mg Se/kg body weight as ^{75}Se-selenite over a period of 200 days. The animals were intially depleted of Se by placing them on a torula yeast diet (0.02 ppm Se) two weeks prior to dosing. In the case of rats dosed with Hg^{+2}, selenite altered the subcellular distribution of Hg in liver and kidney, causing a large increase of Hg levels in nuclei and a corresponding decrease in that of the cytosol (Table 21.5).

Table 21.5   Distribution of Mercury in Subcellular Fractions of Rats Dosed with Inorganic or Methyl Mercury

Tissue and Treatment	Percent of Total Tissue Mercury[a]				
	Nuclei	Mitochondria	Lysosomes	Microsomes	Cytosol
Liver					
Hg	17.5	12.6	5.3	3.0	61.7
Hg+Se	47.9	22.9	8.7	4.6	15.9
Kidney					
Hg	8.0	10.2	11.6	5.7	64.6
Hg+Se	26.6	25.5	13.1	7.5	27.4
Liver					
MeHg	26.5	20.3	6.2	3.0	44.1
MeHg+Se	24.8	21.9	5.0	3.0	44.4
Kidney					
MeHg	19.1	14.3	8.2	7.8	50.7
MeHg+Se	19.7	12.9	10.7	8.9	47.9

[a]Mean of two animals at day 1. [48,49]

These results were similar to those obtained by Chen et al.[32] Selenite treatment also resulted in the accumulation of Hg in the mitochondrial fraction. These Se-induced changes in liver persisted through day 200, whereas after day 1 the kidney values became similar to those seen in the absence of selenite administration. In all cases, there was a gradual decline in the ^{203}Hg content of the liver and kidney cytosol fractions and a slow increase in that of the nuclear fraction over the 200-day experimental period. Addition of 0.5 ppm Se as selenite to the diet at day 46 caused only slight increases in the percentage of [203]Hg in liver and kidney nuclear fractions. Fang[33] noted similar changes in the subcellular distribution of [203]Hg in rats treated orally with Hg^{+2} and either selenomethionine, selenocystine, selenate, or selenite. The first three selenium compounds were more effective than selenite in affecting Hg levels in the subcellular fractions. There was little difference in the [203]Hg content of subcellular fractions from rats dosed with $Me^{203}Hg^+$ whether or not the animals also were given selenite (Table 21.5).

In these experiments, the percentage distribution of [203]Hg from injection of Hg^{+2} or $MeHg^+$ and ^{75}Se from selenite were similar in liver subcellular fractions. In kidney, however, the [203]Hg tended to accumulate to a greater extent in the cell cytosol whereas ^{75}Se concentrated more in the nuclear fraction. This difference may in part be due to the tendency of Hg^{+2} to bind to metallothionein and $MeHg^+$ to hemoglobin, both proteins occurring in the soluble fraction.

Shift Among Cytosol Components

Chen et al.[30] found that injection of ^{75}Se-selenite in rats resulted in a shift of [109]Cd^{+2} bound in the cell cytosol of testis from small protein molecules, molecular weight 10,000 (metallothionein) and 30,000, to one or more high molecular weight proteins that also contained [75]Se (Figure 21.3). These workers speculated that this may be a mechanism by which Se would protect against Cd-induced testicular damage. Chen et al.[31] subsequently confirmed that this Se-induced diversion occurs in the cell cytosol of rat kidney and plasma. A similar shift also occurred with [203]Hg^{+2} in the cytosol of fractions of rat liver, kidney, testis and in plasma.[32] The high molecular weight [203]Hg binding macromolecules also contain ^{75}Se, but they are not of the same size as those that bind [109]Cd and [75]Se. These findings suggest that Hg and Cd may bind specifically to different proteins of high molecular weight. Chen et al.[52] showed that Se failed to affect the proportion of $MeHg^+$ occurring in the cytosol fractions of rat liver, brain, spleen and red blood cells and in plasma. Se treatment caused the disappearance of Hg from the metallothionein peak but no other changes in the gel filtration pattern of the kidney cytosol fraction. Since metallothionein only binds Hg^{+2} and not $MeHg^+$,[43] a Se-induced loss in Hg bound to metallothionein could result from either a diversion of Hg^{+2} to other subcellular fractions or a reduced function of Hg^{+2} from demethylation of $MeHg^+$. This Se effect provides another possible mechanism for protection by Se compounds against Cd^{+2} or Hg^{+2} toxicity. Fang,[33] however, found that oral administration of [203]Hg^{+2} and selenite did not appreciably alter the distribution of Hg in soluble proteins of rat liver and kidney.

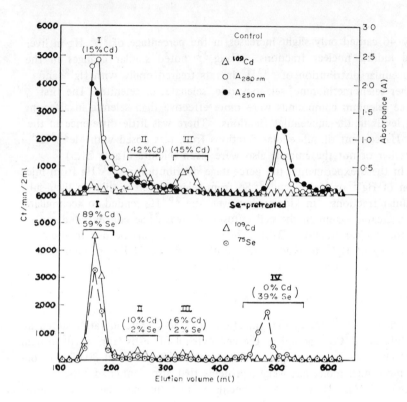

Figure 21.3 Sephadex G-75 chromatography of the soluble fraction from the testis of control or Se-pretreated rats.[30]

Mercury-Selenium Aggregates and Possible Immune Response

Groth *et al.*[13,47] have found from simultaneous feeding of Hg^{+2} and selenate that the mechanism of protection against Hg^{+2} may involve Hg-Se bond formation and aggregation. Black particles containing Hg and Se in a 1:1 molar ratio were seen in lymph nodes, liver, spleen, small intestine, stomach, lung and kidney. The black particles were present in macrophages, in lymph nodes, spleen, lung, liver and kidney. Treatment with tellurate and Hg^{+2}, however, did not cause formation of particles though Te protected better than Se against Hg-induced kidney nephritis. Spallholz and co-workers[50] have shown that dietary selenite enhances the immune response in mice. Phagacytosis thus may play an important role in Se protection against heavy metals.

Biochemical Interactions

Dietary selenite but not vitamin E may decrease mitochondrial swelling caused by Cd^{+2} or Hg^{+2} *in vitro.*[56] Recently, selenite has been shown to accelerate mitochondrial swelling caused by thiols such as cysteine or reduced glutathione.[57] Compounds of Cd^{+2} and Hg^{+2} are potent inhibitors of the selenite catalyzed swelling. Swelling ability paralleled the Se status of the animal and mitochondrial glutathione peroxidase level.[58] Mitochondrial swelling due to reduced glutathione or a combination of reduced and oxidized glutathione is accompanied by a loss of mitochondrial proteins, including glutathione peroxidase.[59]

Levels of glutathione peroxidase, a Se-containing enzyme, in the cell cytosol are sensitive to the Se status of the animal.[60,61] Dietary Ag^{+} and Hg^{+2}, but not Pb^{+2} or Cd^{+2} inhibit activity in Se-adequate animals.[21] Injected Cd^{+2} also was found to cause no inhibition of glutathione peroxidase in plasma, testis, liver and kidney of rats on a purified diet but injected with selenite.[62] Injection of Cd^{+2} into animals with no selenite pretreatment, however, resulted in decreased glutathione peroxidase activity at 1.5 days in plasma and testis but not in liver or kidney.

Changes in enzyme activity prior to testicular damage did not occur. Plasma glutathione peroxidase levels returned to normal by 7 days, but levels in the testis did not. Glutathione peroxidase from testis is more sensitive to Cd^{+2} inhibition *in vitro* than the liver enzyme. Addition of selenomethionine *in vitro* or removal of Cd^{+2} by dialysis could not restore the activity of the testis enzyme.

Any process in which the Se-requiring glutathione peroxidase enzyme is directly involved thus may be sensitive to the Se and heavy metal status of the animal. For instance, glutathione peroxidase has been implicated as a factor that may inhibit the final step of prostaglandin biosynthesis.[63] Se adequacy hence should affect prostaglandin biosynthesis and Hg^{+2} and Ag^{+} would be expected to have antagonistic effects.

CONCLUSIONS

Mechanisms of detoxification of heavy metals by Se are complex and are not identical for all metals or all forms of the same metal. Mechanisms may involve a direct binding between Se and the heavy metal;[13,47] a direct binding between Se, the metal, and another small molecule or macromolecule[24] or an indirect stoichiometric or catalytic effect of Se mediated by other molecules such as an enzyme. The affinity of Hg^{+2}, $MgHg^{+2}$, and Cd^{+2} for sulfhydryl groups is very strong, but the affinity of these metals for the Se analog (R-Se-H) is much greater.[64] In addition, Se can bind to sulfhydryl groups to form R-S-Se-H derivatives.[65,66]

Detoxification may involve redistribution of the metal among tissues,[11-13,30-34,43-46,48,49,52,53] subcellular fractions,[31,33,43,45,48,49,53] or molecules of the same fraction.[30-33,52] Such diversion among tissues or components may be a result of changes in the affinity of molecules for the metal[22,23] but with MeHg^{+2} there may also be Se catalyzed elimination or transport to insensitive storage sites.[49] Thus Se compounds counteract the toxicity of Cd^{+2}, Hg^{+2}, Ag$^+$, and Tl$^+$, yet cause increased retention and decreased elimination of these metals.[1] There is evidence which suggests that Se decreases excretion of MeHg$^+$ in urine and feces,[12] but other findings indicate that Se may be required for elimination of MeHg$^+$ from tissues and blood.[49] Metal levels, therefore, are not a good measure of the degree of intoxication by metals, but can be regarded as an index of previous exposure.

In addition, demethylation of MeHg$^+$ may represent a detoxification route for that biologically important form of Hg, but Se has not been shown to enhance conversion of MeHg$^+$ to Hg^{+2} by liver or kidney preparations *in vitro*.[67]

ACKNOWLEDGMENTS

This work was supported by grants Nos. ES-00210, ES-00887, NS-07413, and AM-19285 from the National Institutes of Health, U.S. Public Health Service. Manuscript issued as Technical Paper No. 4327 from the Oregon Agricultural Experiment Station.

REFERENCES

1. Diplock, A. T. "Metabolic Aspects of Selenium Action and Toxicity," *CRC Crit. Rev. Toxicol.* 5:271-329 (1976).
2. Hoekstra, W. G. "Biochemical Role of Selenium," In: *Trace Element Metabolism in Animals,* Vol. 2. W. G. Hoekstra, J. W. Suttie, H. E. Ganther and W. Mertz, Eds. (Baltimore, Maryland: University Park Press, 1974), pp. 61-77.
3. Stadtman, T. C. "Selenium Biochemistry," *Science* 183:915-922 (1974).
4. Frost, D. V. and P. M. Lish. "Selenium in Biology," *Ann. Rev. Pharm.* 15:259-284 (1975).
5. Kar, A. B., R. P. Das and B. Mukerji. "Prevention of Cadmium-Induced Changes in the Gonads of the Rat by Zinc and Selenium: A Study in Antagonism Between Metals in the Biological System," *Proc. Natl. Inst. Sci. India* Section B, Supplement 26:40-50 (1960).
6. Parizek, J., J. Kalouskova, A. Babicky, J. Benes and L. Pavlik. "Interaction of Selenium with Mercury, Cadmium, and Other Toxic Metals," In *Trace Element Metabolism in Animals,* Vol. 2, W. G. Hoekstra, J. W. Suttie, H. E. Ganther and W. Mertz, Eds. (Baltimore, Maryland: University Park Press, 1974), pp. 119-131.

7. Ganther, H. E., P. A. Wagner, M. L. Sunde and W. G. Hoekstra. "Protective Effects of Selenium Against Heavy Metal Toxicities," In *Sixth Annual Conference on Trace Substances in Environmental Health,* D. D. Hemphill, Ed. (Columbia, Missouri: University of Missouri Press, 1972), pp. 247-252.
8. Ganther, H. E., C. Goudie, M. L. Sunde, M. J. Kopecky, P. Wagner, S. H. Oh and W. G. Hoekstra. "Selenium: Relation to Decreased Toxicity of Methylmercury Added to Diets Containing Tuna," *Science* 175:1122-1124 (1972).
9. Ganther, H. E. and M. L. Sunde. "Effect of Tuna Fish and Selenium on the Toxicity of Methylmercury: A Progress Report," *J. Food Sci.* 39:1-5 (1974).
10. Hill, C. H. "Interrelationships of Selenium with Other Trace Elements," *Fed. Proc.* 34:2096-2100 (1975).
11. Froseth, J. A., R. C. Piper and J. R. Carlson. "Relationship of Dietary Selenium and Oral Methyl Mercury to Blood and Tissue Selenium and Mercury Concentrations and Deficiency-Toxicity Signs in Swine," *Fed. Proc.* 33:660 (1974).
12. Stillings, B. R., H. Lagally, P. Bauersfeld and J. Soares. "Effect of Cystine, Selenium and Fish Protein on the Toxicity and Metabolism of Methylmercury in Rats," *Toxicol. Appl. Pharmacol.* 30:243-254 (1974).
13. Groth, D. H., L. Stettler and G. Mackay. "Interactions of Mercury, Cadmium, Selenium, Tellurium, Arsenic and Beryllium," In *Effects and Dose-Response Relationships of Toxic Metals,* G. F. Nordberg, Ed. (Amsterdam, The Netherlands: Elsevier Scientific Publishing Co., 1976), pp. 527-543.
14. Welsh, S. O. and J. H. Soares, Jr. "The Effects of Selenium and Vitamin E on Methyl Mercury Toxicity in the Japanese Quail," *Fed. Proc.* 34:913 (1975).
15. Kasuya, M. "The Effect of Vitamin E on the Toxicity of Alkyl Mercurials on Nervous Tissue in Culture," *Toxicol. Appl. Pharmacol.* 32:347-354 (1975).
16. Welsh, S. O. "Physiological Effects of Methylmercury Toxicity. Interaction of Methylmercury with Selenium, Tellurium, and Vitamin E," *Diss. Abstr. Int.* 36(B):657-658 (1975).
17. Mason, K. E. "Vitamin E in Early Life," In *Symposium on Nutrition; The Physiological Role of Certain Vitamins and Trace Elements,* R. M. Herriott, Ed. (Baltimore, Maryland: Johns Hopkins Press, 1953), pp. 179-197.
18. Ganther, H. E. "Practical Aspects of Selenium and Mercury Interactions," *Nutri. Notes* 11:4 (1975).
19. El-Bergearmi, M., H. E. Ganther and M. L. Sunde. "Effect of Some Sulfur Amino Acids, Selenium and Arsenic on Mercury Toxicity Using Japanese Quail," *Poult. Sci.* 53:1921 (1974).
20. Martin, J. H., P. D. Elliott, V. C. Anderlini, D. Girvin, S. A. Jacobs, R. W. Risebrough, R. L. Delong and W. G. Gilmartin. "Mercury-Selenium-Bromine Imbalance in Premature Parturient California Sea Lions," *Marine Biol.* 35:91-104 (1976).
21. Whanger, P. D. Unpublished results (1976).

22. Fang, S. C. and E. Fallin. "The Binding of Various Mercurial Compounds to Serum Proteins," *Bull. Environ. Contam. Toxicol.* 15:110-117 (1976).

23. Fang, S. C., R. W. Chen and E. Fallin. "Influence of Dietary Selenite on the Binding Characteristics of Rat Serum Proteins to Mercurial Compounds," *Chem.-Biol. Int.* 15:51-57 (1976).

24. Burk, R. F., K. A. Foster, P. M. Greenfield and K. W. Kiker. "Binding of Simultaneously Administered Inorganic Selenium and Mercury to a Rat Plasma Protein," *Proc. Soc. Exptl. Biol. Med.* 145:782-785 (1974).

25. Cousins, R. J. "Influence of Cadmium on Synthesis of Liver and Kidney Cadmium-Binding Protein," In *Trace Element Metabolism in Animals,* Vol. 2, W. G. Hoekstra, J. W. Suttie, H. E. Ganther and W. Mertz, Eds. (Baltimore, Maryland: University Park Press, 1974), pp. 503-505.

26. Piotrowski, J. K., B. Trojanowska, J. M. Wisniewska-Knypl and W. Bolanowska. "Mercury Binding in the Kidney and Liver of Rats Repeatedly Exposed to Mercuric Chloride: Induction of Metallothionein by Mercury and Cadmium," *Toxicol. Appl. Pharmacol.* 27:11-19 (1974).

27. Day, F. A., B. J. Coles and F. O. Brady. "Post-Induction Actinomycin D Effects on the Levels of Zinc-Thionein and Copper-Chelatin in Rat Liver," *Fed. Proc.* 35:1681 (1976).

28. Bryan, S. E. and H. A. Hidalgo. "Nuclear [115]Cadmium: Uptake and Disappearance Correlated with Cadmium-Binding Protein Synthesis," *Biochem. Biophys. Res. Commun.* 68:858-866 (1976).

29. Bryan, S. E., S. J. Simons, D. L. Vizard and K. J. Hardy. "Interactions of Mercury and Copper with Constitutive Heterochromatin and Euchromatin *In Vivo* and *In Vitro,*" *Biochemistry* 15:1667-1676 (1976).

30. Chen, R. W., P. A. Wagner, G. W. Hoekstra and H. E. Ganther. "Affinity Labeling Studies with 109-Cadmium in Cadmium-Induced Testicular Injury in Rats," *J. Reprod. Fertil.* 38:293-306 (1974).

31. Chen, R. W., P. D. Whanger and P. H. Weswig. "Selenium-Induced Redistribution of Cadmium Binding to Tissue Proteins: A Possible Mechanism of Protection Against Cadmium Toxicity," *Bioinorg. Chem.* 4:125-133 (1975).

32. Chen, R. W., P. D. Whanger and S. C. Fang. "Diversion of Mercury Binding in Rat Tissues by Selenium: A Possible Mechanism of Protection," *Pharmacol. Res. Commun.* 6:571-579 (1974). (1974).

33. Fang, S. C. "Interaction of Selenium and Mercury in the Rat," *Chem.-Biol. Int.* (1977).

34. Koeman, J. H., W. H. M. Peeters, C. H. M. Koudstaal-Hol, P. S. Tjioe and J. J. M. de Goeij. "Mercury-Selenium Correlations in Marine Mammals," *Nature* 245:385-386 (1973).

35. Koeman, J. H., W. S. M. van de Ven, J. J. M. de Goeij, P. S. Tjioe and J. L. van Haaften. "Mercury and Selenium in Marine Mammals and Birds," *Sci. Total Environ.* 3:279-287 (1975).

36. Anas, R. E. "Heavy Metals in the Northern Fur Seal, *Callorhinus ursinus*, and Harbor Seal, *Phoca vitulina Richardi,*" *Fish. Bull.* 72:133-137 (1974).

37. Buhler, D. R., R. R. Claeys and B. R. Mate. "Heavy Metal and Chlorinated Hydrocarbon Residues in California Sea Lions (*Zalophus californianus californianus*)," *J. Fish. Res. Bd. Can.* 32:2391-2397 (1975).

38. Buhler, D. R. and B. R. Mate. "The Fate of $^{14}CH_3$ $^{203}HgCl$ in the California Sea Lion," *Toxicol. Appl. Pharmacol.* 33:189 (1975).

39. Rimerman, R. A. and D. R. Buhler. unpublished results (1976).

40. Swanson, A. B., P. A. Wagner, H. E. Ganther and W. G. Hoekstra. "Antagonistic Effects of Silver and Tri-*o*-Cresyl Phosphate on Selenium and Glutathione Peroxidase in Rat Liver and Erythrocytes," *Fed. Proc.* 33:693 (1974).

41. Rusiecki, W. and J. Brzezinski. "Influence of Sodium Selenate on Acute Thallium Poisonings," *Acta Pol. Pharm.* 23:69-74 (1966).

42. Burch, R. E., R. V. Williams and J. F. Sullivan. "Effects of Se and Co on Tissue Trace Metals," *Fed. Proc.* 32:886 (1973).

43. Chen, R. W., H. E. Ganther and W. G. Hoekstra. "Studies on the Binding of Methylmercury by Thionein," *Biochem. Biophys. Res. Commun.* 51:383-390 (1973).

44. Moffitt, A. E., Jr. and J. J. Clary. "Selenite-Induced Binding of Inorganic Mercury in Blood and Other Tissues in the Rat," *Res. Commun. Chem. Pathol. Pharmacol.* 7:593-603 (1974).

45. Johnson, S. L. and W. G. Pond. "Inorganic vs. Organic Hg Toxicity in Growing Rats: Protection by Dietary Se But Not Zn," *Nutri. Rep. Internat.* 9:135-147 (1974).

46. Potter, S. and G. Matrone. "Effect of Selenite on the Toxicity of Dietary Methyl Mercury and Mercuric Chloride in the Rat," *J. Nutri.* 104:638-647 (1974).

47. Groth, D. H., L. Vignati, L. Lowry, G. Mackay and H. E. Stokinger. "Mutual Antagonistic and Synergistic Effects of Inorganic Selenium and Mercury Salts in Chronic Experiments," In: *Sixth Annual Conference on Trace Substances in Environmental Health,* D. D. Hemphill, Ed. (Columbia, Missouri: University of Missouri Press, 1972), pp. 187-189.

48. Rimerman, R. A., M. C. Henderson and D. R. Buhler. "Selenium and Inorganic Mercury Interactions in the Rat," *Chem.-Biol. Int.* submitted.

49. Rimerman, R. A., M. C. Henderson and D. R. Buhler. "Selenium and Methylmercury Interactions in the Rat," *Chem.-Biol. Int.* submitted.

50. Spallholz, J. E., J. L. Martin, M. L. Gerlach and R. H. Heinzerling. "Immunologic Responses of Mice Fed Diets Supplemented with Selenite Selenium," *Proc. Soc. Exptl. Biol. Med.* 143:685-689 (1973).

51. Lee, S. S., B. R. Mate, K. T. von der Trenck, R. A. Rimerman and D. R. Buhler. "Metallothionein and Subcellular Localization of Mercury and Cadmium in Sea Lion Tissues," *Comp. Biochem. Physiol.,* in press (1977).

52. Chen, R. W., V. L. Lacy and P. D. Whanger. "Effect of Selenium on Methylmercury Binding to Subcellular and Soluble Proteins in Rat Tissues," *Res. Commun. Chem. Pathol. Pharmacol.* 12:297-308 (1975).
53. Iwata, H., H. Okamoto and Y. Ohsawa. "Effect of Selenium on Methylmercury Poisoning," *Res. Commun. Chem. Pathol. Pharmacol.* 5:673-680 (1973).
54. Martin, J. L. and J. A. Hurlbut. "Difference Between the Metabolic Fate of Selenomethionine and Selenocysteine," *Fed. Proc.* 34:924 (1975).
55. Clarkson, T. W. "The Pharmacodynamics of Mercury and Its Compounds with Emphasis on the Short-Chain Alkylmercurials," In: *Proceedings of the Workshop on Mercury in the Western Environment,* D. R. Buhler, Ed. (Corvallis, Oregon: Oregon State University Continuing Education Publications, 1973), pp. 332-360.
56. Morris, V. C. and O. A. Levander. "Effects of Dietary Selenium, Vitamin E, and Crude Diet on Spontaneous, Heavy Metal Induced, or Energy-Linked Swelling of Rat Liver Mitochondria," *Fed. Proc.* 31:691 (1972).
57. Levander, O. A., V. C. Morris and D. J. Higgs. "Acceleration of Thiol-Induced Swelling of Rat Liver Mitochondria by Selenium," *Biochemistry* 12:4586-4590 (1973).
58. Morris, V. C. and D. J. Higgs. "Selenium, Glutathione Peroxidase and Cysteine-Induced Swelling of Rat Liver Mitochondria," *Fed. Proc.* 34:925 (1975).
59. Green, R. C. and P. J. O'Brien. "The Cellular Localization of Glutathione Peroxidase and Its Release from Mitochondria During Swelling," *Biochem. Biophys. Acta* 197:31-39 (1970).
60. Chow, C. K. and A. L. Tappel. "Response of Glutathione Peroxidase to Dietary Selenium in Rats," *J. Nutri.* 104:444-451 (1974).
61. Pedersen, N. D., P. D. Whanger and P. H. Weswig. "Effect of Dietary Selenium Depletion and Repletion on Glutathione Peroxidase Levels in Rat Tissues," *Nutri. Rep. Internat.* 11:429-435 (1975).
62. Omaye, S. T. and A. L. Tappel. "Effect of Cadmium Chloride on the Rat Testicular Soluble Selenoenzyme, Glutathione Peroxidase," *Res. Commun. Chem. Pathol. Pharmacol.* 12:695-711 (1975).
63. Cook, H. W. and W. E. M. Lands. "Mechanism for Suppression of Cellular Biosynthesis of Prostaglandins," *Nature* 260:630-632 (1976).
64. Sillen, L. G. and A. E. Martell. "Stability Constants of Metal-Ion Complexes," *Chem. Soc. London Special Public. No. 17* (1964).
65. McConnell, K. P. "Metabolism of Selenium in the Mammalian Organism," *J. Agric. Food Chem.* 11:385-388 (1963).
66. Ganther, H. E. and H. S. Hsieh. "Mechanisms for the Conversion of Selenite to Selenides in Mammalian Tissues," In: *Trace Element Metabolism in Animals,* Vol. 2, W. G. Hoekstra, J. W. Suttie, H. E. Ganther and W. Mertz, Eds. (Baltimore, Maryland: University Park Press, 1974), pp. 339-353.
67. Fang, S. C. "Induction of C-Hg Cleavage Enzymes in Rat Liver by Dietary Selenite," *Res. Commun. Chem. Pathol. Pharmacol.* 9:579-582 (1974).

CHAPTER 22

EFFECTS OF HEAVY METALS
ON ISOLATED MITOCHONDRIA

G. P. Brierley

Department of Physiological Chemistry
College of Medicine
Ohio State University
Columbus, Ohio 43210

INTRODUCTION

A number of the elements of Group IIB of the periodic table (Zn, Cd, Hg), Group IB (Cu, Ag), and Group IVA (Pb, Sn) react readily with ligands available in proteins. Such strong interactions often result in alteration of conformation, stability, and function of the proteins (see References 1 and 2, for example). It is not surprising, therefore, that the complex and highly integrated activity of mitochondria should be profoundly affected by many of these metals *in vitro*. The heavy metals that presently are considered a toxicological hazard in the environment include lead, mercury and cadmium,[3] and there is at least a reasonable inference from available experiments that the reactivity of these elements with mitochondria *in situ* may be directly related to their toxicity.[4-6] This chapter summarizes some of the observed effects of these heavy metals on isolated mitochondria and discusses the applicability of these *in vitro* studies to conditions that apply *in vivo*.

LOCALIZATION AND INTEGRATION
OF MITOCHONDRIAL ACTIVITIES

Mitochondria are organelles specialized to carry out respiration and oxidative phosphorylation and represent the principle source of ATP for most mammalian cells. Figure 22.1 diagrams the morphology and the flow of components through a typical mitochondrion. The outer membrane is shown as discontinuous, since present evidence suggests that it

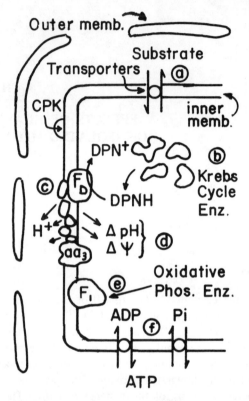

Figure 22.1 Diagram of location of mitochondrial components and possible points of alteration in the presence of heavy metals. See text for explanation and details.

is permeable to K+, sucrose and other molecules of less than 5-10,000 molecular weight. The inner membrane responds as an osmometer to K+ and sucrose and appears to represent the permeability barrier that segregates the mitochondrial components, such as the enzymes of the Krebs cycle, from the cytosol. A substrate, such as pyruvate, would be transported across the inner membrane (from the intermembrane space to the matrix compartment) by one of a series of exchange-diffusion carriers or substrate transporters, which are present (designated "a" in Figure 22.1; see References 7 and 8 for recent reviews).

The pyruvate is then degraded to CO_2 by pyruvic dehydrogenase and the Krebs cycle enzymes ("b") with reducing equivalents conserved as

DPNH. This in turn is oxidized by the DPNH-dehydrogenase and the cytochromes, Fe-S proteins, and other components that make up the electron transport system, "c." These components are embedded in and constitute an integral part of the inner membrane, with the flavoprotein localized on the matrix side, cytochrome c on the cytosol side, and cytochrome oxidase (a-a_3) spanning the membrane. Electron transport activity produces a pH gradient and secondary ion gradients (membrane potential) across the membrane.

It is still not clear whether the H+ ejection is a direct result of electron transport reactions, as postulated by Mitchell,[9] or the result of an H+ pump that utilizes chemical or conformational energy[10] to produce a pH gradient. The pH gradient is converted to ion gradients by the action of the phosphate and substrate transporters of the inner membrane.[7] If the pH gradient and membrane potential are not indeed the basic mechanism for coupling electron transport to ATP synthesis by the F_1-ATPase, "e," as suggested by Mitchell,[9] then these gradients at least reflect the energized state of the mitochondrion. Such being the case, reagents that alter permeability to anions or H+ will affect these gradients and have discernible effects on phosphorylation and respiration (reagents acting at "d" in Figure 22.1). The delivery of ADP to the matrix and ATP to the cytosol is accomplished by the adenine nucleotide transporter, and phosphate enters the matrix by either $HPOH^-$ + H+ symport or $HPOH^-/OH^-$ antiport on the phosphate transporter.[7]

Various reagents have been shown to interfere with mitochondrial activities by acting at each stage in the integrated sequence just outlined. Examples of each type of reagent are given in Table 22.1, along with a partial list of the heavy metals that also seem to act at these points.

Table 22.1

Point of Action (Figure 22.1)	Examples of Classical Reagents	Reactive Heavy Metals
(a) Substrate transporters	Butylmalonate	Pb, Hg
(b) Krebs cycle	Arsenite, malonate	Cd, Pb, Hg
(c) Electron transport system	Cyanide, antimycin	Zn, Pb, Hg
(d) Permeability to K+ –	Valinomycin	Cu, Pb, Zn, Cd, Hg
Permeability to Cl⁻ –		Pb, Hg
Permeability to H+ –	Uncouplers (dinitrophenol)	Hg, Cd
(e) Phosphorylation	Oligomycin	Hg
(f) AN transporter	Atractyloside	(?)
Pi transporter	N-ethylmaleimide	Hg, Cu

It is obvious that mitochondrial activities containing metal-reactive ligands and located on the outer surface of the inner membrane will be the first targets for low concentration of a toxic metal ion. Thus, in isolated mitochondria, the substrate and phosphate transporters and certain portions of the electron transport system are frequently found to be sensitive to metal ions. Activities and components that are sequestered behind the inner membrane will be inhibited only when the heavy metal can gain access to the matrix compartment. Such entrance of metal ions into the matrix could result from the presence of a transport mechanism, from a gradual partitioning of the heavy metal through the membrane by successive reaction with weaker binding sites, or from the complete breakdown of the barrier properties of the membrane as a result of alteration by the heavy metal.

Less extensive alteration of the membrane may also produce alterations in the permeability to K+, anions or protons, and such permeability changes often result in increased passive osmotic swelling of mitochondria suspended in saline media. Another common response is the activation of energy-dependent swelling in acetate or phosphate media by heavy metals. This reaction is thought to depend on the series of events shown in Figure 22.2[9,11] in which a primary respiration or ATP-dependent pH gradient is converted into an anion gradient (membrane potential, $\Delta\Psi$) by membrane anion transporters. Swelling is normally limited by low

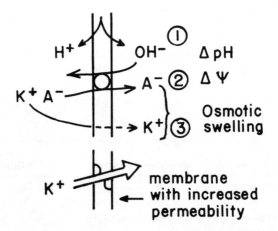

Figure 22.2 Postulated mechanism of energy-dependent osmotic swelling of isolated mitochondria. (1) Respiration or ATP-dependent pH gradient. (2) pH gradient converted to anion gradient in presence of high concentrations of phosphate, acetate or lactate. (3) Electrophoretic cation flow in response to internal negative charge. Swelling will be activated if the membrane is made more permeable to *cations*, but retains the ability to maintain pH and anion gradients.[9,11]

permeability to K+ or other cations, but in an altered membrane a rapid influx of cation will produce extensive osmotic swelling.[11,12] In some cases, such as with Pb and Zn, an energy-dependent uptake of metal into the matrix can be demonstrated,[13,14] and in these cases matrix enzymes such as the Krebs cycle components may be more sensitive to metal inhibition in the energized than in the uncoupled state. Preparation of submitochondrial particles results in inversion of the inner membrane so that the F_1-ATPase and F_D (Figure 22.1) are now oriented to the outside and are readily available for reaction with a metal ion.

With these generalizations in mind, we will now turn to a summary of the experimental evidence for the assignment of points of metal interaction given in Table 22.1.

EFFECTS OF LEAD ON ISOLATED MITOCHONDRIA

Lead provides a good example of the wide variety of effects possible when isolated mitochondria are reacted with a heavy metal, since it has been shown to produce changes in substrate and Pi uptake, Krebs cycle activity, electron transport, and permeability to ions under appropriate experimental conditions.

Uptake of Lead

Isolated heart mitochondria suspended in a KCl medium bind lead almost quantitatively in the concentration range below 50 μM (50 nmol/ mg protein) and show a limiting value near 140 nmol/mg.[13] The bulk of the binding sites are in the protein portion of the membrane.

Scott et al.[13] have reported that considerably less lead is taken up by nonrespiring mitochondria from an acetate medium and the effects of low concentrations of lead can be virtually abolished when 5-10 mM Pi is present in the medium, since precipitates of lead phosphate are formed.[15,16] Other reagents present in the suspending medium also affect the amount of lead bound. Sucrose retards the binding of lead in heart mitochondria,[13] and Parr and Harris[17] have recently noted that both sucrose and dextran increase the apparent toxicity of lead when phosphorylation is measured in isolated liver mitochondria, apparently by permitting increased delivery of soluble lead to the membrane in the presence of phosphate. A similar enhancement of lead toxicity by ATP has also been noted.[18]

Heart mitochondria have been shown to increase the uptake of lead by an energy-dependent mechanism when suspended in K+ acetate.[13] The reaction, which can be followed with murexide as an indicator or by atomic absorption, is sensitive to low levels of lanthanides and is inhibited and reversed by uncouplers of oxidative phosphorylation.[13]   Evidence for uptake of lead into the membrane or the matrix space in a KCl medium is provided by the response of bromthymol blue (Reference 13, Figure 3). This indicator shows an alkalization in the presence of 50 μM lead that closely resembles that with 100 μM Ca^{+2}. Since lead and Ca^{+2} show cross inhibition of the rate of uptake and both are sensitive to La^{+3}, it can be inferred that lead may enter the mitochondrion by way of the endogenous Ca^{+2} transporter present in the membrane.

Walton[19] has also noted the presence of electron-dense granules in rat liver mitochondria incubated with lead *in vitro* under conditions that minimize precipitation of lead salts in the medium. All of these results suggest that lead can probably penetrate the matrix space of the isolated mitochondrion and that all of the reactions outlined in the previous section and Figure 22.1 are potential sites of action for this metal *in vitro*.

Inhibition of Respiration by Lead

Lead inhibits succinate oxidation (succinic dehydrogenase plus the electron transport system) in submitochondrial particles (50% inhibition at 20 μM)[13] and uncoupled, intact beef heart mitochondria[15] at slightly lower concentrations. Succinate oxidation in corn mitochondria[16] is also sensitive to low levels of lead (about 7 μM for 50% inhibition). Iamaccone *et al.*[20] found inhibition of succinic oxidase, DPNH-cyt *c* reductase, cytochrome oxidase, and glutamic dehydrogenase by 0.5 mM Pb *in vitro*. However, the conditions employed (30 min at 37°C followed by two washes) suggest the possibility of considerable secondary alteration and no correlation of degree of inhibition with lead content at the time the enzyme assay was attempted.[20]

Oxidation of DPNH by submitochondrial particles[13] is sensitive to Pb at higher concentrations than succinate (80 μM for 50% inhibition), and Goyer (unpublished studies cited in Reference 4) has found very low levels of Pb inhibitory to pyruvate oxidation *in vitro*. These observations suggest that pyruvic dehydrogenase and possibly other Krebs cycle enzymes are more sensitive to lead than is electron transport. In addition, direct measurement of succinate exchange[13,21] indicates that lead may interfere with the transport of succinate and other substrates into the matrix space in intact mitochondria. The marked stimulation of glutamate respiration by lead under conditions of activated K+ and Cl$^-$ uptake[13] establishes that some respiratory sequences are rather insensitive to lead, however.

Lead and the Permeability of the Mitochondrial Membrane

Lead induces passive osmotic swelling of heart mitochondria suspended in KCl, a result which indicates that the membrane has been made permeable to both K+ and Cl⁻. Rather high levels of bound Pb^{+2} are required (about 75 nmol/mg to produce a ΔA_{546} of 0.1) and a similar level of lead binding produces three to four times as much swelling in K+ nitrate.[13] Since the nitrate anion is already a permeant species, this result suggests that permeability to K+ is induced at lower levels of Pb binding than is permeability to Cl⁻. Direct observation of K+ efflux with a K+ electrode (Reference 13, Figure 7) shows a rapid outflow of endogenous K+ from lead-treated mitochondria, and this outflow is more rapid and extensive from energized mitochondria.

In line with this increased permeability of lead-treated mitochondria to K+, we have noted[13] that lead stimulates the energy-dependent accumulation of K+ acetate when the reaction is supported by a lead-insensitive substrate (glutamate or ascorbate plus tetramethylphenylenediamine). As little as 10 μM lead is effective in stimulating this ion accumulation, and the osmotic swelling that accompanies the reaction and higher levels (100 μM) result in spontaneous reversal of swelling (contraction) after a brief burst of activated uptake (Reference 13, Figures 6 and 9). Of particular interest is the observation that 100 μM Pb is nearly as effective as valinomycin (2 x 10^{-7} M) in the stimulation of glutamate respiration, ejection of protons, and induction of swelling in heart mitochondria suspended in a KCl medium.[13] The activation of K+ uptake by lead and other heavy metals is clearly supportive of an electrophoretic movement of cation in response to a respiration-dependent negative membrane potential as described in Figure 23.2 and Reference 11.

Lead inhibits the accumulation of K+ acetate when succinate is used to support the reaction. In this case, since the uncoupler relieves a portion of the inhibition of respiration, we have suggested that energy-dependent accumulation of lead into the matrix may contribute to the marked inhibition of succinate-dependent reactions observed under these conditions.[13]

Mitochondria and Lead Toxicity *In Vivo*

Isotopic lead administered to intact animals has been localized in mitochondria by electron microscope autoradiography of kidneys,[22] and studies of the distribution of isotopic Pb show significant accumulation in isolated mitochondria from liver and kidney.[23] Goyer[24] noted increased mitochondrial swelling in rat kidneys following extended periods of lead feeding, and mitochondria isolated from these kidneys[25] showed increased swelling compared to controls when suspended in KCl and lower ADP/O and respiratory control ratios with pyruvate as substrate. Succinate-dependent phosphorylation was not affected.

No firm data on the lead content of these mitochondria has been presented, but Goyer[4] has cited unpublished analyses in which lead comparable to the amount necessary to abolish pyruvate respiration *in vitro* was found in kidney mitochondria from lead-fed rats. The experimental situation is complicated by the fact that kidney mitochondria usually show poor respiratory control, low State 3 respiration and phosphorylation and deteriorate rapidly when prepared in the absence of a chelator. Addition of EDTA or EGTA during the preparation improves each of these parameters but raises the possibility of lead removal from the mitochondria of lead-fed rats. In addition, a number of secondary complications may affect mitochondria isolated from lead-intoxicated and other necrotic tissue. One of these would be the presence of excess free fatty acid released by Ca^{+2}- or lead-activated endogenous lipases. A fatty acid vector for mitochondrial deterioation is suggested by the fact that kidney mitochondria prepared in the absence of chelator usually respond favorably to the addition of serum albumin.

At this time a direct relationship between mitochondrial deterioration and the lead content of isolated mitochondria from lead poisoned animals does not appear to have been established, but the presumptive evidence for such a relationship is intriguing. The wide variety of effects of lead on mitochondria that can be demonstrated *in vitro* suggests that, if reasonable amounts of lead reach the mitochondria of a living cell, mitochondrial function will be impaired. The fact that mitochondria can be shown to accumulate lead[13] and that portions of the synthetic pathway for heme are located in the mitochondria may be of significance in the well-documented disruption of heme synthesis in lead poisoning.[26]

EFFECTS OF COPPER ON MITOCHONDRIA

Low concentrations of copper are very toxic to isolated mitochondria. In a typical titration, oxidative phosphorylation and respiratory control with succinate as substrate were abolished at 4 nmol of copper per mg of protein (Reference 27, Figure 10). As copper was increased to 8 nmol/mg, State 4 respiration with succinate was markedly activated, and above about 10 nmol/mg all succinate respiration started to be inhibited.[27] An explanation for this titration behavior is provided by other experiments which show that, at low levels of Cu^{+2}, the phosphate transporter is inhibited (as shown by decreased passive osmotic swelling in isotonic ammonium phosphate, Reference 27), at intermediate Cu^{+2} concentrations the activation of respiration is associated with increased passive permeability to K+ and increased energy-dependent accumulation of K+ salts (as shown by a series of responses that closely resembles those of the K+-specific ionophore valinomycin,[27] and at higher concentrations of Cu^{+2}, electron transport reactions are inhibited. Copper is bound avidly by protein-binding sites in isolated heart mitochondria[27] and low levels of bound Cu^{+2} (relative to Pb^{+2} and other heavy metals with the exception of Hg^{+2}) are effective inducers of passive swelling in KCl media. Since a rather large number of potential binding sites are available (greater than 100 nmol/mg), these results indicate that only a few, rather high-affinity sites are concerned with the specific changes in permeability that permit increased energy-dependent K+ accumulation. In this regard, addition of 3-6 nmol of copper/mg causes increased uptake of K+ acetate and an accompanying osmotic swelling that is both inhibited and reversed by added uncouplers, such as dinitrophenol. Under these conditions copper at 20 nmol/mg induces a very rapid rate of swelling, which is spontaneously-reversed after a short time (Reference 27, Figure 3).

It would seem that as more copper reacted with the membrane, or more copper moved toward the interior of the membrane, or slower re-acting ligands became involved, the membrane became sufficiently altered so that it was unable to maintain the conditions necessary for ion uptake. The permeability to K+ induced by copper exceeds that produced for Na+, so that a measure of K+/Na+ discrimination results when rates of respiration and ATPase are compared.[27] Studies of Cu^{+2}-treated mito-chondria by Hwang et al.[27] also indicate that a given amount of bound Cu^{+2} is more effective in producing altered passive permeability when it is reacted with an energized as opposed to a nonrespiring or uncoupled mitochondrion. This result can be taken to support the suggestion that mitochondrial membrane components undergo considerable alteration in conformation during a transition from the nonenergized to an energized condition.

The high reactivity of Cu^{+2} with isolated mitochondria, combined with the relative nontoxicity of this element in man, suggests that free Cu^{+2} does not come in contact with mitochondria except under unusual cir-cumstances. In this regard, Peters[28] reported that, while Cu^{+2} abolished respiration in isolated mitochondria, similar concentration had no effect on respiration in brain slices, and the toxic effects seemed dependent on inhibition of Na+/K+ ATPase in the plasma membrane. One could specu-late that protective mechanisms have evolved to protect intracellular com-ponents from such a reactive but essential component as Cu^{+2}, whereas the less frequently encountered and more innocuous Pb^{+2} produced no such device, and that the lack of such a protective mechanism is reflected in the present hazard of Pb^{+2} to man.

MERCURY

Organic mercurials exhibit a wide variety of effects on isolated mitochondria that depend to a large extent on whether or not the mercurial can penetrate the inner membrane. Similar responses can often be obtained with inorganic mercury if the appropriate concentration range can be found.[29] The thiol groups of the phosphate transporter are extremely reactive to mercurials and complete inhibition of this activity is seen at less than 10 nmol of mersalyl or p-chloromercuriphenylsulfonate (CMS) per mg protein.[30,31] Blocking the phosphate transporter results in inhibition of oxidative phosphorylation, decreased passive osmotic swelling in isotonic ammonium phosphate, and increased ATP-dependent swelling (since Pi produced by hydrolysis of ATP cannot escape from the matrix and produces a marked increase in interior negative charge).

Inorganic mercury and organic mercurials strongly activate energy-dependent K+ accumulation at levels just above those that inhibit the Pi transporter and at still higher levels a passive osmotic swelling in KCl develops.[32] Polar mercurials, such as CMS, seem to be confined to reaction with the outer surface of the inner membrane in short term experiments (*ca.* 20 nmol/mg maximum) whereas more lipid-soluble reagents such as p-chloromercuribenzoate (CMB) titrate more than 40 nmol of thiols/mg and strongly inhibit matrix enzyme activities.[33] The different responses to these two reagents are exemplified by the fact that CMS reacting with the membrane increases permeability to K+ and strongly activates ATP-dependent K+ accumulation.[33,34] Consequently, a K+-dependent ATPase activity is induced by this mercurial.

In contrast, a like concentration of CMB alters the membrane sufficiently to produce passive permeability to phosphate and other anions and to inhibit ATPase markedly. CMS inhibits succinoxidase at the level of succinate transport,[35] since the inhibition is relieved by disruption of the membrane and respiration with other substrates, such as β hydroxybutyrate, is not inhibited. Again, since CMB is accessible to matrix components, it is strongly inhibitory to respiration with these substrates. Differential effects of these reagents in red blood cell membranes have been described by Rothstein.[36]

The kidney is known to concentrate mercury, a fact that makes it a prime target for damage by this metal, but which permits it to function as a protector for other tissues.[37] A direct link between mitochondrial lesions, such as just described, and mercury toxicity has been suggested.[6] Kidney mitochondria from rats acutely intoxicated with mercury have low P/O ratios and contain significant quantities of Hg^{+2} (3-5 nmol Hg^{+2}/mg).[6]

CADMIUM AND ZINC

Cadmium is known to decrease oxidative phosphorylation *in vitro* to a greater extent than it does respiration,[38] and it has recently been reported that liver mitochondria from Cd^{+2}-intoxicated rats have diminished respiratory control.[5] Succinate respiration *in vitro* was markedly stimulated in the concentration range from 1 to 10 μM Cd^{+2}.[5] Since Cd^{+2} is known to activate the respiration-dependent uptake of K^+[39] and Mg^{+2}[40] by isolated heart mitochondria, it would appear that activation of respiration and decreased phosphorylation could be explained by a Cd^{+2}-dependent increase in permeability to cations (cf. Reference 12).

Zinc is much more inhibitory to electron transport reactions, showing a 50% inhibition of succinoxidase in uncoupled mitochondria at 3 μM.[41] The point of inhibition seems to be located between cytochrome b and CoQ.[41] Zn^{+2}, like Cd^{+2}, strongly activates K^+ and Mg^{+2} uptake in the presence of a respiratory substrate such as ascorbate-tetramethyl-phenylenediamine, which is relatively insensitive to the metal.[14,39,40] These effects of Zn^{+2} *in vitro* require the presence of Pi even though insoluble Zn-phosphate salts precipitate,[14] and it appears that the precipitate is absorbed to the mitochondrial membrane in such a way as to make Zn^{+2} readily available. Passive permeability can be demonstrated only after a period of respiration[42] and Zn^{+2} can be shown to be taken up by an energy-dependent process.[14] It seems, therefore, that the permeability changes produced by Zn^{+2} depend on the metal reaching sites that are available to it only in the energized membrane.

RELEVANCE OF MITOCHONDRIAL STUDIES
TO HEAVY METAL TOXICITY

It is clear from the above considerations that a number of different responses can be obtained when isolated mitochondria are challenged with a heavy metal ion *in vitro*. The observed results will reflect an interplay between the following factors: (1) The composition of the suspending medium, since sucrose, buffers, ATP, Pi, and salts (such as acetate) all control the amount of heavy metal that will be available to the mitochondrion to one degree or another. (2) The choice of substrate (*i.e.,* respiration with pyruvate is inhibited by lead, whereas that with ascorbate or glutamate is activated). (3) The state of the mitochondria, since uncoupled succinate respiration is less sensitive to lead than is State 4 respiration. (4) The pH. (5) The order of addition of components, since formation of ATP from ADP and Pi promotes lead toxicity.[18]

Manipulation of these factors can result in the production of quite varied effects *in vitro* by a given concentration of metal. It is well to keep in mind that all of the effects of heavy metals that have been described represent deviations from normal mitochondrial activity, however. It would seem likely that whenever significant amounts of a toxic metal ion reach the mitochondrial population of a cell *in vivo*, mitochondrial activity will be compromised. Whether this alone will result in irreversible damage to the cell will depend on such factors as the strength of binding to mitochondrial components (reversibility), the residence time of metal in the mitochondria (clearance), the availability of alternative metabolic pathways (increased glycolysis), possible compensatory mechanisms (shifting to a different substrate) and the biosynthesis of new mito-chondria. The possibility of secondary damage to mitochondria by such components as free fatty acids has already been mentioned and this appears to occur frequently in damaged cells. In addition, other secondary effects such as metal-catalyzed membrane peroxidation and mitochondrial swelling due to accumulation of lactate or phosphate,[43] appear to be possible in metal ion-intoxicated cells. Studies of the effect of heavy metals on isolated mitochondria have shown us many of the possibilities for the reaction of the components *in vivo*, but further clarification of the exact status of the cell at each stage of toxicity will be necessary to spell out the relationship of mitochondrial damage by these agents to cell death.

ACKNOWLEDGMENTS

Experimental studies in my laboratory were supported in part by U.S. Public Health Services Grant HL09364 and by a Grant in Aid from the Central Ohio Heart Association. Many stimulating and helpful discussions with Dr. A. Krall are gratefully acknowledged.

REFERENCES

1. Passow, H., A. Rothstein and T. W. Clarkson. "The General Pharmacology of the Heavy Metals," *Pharmacol. Rev.* 13:185-224 (1961).
2. Friedberg, F. "Effects of Metal Binding on Protein Structure," *Quart. Rev. Biophys.* 7:1-33 (1974).
3. Hammond, P. B. "Metabolism and Metabolic Action of Lead and Other Heavy Metals," *Clin. Toxicol.* 6:353-365 (1973).
4. Goyer, R. A. "Lead Toxicity: A Problem in Environmental Pathology," *Amer. J. Pathol.* 64:167-181 (1971).
5. Diamond, E. M. and J. E. Keneh. "Effects of Cadmium on the Respiration of Rat Liver Mitochondria," *Environ. Physiol. Biochem.* 4:280-283 (1974).

6. Southard, J., P. Nitisewojo and D. E. Green. "Mercurial Toxicity and the Perturbation of the Mitochondrial Control System," *Fed. Proc.* 33:2147-2153 (1974).

7. Klingenberg, M. "Metabolite Transport in Mitochondria: An Example of Intracellular Membrane Function," *Essays in Biochem.* 6:119-159 (1970).

8. Meijer, A. J. and K. Van Dam. "The Metabolic Significance of Anion Transport in Mitochondria," *Biochim. Biophys. Acta* 346: 213-244 (1974).

9. Mitchell, P. "Protonmotive Function of Cytochrome Systems," In *Electron Transfer Chains and Oxidative Phosphorylation*, E. Quagliariello, *et al.*, Eds. (Amsterdam: North Holland Pub. Co., 1975), pp. 305-316.

10. Slater, E. C. "Electron Transfer and Energy Conservation," In *Dynamics of Energy-Transducing Membranes*, L. Ernster, R. W. Estabrook and E. C. Slater, Eds. (Amsterdam: Elsevier, 1974), pp. 1-20.

11. Brierley, G. P. "The Uptake and Extrusion of Monovalent Cations by Isolated Heart Mitochondria," *Mol. Cell. Biochem.* 10:41-62 (1976).

12. Brierley, G. P. "Passive Permeability and Energy-Linked Ion Movements in Isolated Heart Mitochondria," *Ann. N. Y. Acad. Sci.* 227: 298-411 (1974).

13. Scott, K. M., K. M. Hwang, M. Jurkowitz and G. P. Brierley. "Ion Transport by Heart Mitochondria, XXIII. The Effects of Lead on Mitochondrial Reactions," *Arch. Biochem. Biophys.* 147:557-567 (1971).

14. Brierley, G. P. and V. A. Knight. "Ion Transport by Heart Mitochondria, X. The Uptake and Release of Zn^{+2} and Its Relation to the Energy-Linked Accumulation of Mg^{+2}," *Biochem.* 6:3892-3902 (1967).

15. Cardona, E., M. A. Lessler and G. P. Brierley. "Mitochondrial Oxidative Phosphorylation Interaction of Lead and Inorganic Phosphate," *Proc. Soc. Exp. Biol. Med.* 136:300-304 (1971).

16. Koeppe, D. E. and R. J. Miller. "Lead Effects on Corn Mitochondrial Respiration," *Science* 167:1376-1378 (1970).

17. Parr, D. R. and E. J. Harris. "Effects of Sucrose and Dextran on the Toxicity of Lead to Mitochondria in the Presence of Inorganic Phosphate *In Vitro*," *Biochem. Soc. Trans.* 3:951-953 (1975).

18. Parr, D. R. and E. J. Harris. "Enhancement by Chelating Agents of Lead Toxicity to Mitochondria in the Presence of Inorganic Phosphate," *FEBS Letters* 59:92-95 (1975).

19. Walton, J. R. "Granules Containing Lead in Isolated Mitochondria," *Nature* 243:100-101 (1973).

20. Iannaccone, A., P. Boscolo, E. Bertoli and G. Bombardieri. "*In Vitro* Effects of Lead on Enzymatic Activities of Rabbit Kidney Mitochondria," *Experientia* 30:367 (1974).

21. Krall, A. R., T. T. Meng, S. J. Harmon and W. J. Dougherty. "Uncoupling of NADH-CoQ Coupled Phosphorylation and Inhibition of Substrate Exchange in Kidney Mitochondria by Lead," *Fed. Proc.* 30:1285 Abs. (1971).

22. Murakami, M. and K. Hirosawa. "Electron Microscope Autoradiography of Kidney after Administration of ^{210}Pb in Mice," *Nature* 245:153-154 (1973).

23. Baltrop, D., A. J. Barrett and J. T. Dingle. "Subcellular Distribution of Lead in the Rat," *J. Lab. Clin. Med.* 77:705-712 (1971).

24. Goyer, R. A. "The Renal Tubule in Lead Poisoning, I. Mitochondrial Swelling and Aminoaciduria," *Lab. Invest.* 19:71-77 (1968).

25. Goyer, R. A., A. Krall and J. P. Kimball. "The Renal Tubule in Lead Poisoning, II. *In Vitro* Studies of Mitochondrial Structure and Function," *Lab. Invest.* 19:78-83 (1968).

26. Goyer, R. A. and B. Rhyne. "Pathological Effects of Lead," *Int. Rev. Exptl. Path.* 12:1-77 (1973).

27. Hwang, K. M., K. M. Scott and G. P. Brierley. "Ion Transport by Heart Mitochondria, XXIV. The Effects of Cu^{+2} on Membrane Permeability," *Arch. Biochem. Biophys.* 150:746-756 (1972).

28. Peters, R. A. "A Study of the Toxic Action of Copper on Brain Tissue *In Vivo* and *In Vitro*," In: *The Biochemistry of Copper*, J. Peisach, P. Aisen and W. E. Blumberg, Egs. (New York: Academic Press, 1966), pp. 175-182.

29. Brierley, G. P., V. A. Knight and C. T. Settlemire. "Ion Transport by Heart Mitochondria, XII. Activation of Monovalent Cation Uptake by Sulfhydryl-Group Reagents," *J. Biol. Chem.* 243:5035-5043 (1968).

30. Tyler, D. D. "Evidence of a Phosphate-Transporter System in the Inner Membrane of Isolated Mitochondria," *Biochem. J.* 111:665-678 (1969).

31. Fonyo, A., F. Palmieri, J. Ritvay and E. Quagliariello. "Kinetics and Inhibitor Sensitivity of the Mitochondrial Phosphate Carrier," In: *Membrane Proteins in Transport and Phosphorylation*, G. F. Azzone, *et al.*, Eds. (Amsterdam: North Holland Pub. Co., 1974), pp. 283-286.

32. Scott, K. M., V. A. Knight, C. T. Settlemire and G. P. Brierley. "Differential Effects of Mercurial Reagents on Membrane Thiols and on the Permeability of the Heart Mitochondrion," *Biochem.* 9:714-724 (1970).

33. Brierley, G. P., K. M. Scott and M. Jurkowitz. "Ion Transport by Heart Mitochondria, XXI. Differential Effects of Mercurial Reagents on ATPase Activity and on ATP-Dependent Swelling and Contraction," *J. Biol. Chem.* 246:2241-2251 (1971).

34. Brierley, G. P., M. Jurkowitz and K. M. Scott. "Ion Transport by Heart Mitchondria, XXVII. The Relation of Mercurial-Dependent ATPase Activity to Ion Movements," *Arch. Biochem. Biophys.* 159:742-756 (1973).

35. Scott, K. M., M. Jurkowitz and G. P. Brierley. "Ion Transport by Heart Mitochondria, XXVI. Carrier-Mediated Anion Transport by Isolated Beef Heart Mitochondria," *Arch. Biochem. Biophys.* 153:682-694 (1972).

36. Rothstein, A. "Mercaptans, the Biological Targets for Mercurials," In: *Mercury, Mercurials and Mercaptans*, M. W. Miller and T. W. Clarkson, Eds. (Springfield, Illinois: C. C. Thomas, 1973), pp. 68-92.

37. Magos, L. "Factors Affecting the Uptake and Retention of Mercury by Kidneys in Rats," In: *Mercury, Mercurials and Mercaptans,* M. W. Miller and T. W. Clarkson, Eds. (Springfield, Illinois C. C. Thomas, 1973), pp. 167-184.

38. Jacobs, E. E., M. Jacob, D. R. Sanadi and L. B. Bradley. "Uncoupling of Oxidative Phosphorylation by Cadmium," *J. Biol. Chem.* 223: 147-156 (1956).

39. Brierley, G. P. and C. T. Settlemire. "Ion Transport by Heart Mitochondria, IX. Induction of the Energy-Linked Uptake of K+ by Zinc Ion," *J. Biol. Chem.* 242:4324-4328 (1967).

40. Brierley, G. P. "Ion Transport by Heart Mitochondria, VII. Activation of the Energy-Linked Accumulation of Mg^{+2} by Zn^{+2} and Other Cations," *J. Biol. Chem.* 242:1115-1122 (1967).

41. Kleiner, D. "The Effect of Zn^{+2} on Mitochondrial Electron Transport," *Arch. Biochem. Biophys.* 165:121-125 (1974).

42. Brierley, G. P., C. T. Settlemire and V. A. Knight. "Ion Transport by Heart Mitochondria, XI. The Spontaneous and Induced Permeability of Heart Mitochondria to Cations," *Arch. Biochem. Biophys.* 126:267-288 (1968).

43. Jurkowitz, M., K. M. Scott, R. A. Altschuld, A. J. Merola and G. P. Brierley. "Retention and Loss of Energy-Coupling in Aged Heart Mitochondria," *Arch. Biochem. Biophys.* 165:98-113 (1974).

CHAPTER 23

NEUROTRANSMITTER MECHANISMS IN INORGANIC LEAD POISONING

A. M. Goldberg

The Johns Hopkins University
Department of Environmental Health Sciences
School of Hygiene and Public Health
Baltimore, Maryland 21205

INTRODUCTION

The administration of inorganic lead during critical periods of development can lead to behavioral dysfunction in experimental animals. These
behavioral changes have been described in mice,[1] rats[2,3] and monkeys.[4]
The major behavioral effects described have been changes in spontaneous
motor activity, aggressiveness, arousal, patterning of behavior, and vocaliza-
tion. Although we might not totally agree semantically as to the behavioral deficit, a behavioral dysfunction has been observed in several species
and several laboratories, and thus I feel justified in accepting that lead
does produce a behavioral deficit.

In this chapter, I will summarize the available information on neurochemical mechanisms associated with lead poisoning. The major emphasis
will be on cholinergic mechanisms, and the interaction between cholinergic
and aminergic function. The studies that I will report on from my
laboratory have been carried out mainly in collaboration with Drs. Ellen
Silbergeld and Paul Carroll.

THE ANIMAL MODEL OF LEAD EXPOSURE

Pregnant CD-1 mice (Charles River Laboratories) weighing between
25-35 g were obtained 15-17 days after impregnation. The method of

lead exposure has been previously reported.[1,5] Briefly, lead is administered to the mothers after littering and via her milk to the nursing offspring that are the subjects of study. The mothers are exposed, via the drinking water, to a solution of lead acetate (2, 5, or 10 mg/ml). The 5 mg/ml exposure level was used unless otherwise stated. Within 24 hr litters were reduced to six animals. After weaning, which is delayed as a result of the lead exposure, the offspring were then exposed to the same concentrations of lead in their drinking water as the mothers had received during nursing.

The animals were between 30-70 days of age unless otherwise indicated and control animals, age matched, were always run simultaneously (Figure 23.1).

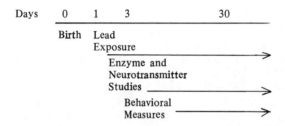

Figure 23.1   Experimental protocol.

RESULTS AND DISCUSSION

The developmental aspects of the animals have previously been described as well as the resultant hyperactivity (increases in spontaneous locomotor activity). I would like to emphasize that in this model increases in exposure do not produce increases in the behavior but do induce other sequela of lead poisoning. Further, animals exposed to lead only at later times in development have not been reported to evince the behavioral dysfunction of hyperactivity seen with early exposure but do manifest other behavioral changes.

Not all laboratories have specifically seen hyperactivity. I think there are many reasons for this and feel that a discussion of these may help clarify the differences reported, although this will not be the major topic of my presentation. Concerning the mouse, there are reports from two different laboratories that describe either hyperactivity or overactivity.[1,6] With the rat, the picture becomes even more complex. Hyperactivity in this species has been reported by Sauerhoff and Michaelson,[2] Golter and Michaelson,[7] Shih et al.,[3] and Grant et al.[8] Sobotka,[9] Modak et al.[10]

and Grant *et al.*[11] have not observed this effect. There are a few aspects of these apparent contradictions that should be noted but these are not the only differences between these studies. First, the route and level of exposure have, in most cases, been different. Second, the methods of measuring the animal's activity (an imprecise technique in itself) has not been standardized. Third, the nutritional status of the animals has not been controlled between laboratories, either as regards caloric intake or other nutritional factors, such as other trace metals. Last, the litter size and thus both nutritional factors and psychological factors have not been uniform. With this lack of uniformity it is most difficult to compare directly the studies that have been reported. However, it should be noted that the effect of drugs, which is "paradoxical," originally observed in mice,[5] has been observed in the rat independent of the appearance of hyperactivity.[3,9]

What evidence do we have for even suggesting that lead poisoning affects neurotransmitter systems? At the pharmacological level, we have evidence that lead modifies the response to a wide array of pharmacological agents. At the physiological level we know that lead, *in vitro,* interferes with neuromuscular and ganglionic transmission. One advantage or disadvantage, depending on how one looks at it, is that both of these systems are cholinergic, *i.e.,* ACh is the suspected transmitter. At the neurochemical level, I will summarize the data suggesting an aminergic imbalance and will present evidence showing effects of inorganic lead on the release of ACh from brain tissue.

We chose to study the pharmacology of lead-exposed animals by comparing the effects of various drugs on lead-induced hyperactivity. The compounds chosen were not selected because of their effects on activity or behavior but because of their major effects on neurochemical systems. It was anticipated that by this approach we might be able to make a first approximation as to the neurochemical systems involved. An abbreviated summary of drugs used is shown in Table 23.1. A number of conclusions can be suggested: (1) drugs that increase the functional capacity, if we use the term loosely, of acetylcholine (ACh) tend to calm these animals, and (2) drugs that increase the functional capacity of norepinephrine and dopamine tend to exacerbate either the activity or reactivity of these animals.

Measurements have been made in lead-poisoned rats and mice of steady state levels of several neurotransmitters and the activities of associated enzymes that are directly or indirectly associated with neurotransmitter function (Tables 23.2, 23.3, 23.4). In a general way, it could be stated that these systems are essentially unaffected. Many authors, ourselves included, have reported changes of up to 30% in specific brain enzymes.

Table 23.1 Effect of Drugs on Lead-Induced Hyperactivity

Drug	Effect on Activity[a]	
	Lead-Treated Hyperactive	Control
d-Amphetamine (10 mg/kg)	− −	+ +
Dimethylaminoethanol (200 mg/kg)	− −	+
Methylphenidate (40 mg/kg)	− −	+ +
Oxotremorine (0.08 mg/kg)	−	0
Physostigmine (0.1 mg/kg)	− −	0
Apormorphine (10 mg/kg)	0	−
Benztropine (15 mg/kg)	+	0
l-Dopa (50 mg/kg)	+ +	0

+ = increase in activity
− = decrease in activity
0 = no change in activity

[a]Data from Silbergeld and Goldberg.[24]

Table 23.2 Steady State Levels of Neurotransmitters and Related Systems

System[a]	Species	References
Acetylcholine	Mouse	19
	Rat	10
Choline	Mouse	19
Dopamine	Mouse	14
	Rat	7
	Rat	9
	Rat	11
Gamma aminobutryic acid	Rat	25
5-Hydroxyindole acetic acid	Rat	9
Serotonin	Rat	25
		9

[a]There is no difference between control and lead-treated groups except in ACh in the diencephalon in the rat.

Table 23.3   Effects of Inorganic Lead on Brain Enzymes

	% of Control (Reference)	
	Choline Acetyltransferase	Acetylcholinesterase
Mouse		
Whole brain	NS (19,27)	NS (19.27)
Striatum	NS (27)	—
Cortex	NS (27)	—
Cerebellum	NS (27)	—
Rat		
Cerebellum	NS (10)	NS 70 (10,9)
Medulla-pons	115 (10)	89 (10)
Diencephalon	NS (10)	89 (10)
Hippocampus	117 (10)	NS (10)
Striatum	NS (10)	NS (10)
Cortex	118 (10)	NS (10)
Midbrain	—	87 (10)
Telencephalon	—	70 (9)

NS = Not statistically significant

Table 23.4   Effects of Inorganic Lead on Brain Enzymes

Enzyme	Region of Mouse Brain	% of Control	Reference
Choline phosphokinase	Whole brain	NS	19
Glutamic acid	Whole brain	NS	27
Decarboxylase	Cerebellum	NS	27
	Cortex	NS	27
MAO	Whole brain	120	26
Tyrosine hydroxylase	Whole brain	NS	27
	Striatum	NS	27
Tryptophane hydroxylase	Whole brain	NS	27

NS = Not statistically significant

Since the enzymes that are changed are not rate-limiting enzymes, it is difficult to consider that there is any biological significance to the changes reported. Further, in most of the studies the enzymes were measured at a time after the behavioral change, if any change had occurred.

It has been observed that in severe undernutrition there is a decrease in acetylcholinesterase.[12] Acetylcholinesterase of lead-poisoned animals has been reported as not changed or slightly decreased. Additionally, Maker et al.[6] concluded that undernutrition was not the major factor in their studies as varying litter size did not modify the effects of lead. These results militate against undernutrition as being the major factor in the results obtained in lead poisoning.

A number of studies have been reported dealing with the effects of lead exposure on catecholaminergic function in the brains of both rats and mice (Table 23.5). These include increases in the turnover[13] and the steady state levels of norepinephrine.[7,14] Further, there are increases in

Table 23.5   Effects of Inorganic Lead on Brain Norepinephrine

System	Species	Results (Reference)
Turnover	Rat	Increased (13)
Steady-state levels	Mouse	27% increase (14)
	Rat	13% increase (17)
	Rat	No change (9)
	Rat	No change (11)
	Mouse	No change (27)
Vanillylmandelic acid	Mouse	48% increase (15)

the brain levels of vanillylmandelic acid (VMA), a metabolite of norepinephrine.[15] The levels of dopamine are unchanged although homovanillic acid (HVA) is increased in brain. In addition, the urinary excretion of VMA and HVA are increased in lead-exposed animals and children.[15] All of the above results have been interpreted to indicate an increase in aminergic function and/or metabolism in lead poisoning. In contradistinction, Grant et al.[11] and Sobotka[9] were unable to observe any change in the steady-state levels of norepinephrine in rats. Again, all of these animals were different strains, ages, and on different lead regiments. It would be desirable, however, if the increase in aminergic function hypothesis could be tested directly. Unfortunately, these data are unavailable.

Evidence that lead can affect cholinergic function is derived from three types of studies. The first type, already discussed, is the pharmacological response to widely different drugs. The second studies include the effects of lead added *in vitro* to several physiological preparations, and the third is obtained by studying cholinergic parameters in brain tissues derived from lead-poisoned animals.

Kostial and Vouk,[16] using the superior cervical ganglion of the cat, demonstrated that lead added *in vitro* blocked ganglionic transmission and produced a decrease in the release of ACh. Further, they demonstrated that this effect of lead appears to be related to the interaction of lead and calcium. Manalis and Cooper,[17] using a frog sartorius muscle preparation, demonstrated that lead increases miniature end plate potential (mepp) frequency and decreases end plate potential (epp) amplitude. Silbergeld, Fales and Goldberg[18] demonstrated that *in vitro* lead can decrease the force of contraction of the diaphragm when the phrenic nerve is stimulated. The ability of lead to decrease epp amplitude and the force of muscle contraction cannot be explained by a postsynaptic inhibition since it does not alter the postsynaptic sensitivity to ACh.[17,18] All of these results are consistent with the suggestion that lead, added *in vitro*, decreases the release of ACh.

In the mouse model described, we looked at the potassium-induced release of ACh from brain tissue to find if the inhibition of ACh release by lead *in vitro* was a general property of lead and if the paradoxical pharmacology seen in lead-induced hyperactivity was the result of cholinergic stimulation by these drugs. The experimental protocol[19] consisted of pairing control and lead-treated animals for up to 70 days of age. Acetylcholine release was induced, *in vitro*, by exposing the brain minces to elevated K^+, 35 mM, for periods of up to 1 hr. As previously shown,[20] the release of ACh is linear for at least 1 hr and is calcium dependent. The results presented in Table 23.6 show that chronic lead exposure inhibits the potassium-induced release of ACh and that there is no dose-response relationship. It is interesting to note that the three doses used in this study have been previously reported to produce a dose-independent hyperactivity.[1] Since the effect observed in animals exposed to lead and *in vitro* lead exposure produce the same effects, it is possible to tentatively conclude that this is a direct effect of lead and not a secondary consequence of the lead exposure.

As stated earlier, methylphenidate and amphetamine produce a paradoxical response in lead-treated animals. Although these drugs are generally thought of as aminergic stimulants, they possess many additional properties not related to their catechoaminergic effects. Amphetamine has been shown to increase ACh release from brain. In attempting to see whether

Table 23.6   Effect of Chronic Lead Administration on Potassium-Induced Release of ACh[a]

Lead Exposure[b] (N)	Control	Lead	Lead & Methylphenidate
	(nmol/g tissue/hr ± S.E.M.)		
2 mg/ml (9)	249 ± 22	208 ± 23[c]	
5 mg/ml (11)	290 ± 32	201 ± 21[c]	
5 mg/ml (5)		158 ± 21	311 ± 51[d]
10 mg/ml (5)	282 ± 17	225 ± 17[c]	

[a]Data of Carroll et al.[19]
[b]See text for experimental protocol.
[c]$p < 0.05$ as compared to control.
[d]$p < 0.05$ as compared to lead.

methylphenidate also had a cholinergic action we did the following experiment. Lead-exposed animals were treated with 40 mg/kg methylphenidate and killed 2 hr later. This is the dose and time period previously shown to reverse the lead-induced hyperactivity. The brains from control, lead-exposed and lead-exposed animals given methylphenidate were removed and the K^+-induced release of ACh measured (Table 23.6). As in the previous experiments lead-exposed animals had a decrease in the release of ACh, and this decrease was completely reversed in the methylphenidate-treated animals. These data suggest a cholinergic link in the mechanism of action of methylphenidate.[19] Further, evidence to support a cholinergic effect of methylphenidate has been reported.[21]

A NEUROCHEMICAL MODEL

The results presented suggest that in lead poisoning there exists an imbalance in central aminergic and cholinergic systems. In many behavioral studies,[22] a correlation can be made between decreased cholinergic function and increased motor activity. Further, Gordon and Shellenberger[23] have demonstrated that increased aminergic function is associated with increased motor activity. We have previously proposed that the primary neurochemical defect in lead poisoning is a decrease in a cholinergic inhibitory system with a corresponding increase in central aminergic function (Figure 23.2). Therefore, in lead-induced hyperactivity, aminergic function is disinhibited and its activity increases above control as a result of impairment of the cholinergic system. The alterations in these systems modify the pharmacological response to many drugs since both aminergic

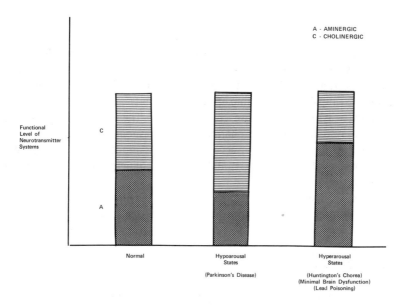

Figure 23.2   Neurotransmitter interactions.

and cholinergic systems are affected by these stimulant drugs. Therefore we have suggested that in lead poisoning an imbalance exists in both an excitatory aminergic system and an inhibitory cholinergic system, the final result is hyperarousal. A similar neurochemical dysfunction has been presented in choreiform diseases and the neurochemical mirror image for Parkinson-like diseases.[24] Thus, drugs previously thought to act paradoxically, might in actuality be acting in a predictable manner. The CNS stimulants, amphetamine and methylphenidate, are acting not only on catecholaminergic systems but are also acting on cholinergic systems. These drugs may then be restoring a more normal neurochemical balance, thus reducing the hyperactive state.

CONCLUSIONS

Lead is capable of stimulating aminergic function and inhibiting cholinergic function. The inhibition of cholinergic function is supported by pharmacological studies in animals, physiological studies using isolated tissue preparations, and *in vivo* in chronically treated animals. In addition, inorganic lead administered during critical periods of development produces an increase in spontaneous motor activity. Reversal of the behavioral effects of lead by methylphenidate also reverses the inhibition of

ACh release. It is suggested that lead-induced hyperactivity is, at least in part, the result of a decrease in central cholinergic metabolism.

In the normal condition there is a balance between cholinergic and aminergic function. In the lead-treated animal a cholinergic inhibitory system is impaired. This impairment disinhibits aminergic function and its activity is increased above control levels. The resulting imbalance in the two systems alters the pharmacological response of these animals to stimulant drugs. Therefore, according to this model, the CNS stimulants produce a relatively greater stimulation of cholinergic function and tend to reset the normal balance.

Thus, we have demonstrated a behavioral change associated with lead exposure and have suggested a neurochemical mechanism to explain these changes.

REFERENCES

1. Silbergeld, E. K. and A. M. Goldberg. "A Lead-Induced Behavioral Disorder," *Life Sci.* 13:1275-1283 (1973).
2. Sauerhoff, M. W. and I. A. Michaelson. "Hyperactivity and Brain Catecholamine in Lead-Exposed Developing Rats," *Science* 182: 1022-1024 (1973).
3. Shih, T.-M., Z. S. Khachaturian, K. L. Reisler, M. M. Rizk and I. Hanin. "Methylphenidate as a Cholinergic Agonist: Further Observations," *Fed. Proc.* 35:307 (1976).
4. Allen, J. R., P. J. McWay and S. J. Suomi. "Pathophysiological and Behavioral Changes in Rhesus Monkeys Exposed to Lead," *Environ. Health Persp.* 7:239-246 (1974).
5. Silbergeld, E. K. and A. M. Goldberg. "Lead-Induced Behavioral Dysfunction: An Animal Model of Hyperactivity," *Expl. Neurol.* 42:146-157 (1974).
6. Maker, H. S., G. M. Lehrer and D. J. Silides. "The Effect of Lead on Mouse Brain Development," *Environ. Res.* 10:79-91 (1975).
7. Golter, M. and I. A. Michaelson. "Growth, Behaviour, and Brain Catecholamines in Lead-Exposed Neonatal Rats: A Reappraisal," *Science* 178:359-361 (1975).
8. Grant, L. D., J. L. Howard, S. Alexander and M. R. Krigman. "Low Level Lead Exposure: Behavioral Effects," *Environ. Health Persp.* 10:267 (1975).
9. Sobotka, T. J., R. E. Brodie and M. P. Cook. "Psychophysiologic Effects of Early Lead Exposure," *Toxicol.* 5:175-191 (1975).
10. Modak, A. T., S. T. Weintraub and W. B. Stavinoha. "Effect of Chronic Ingestion of Lead on the Central Cholinergic System in Rat Brain Regions," *Toxicol. Appl. Pharmacol.* 34:340-347 (1975).
11. Grant, L. D., J. L. Breese, J. L. Howard, M. R. Krigman and P. Mushak. "Neurobiology of Lead-Intoxication in the Developing Rat," *Fed. Proc.* 35:503 (1976).

12. Adlard, B. P. F. and J. Dobbing. "Elevated Acetylcholinesterase Activity in Adult Rat Brain After Undernutrition in Early Life," *Brain Res.* 30:198-199 (1974).

13. Michaelson, I. A., R. D. Greenland and W. Roth. "Increased Brain Norepinephrine Turnover in Lead Exposed Hyperactive Rats," *The Pharmacologist* 16:250 (1974).

14. Silbergeld, E. K. and A. M. Goldberg. "Pharmacological and Neurochemical Investigations of Lead-Induced Hyperactivity," *Neuropharmacol.* 14:431-444 (1975).

15. Silbergeld, E. K. and J. J. Chisholm, Jr. "Lead Poisoning: Altered Urinary Catecholamine Metabolited as Indicators of Intoxication in Mice and Children," *Science* 192:153-154 (1976).

16. Kosital, K. and V. B. Vouk. "Lead Ions and Synaptic Transmission in the Superior Cervical Ganglion of the Cat," *Brit. J. Pharmacol.* 12:219-222 (1957).

17. Manalis, R. S. and G. Cooper. "Presynaptic and Postsynaptic Effects of Lead at the Frog Neuromuscular Junction," *Nature* 243: 5406, 345-356 (1974).

18. Silbergeld, E. K., J. T. Fales and A. M. Goldberg. "The Effect of Inorganic Lead on the Neuromuscular Junction," *Neuropharmacol.* 13:795-801 (1974).

19. Carroll, P. T., E. K. Silbergeld and A. M. Goldberg. "Alterations of Central Cholinergic Function in Lead-Induced Hyperactivity," *Biochem. Pharmacol.* (in press (1976).

20. Carroll, P. T. and A. M. Goldberg. "Relative Importance of Choline Transport to Spontaneous and Potassium Depolarized Release of ACh," *J. Neurochem.* 25:523-527 (1975).

21. Shih, T. M., Z. S. Khachaturian, H. Barry, III and I. Hanin. "Cholinergic Mediation of the Inhibitory Effect of Methylphenidate on Neuronal Activity in the Reticular Formation," *Neuropharmacol.* 15:55-60 (1976).

22. Hingtgen, J. N. and M. H. Aprison. "Behavioral and Environmental Aspects of the Cholinergic System," In *Biology of Cholinergic Function*, A. M. Goldberg and I. Hanin, Eds. (New York: Raven Press, 1976).

23. Gordon, J. H. and M. K. Shellenberger. "Regional Catecholamine Content in the Rat Brain: Sex Differences and Correlation with Motor Activity," *Neuropharm.* 13:129-137 (1974).

24. Silbergeld, E. K. and A. M. Goldberg. "Hyperactivity," In: *Biology of Cholinergic Function*, A. M. Goldberg and I. Hanin, Eds. (New York: Raven Press, 1976).

25. Sauerhoff, M. W. and I. A. Michaelson. "Effect of Inorganic Lead on Monoamines in Brain of Developing Rat," *The Pharmacologist* 15:165 (1973).

26. Silbergeld, E. K., P. T. Carroll and A. M. Goldberg. "Monoamines in Lead-Induced Hyperactivity," *The Pharmacologist* 17:212 (1975).

27. Data obtained in collaboration with P. McGeer and E. McGeer.

CHAPTER 24

EFFECTS OF TRACE METALS AND THEIR DERIVATIVES ON THE CONTROL OF BRAIN ENERGY METABOLISM

R. J. Bull

U. S. Environmental Protection Agency
Health Effects Research Laboratory
Cincinnati, Ohio 45268

INTRODUCTION

Many toxic metals are known to interfere with mitochondrial metabolism. Several essential metals, particularly calcium, magnesium, manganese, iron and copper, are intimately involved in mitochondrial function. Therefore, it is not surprising that they bind related toxic metals with relatively high affinities. However, some difficulty is encountered conceptually if an attempt is made to explain organ-specific effects of a toxic metal on the basis of mitochondrial metabolism. This is particularly true of metals having some specificity for the nervous system. The concentrations of these metals in brain rarely approach the concentrations measured in other organs. If it is assumed that mitochondria function similarly despite their source, specificity is difficult to rationalize. The situation is further complicated by the fact that mitochondria from brain are rarely used for studying mitochondrial metabolism or for assessing the effects of environmental chemicals on mitochondria. This is primarily attributable to the difficulty of preparing brain mitochondria with good respiratory control ratios and even the greater difficulty involved in obtaining mitochondria from this source with any degree of purity.[1] Consequently differences in brain mitochondria from those of other sources that might account for differing sensitivities to toxic metals have not been documented.

Brain, however, does differ considerably from other organs in terms of its metabolic organization. Best known is the distinct dependence of brain upon glucose as substrate for its energy metabolism.[2] This difference appears to be intrinsic to the tissue rather than simply a question of permeability, as was previously supposed.[3] Consideration must also be given to the rather unique emphasis on relationships of amino acid metabolism and TCA cycle oxidations in the brain relative to other tissues. Third, the intimate involvement of currents carried by ions across cell membranes places more emphasis on the mitochondrial capabilities for concentrating and releasing cations in brain relative to nonexcitable tissues.

To determine the extent to which effects of certain metals on the nervous system might involve energy metabolism, our laboratory has concentrated upon methods that can be applied at a tissue level of organization. In addition to avoiding the problems involved in the preparation of isolated brain mitochondria, certain other benefits result. Most important, isolated slices of brain tissue retain many of their *in vivo* functional properties.[2] This allows observations to be made on the control of energy metabolism in the cellular environment rather than the artificial environment necessary for work on isolated mitochondria. The disadvantage, of course, is that less precise control can be exerted over the experimental conditions, and indirect means of changing mitochondrial energy states must be employed. In the present work elevations in the media potassium concentrations have been employed. This brings about a metabolic transient, somewhat analogous to a state 4 to state 3 transition in isolated mitochondria, which is followed by a change in the tissue's steady-state metabolism.[4,5]

The purpose of this chapter is to summarize research using this approach with *in vivo* treatments of lead and methyl mercury. In addition, some findings that compare the effects of dialkyltin compounds used as stabilizers in PVC pipe with triethyltin, *in vitro*, are presented.

METHODS

Animals

Lead and methyl mercury were administered by intraperitoneal injection to Sprague-Dawley derived Charles River rats (200-400 g). The chloride salt of lead was administered in doses of 0.5, 2, and 10 mg Pb/kg body weight in 2.0 ml distilled water/kg six times over a two-week period for total doses of 3, 12, and 60 mg/kg. Animals were sacrificed 14 days following the first injection and 2 days following the last injection. Methyl mercuric chloride was injected daily in 1.0 ml distilled water/kg at doses of 0.01, 0.05, 0.15, 0.5 and 2 mg/kg (as the chloride) for 14 days. These animals were sacrificed on the 15th day.

Metabolic Measurements

Slices of tissue were taken only from the first layer of the cerebral cortex and averaged 0.34 ± 0.02 mm in thickness. Preparation and incubation of these tissues for measurements of respiration, glycolytic rate and redox state of electron transport intermediates has been previously described.[3,4] The incubation media was (mM): NaCl, 127; $MgCl_2$, 1.3; NaH_2PO_4, 1.3; $CaCl_2$, 0.75; $NaHCO_3$, 26; KCl, 3.0. The media was continuously oxygenated with 95% O_2, 5% CO_2. Where indicated the media concentration of potassium was increased to 30 mM at 30 min of incubation to produce metabolic transients in the tissues. Temperature was maintained at 37.0°C in the tissue chambers. Tissues treated *in vitro* with alkyltin derivatives were prepared and incubated in the same manner for measuring metabolic responses to potassium. The tin compounds were added at 10 min of incubation, 20 min prior to the addition of potassium. Addition of the alkyltin compounds were made in 0.3 μl ethanol/ml of media, and the same volume of ethanol was added to control incubations.

Turnover of Tissue Ca^{++}

Tissues taken from control of lead-treated rats were preloaded with ^{45}Ca (5 μCi/ml of incubation media) under static conditions of incubation. The tissues were transferred to a superfusion cell, similar in design to that previously described for measurements of O_2 consumption, but with a smaller tissue chamber.[4] The loss of ^{45}Ca was monitored in the outflow of the cell. For the first 10 min, the perfusion rate was maintained at 2.0 ml/min to quickly wash out adhering media. Thereafter, flow was maintained at 0.20 ± 0.01 ml/min, which gave a calculated turnover time for media in the tissue chamber (volume = 0.32 ml) of 1.6 min, slightly longer than that used for metabolic measurements (1.25 min). The potassium concentration was increased from 3 to 30 mM after 30 min in the perfusions system and maintained at this level throughout the remainder of the experiment. ^{45}Ca lost from the tissue was determined in 1-min aliquots of the chamber effluent, diluted to 1.0 ml with distilled water placed in 10 ml of a commercially prepared scintillation cocktail.

At the end of the experiment, tissues were solubilized with 1.0 ml Soluene (Packard) and the ^{45}Ca content quantified by liquid scintillation counting. Quench was determined to be virtually identical for the aqueous effluents and the solubilized tissues using an internal standard of ^{14}C-toluene.

Consequently, the data were normalized by calculating the percentages of ^{45}Ca lost from the tissue per min, based upon the total counts associated with the tissue at each given time interval. A tissue from a lead-treated animal was always run simultaneously with a control tissue. Both tissues received their media from a common reservoir to maintain conditions between control and experimental tissues as constant as possible.

Metal Analysis

Analysis of brain tissue for lead was done by standard additions using an atomic absorption spectrophotometer fitted with a graphite furnace (Ulmer, manuscript in preparation). Mercury content of the cerebral cortex was determined by flameless atomic absorption spectrophotometry as previously described.[6]

RESULTS

Lead

Lead concentrations in the cerebral cortex of treated rats were measured to confirm that lead was being translocated to the brain and to compare the levels achieved with data obtained from human autopsy studies. Figure 24.1 depicts these results. Whereas increasing the total dose given

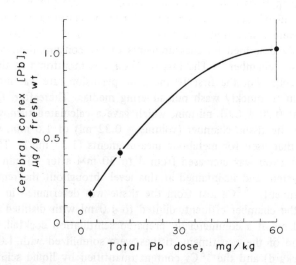

Figure 24.1 Concentrations of Pb achieved in the cerebral cortex of rats subjected to i.p. administration of PbCl$_2$. Amounts of Pb indicated are the total doses administered over a 2-week period. Values are indicated ± SEM.

to the animals from 3 to 12 mg Pb/kg increased the brain concentrations of lead 0.6 times for each multiple of the lead dose, the increase was only 0.5 times between 12 and 60 mg Pb/kg. This resulted in a non-linear relationship between lead dosage and the concentration of lead achieved in the cerebral cortex. This finding appears to be explained by the fact that animals injected on the high dosage schedule were found to have variable amounts of a white precipitate in their peritoneal cavity, presumably consisting of carbonate or phosphate salts of lead. This was not observed in animals receiving the lower doses. Individual values were considerably more variable at the high dose level as a result. Therefore, it appeared that a practical limit for achieving increases in brain lead concentration had been reached within the time frame of the treatment schedule used.

The normal responses of isolated cerebral cortex slices to elevated potassium concentrations and the accompanying changes in tissue respiration, aerobic glycolytic rate and adenine nucleotide changes have been described previously.[4,5] Upon increasing the media potassium concentration from 3 to 30 mM, a metabolic transient is induced, which involves a large increase in the rate of respiration that is accompanied by an oxidation of the electron transport intermediates and decreases in the tissue content of ATP and phosphocreatine. The respiratory change has a limited time course, returning to near the prestimulation baseline within 4-5 min. Cessation of the respiratory burst is accompanied by reduction of the electron carriers, substantial recovery of the tissue ATP and phosphocreatine concentrations and an increase in the rate of aerobic glycolysis, despite the fact that the media potassium concentration is maintained at 30 mM.

Cerebral cortex slices taken from animals receiving total doses of lead of 12 and 60 mg/kg displayed altered metabolic responses to potassium (Figure 24.2). A total dose of 3 mg Pb/kg produced no significant alterations in the response. Spectrally, alterations induced by lead treatment involved a greatly increased rate of NAD(P) reduction relative to control that was dose-dependent. This resulted in an accumulation of NAD(P)H* at approximately twice the control level in both the 12 and 60 mg/kg doses. Tissue respiration in lead-treated animals very closely approximated control animals prior to addition of potassium (1.63 ± 0.19 μmol/g per min for controls vs. 1.60 ± 0.31 for lead-treated animals). However, a significant depression in the respiratory response to potassium was observed. This inhibition of oxygen uptake was most marked at 2 to 3 min

---

*The term NAD(P)H is used to refer to both NADH and NADPH since they cannot be differentiated spectrally. NADH is the predominant dinucleotide present in brain tissue, however.

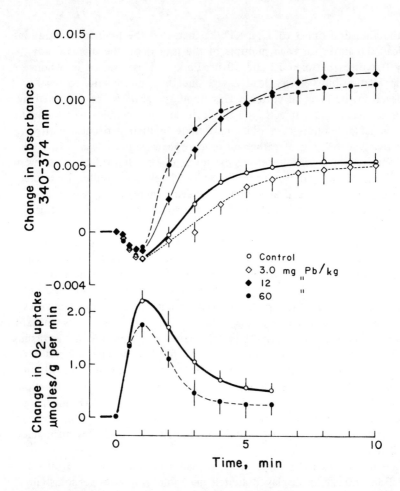

Figure 24.2 Effect of Pb on the metabolic responses of cerebral cortical slices to
elevated potassium. Upper figure represents redox changes in tissue NAD(P)H,
a downward deflection indicating an oxidation of the intermediate. The lower
figure depicts the respiratory responses to potassium. Potassium concentration
was increased from 3 to 30 mM at 0 time. Administration of Pb was
the same as indicated in Figure 24.1. Values are indicated ± SEM.

after the addition of potassium, correlating closely with the time at which
the accelerated reduction of NAD(P) was observed. These data indicate
that the accumulation of NAD(P)H results from a decreased rate of
electron transport rather than an enhancement of NAD(P) reduction. No
significant alterations were observed in the lactic acid produced by the
tissues either before or after the addition of potassium.

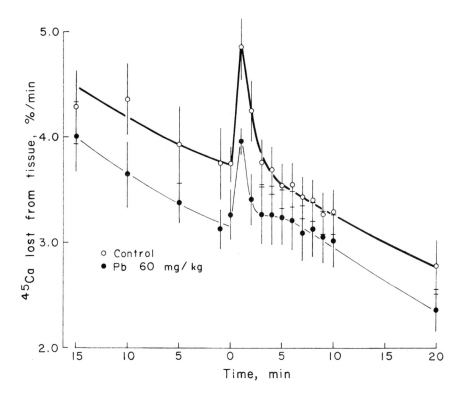

Figure 24.3   Turnover of tissue calcium in cerebral cortical slices taken from rats treated with lead as in Figure 24.1. Potassium concentration of the incubation media was increased from 3 to 30 mM at 0 time.   Data is expressed as the percentage of the tissue ^{45}Ca lost per min ± SEM.   Six individual animals were used in each group.

In conjunction with the metabolic alterations, tissues taken from lead-treated animals were found to differ from control animals in terms of their calcium turnover (Figure 24.3).   The efflux of calcium from tissues was depressed by about 10% under nonstimulated conditions in the lead-treated group, but this difference was not statistically different at P = 0.05.   However, the transient increase in calcium efflux induced by potassium was significantly depressed by lead treatment (P < 0.01).   Note should be taken of the fact that this difference may be more closely related to the time course of the release rather than the absolute amount of calcium released.   Although the peak of calcium release was depressed with lead treatment, there was a tendency for the rate of calcium release to remain above prestimulation levels.   This was not observed in control tissues.

Methyl Mercury

Animals subjected to intraperitoneal injections of methyl mercuric chloride achieved levels of Hg in the cerebral cortex proportional to the dose of methyl mercury administered (Figure 24.4). Spectral responses

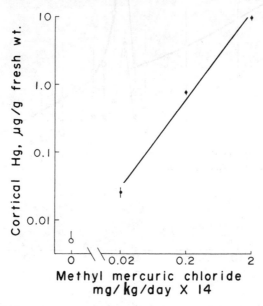

Figure 24.4 Cerebral cortical Hg content following the daily i.p. injection of the doses indicated for a 14-day period. Values are indicated ± SEM.

of tissues taken from animals injected with doses of 0.05 mg methyl mercuric chloride/kg per day displayed alterations in the spectral responses to potassium substantially similar to those observed with lead (Table 24.1). Higher doses produced similar effects, although there was a tendency for the magnitude of the effect to decrease with dose. This modification of the effect seen at low doses appeared to be related to an impaired capability for aerobic glycolysis in response to elevated potassium at higher doses.[6] At the higher doses a progressive inhibition of the initial oxidative phase of the response to potassium was also observed, although this effect did not become statistically significant ($P < 0.05$) until a dose of 2 mg methyl mercuric chloride/kg per day was reached.

Table 24.1 Methyl Mercury-Induced Alterations in the Metabolic Responses of Brain Slices to Elevated Potassium

Methyl Mercuric Chloride mg/kg/day x 14 days	Change in Absorbance, 340-374 nm	
	60 sec	600 sec
0	-0.0029 ± 0.0003	+0.0045 ± 0.0006
0.01	-0.0031 ± 0.0004	+0.0050 ± 0.0009
0.05	-0.0030 ± 0.0006	+0.0092 ± 0.0015[a]
0.15	-0.0027 ± 0.0005	+0.0083 ± 0.0024[a]
0.5	-0.0024 ± 0.0003	+0.0056 ± 0.0007
2.0	-0.0017 ± 0.0003[a]	+0.0070 ± 0.0013[a]

Values shown ± SEM of not less than 6 animals
[a]Significantly different from control ($P < 0.05$).

Alkyltins

In vitro incubation of cerebral cortical tissue with triethyltin results in substantially different effects than previously observed with lead and methyl mercury. Rather than an enhanced reduction of NAD(P) following potassium, triethyltin inhibits the reductive phase of the response (Figure 24.5). Two dialkyltin compounds—dimethyltin dichloride and dibutyltin dichloride—were found to produce the same effect. Comparisons of the potency of these compounds with triethyltin are shown in Table 24.2. Half-maximal inhibition was observed to occur at 1.1 μM triethyltin, whereas the same degree of inhibition required 66 μM and 45 μM concentrations of dimethyltin and dibutyltin, respectively.

The response of cerebral cortical tissues' aerobic glycolytic rate to potassium correlates closely with the reductive aspect of the spectral responses in time course.[4] Lactic acid production by tissues incubated with 33 μM triethyltin were altered both in terms of rate and in terms of the pattern of the response to elevated potassium concentrations (Figure 24.6). The rate of lactic acid production was more than double prior to the addition of potassium and the response to potassium displayed an initial but transient increase in the rate. Within 5 min, the lactic acid production returned to the prestimulation baseline. The time course of the lactic acid response in controls did not show the initial lag and followed a somewhat faster time course than had been previously reported or shown in the lead results.

Subsequent to these experiments it was determined that a design change in the tissue chamber allowed streaming of media through the chamber before proper mixing of the chamber contents had occurred, cutting down

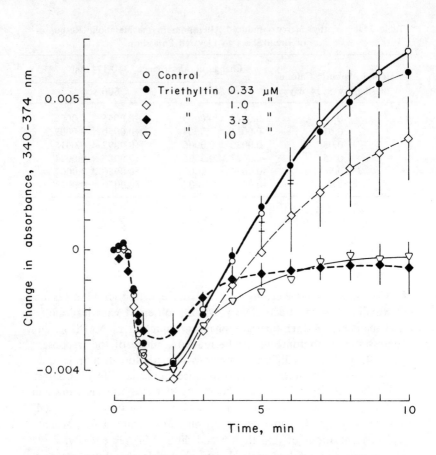

Figure 24.5 Effect of triethyltin, *in vitro,* on the responses of cerebral cortical slice NAD(P)H to an elevation in the media potassium concentration. A downward deflection represents an oxidation of the intermediate. The media potassium concentration was increased from 3 to 30 mM at 0 time. Values indicated are the averaged responses of 6 tissues ± SEM.

on the transit time through the system. Although somewhat distorted in time course as a result, the control response was still representative and typified by a shift from one steady-state rate of aerobic glycolysis to a higher rate that is maintained over time. The principal difference is that tissues treated with triethyltin are not capable of maintaining a higher steady-state rate of aerobic glycolysis after potassium relative to the prepotassium baseline in distinct contrast with control tissues.

Table 24.2   Effects of Alkyltin Derivatives on K^+-Induced Reduction of NAD(P) in Isolated Rat Cerebral Cortex Slices

Compound	Concentration (x 10^{-6} M)	% Inhibition	I_{50} (x 10^{-6} M)
Triethyltin bromide			1.1
	0.33	10.6	
	1.0	43.9	
	3.3	107.8	
	10	103.0	
Dimethyltin dichloride			66
	33	0	
	66	65.9	
	100	72.9	
Dibutyltin dichloride			45
	33	39.3	
	100	82.1	

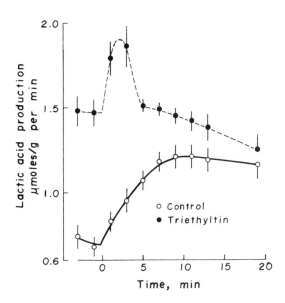

Figure 24.6   Effect of triethyltin, 33 μM, on the aerobic glycolytic rate of cerebral cortical slices. The media potassium concentration was increased from 3 to 30 mM at 0 time. Values ± SEM of 6 tissues.

DISCUSSION

Data has been developed to varying degrees suggesting that lead, methyl mercury and alkyltin compounds produce effects on brain energy metabolism. Deficits in brain function resulting in changes induced in mitochondrial metabolism would undoubtedly vary depending upon the aspect of mitochondrial function interfered with and the brain area principally involved. There is no doubt that energy metabolism of brain is critical to the continued normal function of the organ. This is illustrated by the profound and permanent damage to brain function that can be produced by short periods of anoxia or decreased availability of blood glucose.[2]

The alterations produced by lead and methyl mercury first occurred at levels averaging 0.41 μg Pb/g and about 0.1 μg Hg/g in the cerebral cortex. These values can be compared to levels of 0.1 μg Pb/g in non-exposed and 0.65 μg Pb/g in workers occupationally exposed to lead.[7] These workers were apparently without overt signs of lead poisoning. The critical brain concentration of Hg, administered as methyl mercury, to produce the overt neurological deficits has been estimated between 5 and 10 μg/g.[8] It is clear that the concentrations of both lead and methyl mercury required in the brain to produce alterations in metabolic responses are below those required for overt toxicity in humans. The changes occur prior to overt damage and could, therefore, be intimately involved in the central nervous system effects produced by these metals.

It is reasonably clear in the case of lead that an effect on energy metabolism is responsible for the changes observed in the responses to potassium. First, the accumulation of NAD(P)H was accompanied by a decrease in oxygen uptake by the tissue. This demonstrates that the increased rate of NAD(P)H reduction was the result of reduced electron transport rather than a true enhancement of the rate. Second, the effect appears to be selective for substrates that donate a cytosolic reducing equivalent.[9] The effect was absent when pyruvate served as substrate, but present when glucose or lactate were being utilized with both *in vitro* and *in vivo* exposures to lead. These results led to the conclusion that lead interfered with the oxidation of cytosolic reducing equivalents.[9]

The concomitant effect of lead treatment on calcium turnover of the tissues suggests that a calcium-dependent function of mitochondria may be involved for the alterations in the metabolic response. Chance's laboratory[10] has shown that calcium influences the compartmentation and oxidation of NADH in isolated mitochondria. Gazzoti[11] has observed a calcium-induced oxidation of exogenous NADH in isolated liver mitochondria. Similarly, calcium has been shown to activate glycerophosphate dehydrogenase in isolated lung mitochondria.[12] Scott *et al.*[13] have shown that lead is taken up by isolated mitochondria, apparently by the same mechanism by which mitochondria concentrate calcium. Thomas *et al.*[14] and Bouldin *et al.*[15] reported that animals treated with lead display an increase in brain calcium concentrations. Our laboratory has shown that the metabolic responses to potassium in isolated brain slices possess a calcium-dependent, ouabain-insensitive component.[16] This circumstantial data, plus the compatibility of the time course of calcium release and the respiratory burst by the tissue, indicate that it is not unreasonable to presume that they are related.

Decreased turnover of tissue calcium in lead-treated animals has implications that go beyond a possible involvement in energy metabolism. Calcium is intimately involved in a variety of functions of the nervous system, including neurotransmitter release. Alterations in the release of acetylcholine has been observed in minces taken from lead-treated animals.[17] In addition, alterations in catecholamines levels and turnover *in vivo* have been reported both in lead-treated animals and in young children with excessive blood lead concentrations.[18,19] An increase in the intracellular free calcium concentration could account for these effects since they are both calcium-dependent processes.

Spectrally, methyl mercury produces effects quite similar to those observed with lead, particularly at low doses. Attempts to measure concomitant changes in oxygen consumption by the tissues failed to show a difference.[6] However, the apparatus used at that time was crude and only peak rates were recorded. It is relevant to point out that the peak rate of respiration was not significantly affected by lead either (Figure 24.2) and only by comparing the whole time course of the response was the effect evident. Methyl mercury, at higher doses, does interfere with the glycolytic response to elevated potassium,[6] a property not shared by lead. This observation coupled with the spectral results is consistent with the observations that methyl mercury appears to interfere rather specifically with the conversion of glucose to CO_2[20] and the altered levels of glycolytic intermediates observed in the brains of animals exposed to low doses of methyl mercury.[21,22]

Organotin derivatives, *in vitro*, produced dramatic changes in the metabolic responses to increased potassium. Rather than an accumulation of NAD(P)H following potassium, the net reduction of NAD(P) produced by potassium was completely inhibited by the alkyltin compounds. As might have been expected from the *in vivo* toxicity of these compounds,[23] triethyltin was considerably more potent than dimethyltin and dibutyltin. These latter two compounds are stabilization reaction products of organotin compounds, which have been promoted for use as stabilizers in PVC pipe to be used in potable water systems in the U.S.[24]   In contrast, European manufacturers of PVC pipe have continued to use lead compounds to stabilize PVC pipe. Although there are some indications that dialkyltin compounds do not produce the gross interstitial edema typical of tri-ethyltin intoxication, the possibility of producing less severe or differing forms of central nervous system damage has received virtually no atten-tion. It is clear from the present work that these compounds do possess some of the same properties as triethyltin in isolated brain tissue. Al-though the effects of these compounds in brain tissue are different from those of lead, they are at least as potent as inorganic lead in vitro.[9]

The lack of a net reductive response of tissue NAD(P) in the presence of organotin compounds was in distinct contrast to the effects observed with lead and methyl mercury. The rate of lactic acid production in tissue was markedly increased prior to the addition of potassium, sug-gesting that the lack of a reduction of NAD(P) was related to an already elevated cytosolic redox potential. Although the glycolytic pathway appeared to remain sensitive to the energy demand immediately after potassium, a net increase in the rate was not maintained. Previous work has shown that the net reduction of NAD(P) is observed with glucose as substrate, but not with pyruvate,[4] and that this reduction is dependent upon the tissue's ability to concentrate potassium. Cremer[25] has shown that tissues treated with triethyltin have an impaired ability to concen-trate potassium. Consequently, in addition to the possible limit imposed by an already elevated cytosolic redox potential, a decreased net uptake of potassium may also contribute to the lack of a net reduction of NAD(P) following potassium.

Although the effects of alkyltin compounds differ from those of lead, they do share one common property. Cremer[26] and Lock[27] have shown that respiration of brain slices supported by glucose is much more sensi-tive to triethyltin than that supported by pyruvate. A similar specificity has already been noted for lead.[9] Glucose is the only substrate that will adequately serve the metabolic demands of adult brain, in vivo[2] and in vitro.[3] These findings emphasize the fact that organ specific effects of chemicals are expressed in the peculiarities of a tissue's metabolic or-ganization. This specialization of a tissue's metabolism is not simply expressed and is not evident in a single enzyme activity, any one sub-cellular compartment, or even in one specialized functional property of a tissue. For proper evaluation of the risks associated with environmental chemicals, it is essential that effects on these properties of target tissues be studied. To adequately get at this problem, more work is required at a tissue level of organization, an area that has been neglected in biochem-istry in recent years in favor of studies on isolated enzyme activities.

Reductionism is fine when in pursuit of a specific problem based upon logical extensions of data at higher levels of metabolic organization. However, emphasis on such minute entities before preliminary testing has been completed fragments efforts beyond the point of being able to evaluate the risks associated with environmental chemicals and to synthesize rationale environmental standards.

REFERENCES

1. Moore, C. L. and P. M. Strasberg. In: *Handbook of Neurochemistry*, Vol. 3, *Metabolic Reactions in the Nervous System*, A. Lajtha, Ed. (New York: Plenum Press, 1970), pp. 53-85.
2. McIlwain, H. and H. S. Bachelard. *Biochemistry and the Central Nervous System*, 4th ed. (London: Churchill Livingstone, 1971), pp. 8-31.
3. Bull, R. J. "Cytochrome Redox Potential Dependence on Substrate in Rat Cerebral Cortex Slices: Importance of Cytoplasmic NAD(P)H and Potassium," *J. Neurochem.* 26:149-156 (1976).
4. Bull, R. J. and S. D. Lutkenhoff. "Early Changes in Respiration, Aerobic Glycolysis and Cellular NAD(P)H in Slices of Rat Cerebral Cortex Exposed to Elevated Concentrations of Potassium," *J. Neurochem.* 21:913-922 (1973).
5. Bull, R. J. and J. J. O'Neill. "Spectral Changes in the Respiratory Chain of Cerebral Cortex Slices. Correlation with the Energy Status of the Tissue," *Psychopharmacol. Commun.* 1:109-115 (1975).
6. Bull, R. J. and S. D. Lutkenhoff. "Changes in the Metabolic Responses of Brain Tissue to Stimulation, *In Vitro,* Produced by *In Vivo* Administration of Methyl Mercury," *Neuropharmacol.* 14: 351-359 (1975).
7. Barry, P. S. I. "A Comparison of Concentrations of Lead in Human Tissues," *Brit. J. Ind. Med.* 32:119-139 (1975).
8. *Methyl Mercury in Fish. A Toxicologic-Epidemiologic Evaluation of Risks.* Nordisk Hygienisk Tidskrift Suppl. 4 (1971), pp. 155-198.
9. Bull, R. J., P. M. Stanaszek, J. J. O'Neill and S. D. Lutkenhoff. "Specificity of the Effects of Lead on Brain Energy Metabolism for Substrates Donating a Cytoplasmic Reducing Equivalent," *Environ. Health Persp.* 12:89-95 (1975).
10. Vinogradov, A., A. Scarpa and B. Chance. "Calcium and Pyridine Nucleotide Interaction in Mitochondrial Membranes," *Arch. Biochem. Biophys.* 152:646 (1972).
11. Gazzotti, P. "The Effect of Ca^{2+} on the Oxidation of Exogenous NADH by Rat Liver Mitochondria," *Biochem. Biophys. Res. Comm.* 67:634 (1975).
12. Fisher, A. B., A. Scarpa, K. F. LaNoue, D. Bassett and J. R. Williamson. "Respiration of Rat Lung Mitochondria and the Influence of Ca^{2+} on Substrate Utilization," *Biochemistry* 12:1438 (1973).
13. Scott, K. M., K. M. Hwang, M. Jurkowitz and G. P. Brierley. "Ion Transport by Heat Mitochondria, XXIII. The Effects of Lead on

Mitochondrial Reactions," *Arch. Biochem. Biophys.* 147:557 (1971).

14. Thomas, J. A., F. D. Dallenbach and M. Thomas. "Considerations on the Development of Experimental Lead Encephalopathy," *Virchows Arch. Abt A Path Anat.* 352:61-74 (1971).

15. Bouldin, T. W., P. Mushak, L. A. O'Tuama and M. R. Krigman. "Blood-Brain Barrier Dysfunction in Acute Lead Encephalopathy: A Reappraisal," *Environ. Health Persp.* 12:81 (1975).

16. Bull, R. J. and J. T. Cummins. "Influence of Potassium on the Steady-State Redox Potential of the Electron Transport Chain in Slices of Rat Cerebral Cortex and the Effect of Ouabain," *J. Neurochem.* 21:923 (1973).

17. Carroll, P. T., E. K. Silbergeld and A. M. Goldberg. "The Effect of Chronic Lead Treatment on Spontaneous and Evoked Release of ACH from Brain Tissue," *Neurosci. Abstr.* 1:389 (1975).

18. Golter, M. and I. A. Michaelson. Behavior and Brain Catecholamines in Lead-Exposed Neonatal Rats: A Reappraisal," *Science* 187:359 (1975).

19. Silbergeld, E. K. and J. J. Chisholm, Jr. "Lead Poisoning: Altered Urinary Catecholamine Metabolites as Indicators of Intoxication in Mice and Children," *Science* 192:153 (1976).

20. Menon, N. K. and R. A. P. Kark. "Inhibition of Oxidation in Chronic Alkyl-Mercury Poisoning," *Trans. Amer. Soc. Neurochem.* 7:159 (1976).

21. Paterson, R. A. and D. R. Usher. "Acute Toxicity of Methyl Mercury on Glycolytic Intermediates and Adenine Nucleotides of Rat Brain," *Life Sci.* 10:121 (1971).

22. Salvaterra, P., B. Lown, J. Morganti and E. J. Massaro. "Alterations in Neurochemical and Behavioural Parameters in the Mouse Induced by Low Doses of Methyl Mercury," *Acta Pharmacol. et Toxicol.* 33:177 (1973).

23. Stoner, H. B., J. M. Barnes and J. I. Duff. "Studies on the Toxicity of Alkyl Tin Compounds," *Brit. J. Pharmacol.* 12:16 (1955).

24. Piver, W. T. "Organotin Compounds: Industrial Applications and Biological Investigation," *Environ. Health Persp.* 4:61 (1973).

25. Cremer, J. E. "Studies on Brain-Cortex Slices. The Influence of Various Inhibitors on the Retention of Potassium Ions and Amino Acids with Glucose or Pyruvate as Substrate," *Biochem. J.* 104: 223 (1967).

26. Cremer, J. E. "Studies on Brain-Cortex Slices. Differences in the Oxidation of ^{14}C-Labelled Glucose and Pyruvate Revealed by the Action of Triethyltin and Other Toxic Agents," *Biochem. J.* 104: 212 (1967).

27. Lock, E. A. "The Action of Triethyltin on the Respiration of Rat Brain Cortex Slices," *J. Neurochem.* 26:887 (1976).

CHAPTER 25

EVALUATION OF ANIMAL MODELS USED TO STUDY EFFECTS OF LEAD ON NEUROCHEMISTRY AND BEHAVIOR

R. L. Bornschein, I. A. Michaelson, D. A. Fox and R. Loch
Laboratories of Behavioral and Neurochemical Toxicology
Division of Toxicology
Department of Environmental Health
University of Cincinnati College of Medicine
Cincinnati, Ohio 45267

INTRODUCTION

The animal literature on cerebral dysfunction resulting from lead exposure is meager, largely due to the inability to produce unequivocal neurological changes in laboratory animals comparable to human clinical cases of lead encephalopathy. Adult animals show resistance to the central nervous system effect of lead poisoning. The major criticism of most experimental models is that very large doses of lead are required to produce even marginal toxicity and that often there is a paucity or even absence of clinical manifestations of central nervous system toxicity in these models.

An experimental model exhibiting the morphological alterations similar to those occurring in children with lead encephalopathy has been described by Pentschew and Garro.[1,2] They showed that lesions of the central nervous system of neonatal rats can be produced when lead, fed to a lactating rat, is transmitted to the suckling young via the maternal milk. Replication of the Pentschew model of lead encephalopathy has been reported by Lampert et al.,[3] Thomas et al.,[4] Michaelson,[5] Krigman et al.,[6] and Clasen et al.[7] in the rat, and by Rosenblum and Johnson[8] in the mouse. The mouse model was modified slightly by Silbergeld and

441

Goldberg.[9] They utilized lower concentrations of lead and administered the lead via the dam's drinking water instead of her food supply. These models, or some modification thereof, are being used with increasing frequency for studies on the effect of lead on morphology and chemistry of the brain as well as neurotransmitter metabolism and behavior.

NEUROCHEMICAL STUDIES

Experimental protocols used in studies on neurochemical effects of lead in the developing young rodent are listed in Table 25.1. The range of neurochemical parameters examined is not extensive. While there are several isolated studies reporting the effects of lead exposure on DNA, RNA, protein, lipids and trace metals,[5-7,24] the preponderance of studies have dealt with various aspects of neurotransmitter metabolism. There is little agreement as to the effects of lead. For example, Modak[20] reports a significant decrease in acetylcholine concentration of lead-exposed neonatal mice whereas others find no change in brain ACh.[21] Silbergeld and Goldberg[21,25] report increases in norepinephrine but not in dopamine levels, while Grant et al.[12] report no change in either amine. Sobotka et al.[19] report no change in regional brain levels of 5-hydroxytryptamine, 5-hydroxyindoleacetic acid, norepinephrine or dopamine following lead exposure, but Michaelson et al.[26] report increased concentration and enhanced turnover of whole brain norepinephrine.[27]

BEHAVIORAL STUDIES

Some of these studies also report behavioral alterations as a result of the lead exposures. While a few investigators have examined learning processes,[19,28-32] by far the most commonly employed behavioral measure has been activity. Several laboratories have reported increased locomotor activity in rats[18,33-35] and mice.[9,36] Other laboratories have failed to observe hyperactivity[12,32] and still others have observed hypoactivity.[35] These differences may be attributable to different techniques used in different laboratories.

Silbergeld[9,36] assessed the activity of individual adult male mice for 3- or 4-hr periods following transfer from the home cage to a similar cage equipped with electrosensitive plates. With the aid of an electromagnetic field Selective Activity meter, Sauerhoff and Michaelson[18] measured the 24-hr activity of six weanling littermates housed in their home cage. Sobotka and Cook[32] used a photoactometer to obtain 30-min measures of individual weanling rat activity. Reiter et al.[35] recorded hourly activity of 120-day-old male rats in a residential maze for periods of up to 5 days.

Table 25.1 Protocols Used to Study Effects of Lead on Brain Chemistry of Rat (R) and Mouse (M)

Reference No.			Lactation Dam	Neonate	Weanling	Adult	Pb Concentration, μg% Blood	Brain	Milk	Brain Chemistry
Bull	10	R				$3,12,60^c$	10-1040	10-178		K±NAD(P)H-REDOX
Brown	11	R		4.1^c (10 days)						AChE
Clasen	7	R	$21,800^a$ Start day 4		$21,000^a$					Fe, Na, K, Albumin Cl
Grant	12	R		$25,100,200^d$			23-72	32-79		Dopamine, Norepinephrine
Goldstein	13	R	$31,000^a$ Start day 12		$31,000^a$		600	600		Na, K, Na/K-ATPase
Holtzman	14	R	$31,000^a$		$31,000^a$					Mitochondrial Respiration
Krall	15	R	$21,800^a$		$21,000^a$					NE, MAO Mitochondrial Phosphor.
Krigman	6	R	$31,000^a$		$31,000^a$			920		DNA, Protein, Lipids
Millar	16	R	$21,800^a$		$21,000^a$		450	400		ALA-D
Modak	17	R	$5,500^a$		$5,500^b$					AChE, CAT, ACh
Michaelson	5,24	R	$27,300^a$		$27,300^a$		202-288	1200		RNA, DNA, Protein Fe, Zn, Cu, Ca, Na & K
Sauerhoff	18	R	$27,300^a$		400^a			50-80		NE, DA, 5HT, GABA
Sobotka	32	R		$5,15,44^d$			17-83		2500	AChE, ALA-D, NE DA, 5HT, 5HIAA
Thomas	4	R	$34,000^a$		$34,000^a$		300	1150		Ca
Modak	20	M	$1366-5500^b$		$1366-5500^b$					ACh
Silbergeld	21,22	M	$1090-5500^b$		$1090-5500^b$	$1090-5500^b$	70-194			ACh, NE, DA, HVA, VMA
Gerber	23	M				$0.05-546^b$				5HT

[a] ppm of Pb in diet	Acetylcholinesterase (AChE)	Aminolevulinic Acid-Dehydratase (ALA-D)	Gamma Aminobutyric Acid (GABA)
[b] ppm of Pb in water	Dopamine (DA)	Cholineacetyltransferase (CAT)	5-Hydroxyindoleacetic Acid (5HIAA)
[c] mg/kg i.p.	Norepinephrine (NE)	Acetylcholine (ACh)	Homovanillic Acid (HVA)
[d] mg/kg p.o.	Monoamine Oxidase (MAO)	5-Hydroxytryptamine (5HT)	Vanylmandelic Acid (VMA)

It is not surprising that contradictions exist among the various investigators. In fact, it is surprising to find areas of agreement, considering the species and strain differences, the diversity of behavioral testing procedures and the diversity of exposure techniques (level, route, duration and timing with respect to age). Only those using the direct route have knowledge of the external exposure. None using the indirect route via dam's milk have offered information as to actual exposure to the neonate while suckling. Few have bothered to ascertain the internal dose by providing the blood and/or brain lead values during, or after, exposure.

EVALUATION OF RODENT MODELS

Before attempting to interpret the findings from these diverse studies, it may be beneficial to evaluate the animal models. Only a few investigators[33,34,37] using the lactating dam as a vehicle for administering lead to the neonate report the effects of lead ingestion on the dam. We have documented such effects on the eating and drinking behavior of rats ingesting 5% lead acetate in their diet and of mice drinking 0.5% lead acetate containing water.

A brief survey of Table 25.1 indicates that most of the animals are being subjected to very high levels of lead. Rats eating a 4% lead carbonate diet take in 3 to 5 g of lead per kg body weight. Mice drinking 0.5% lead acetate in water take in excess of 1 g/kg. These levels have profound effects on ingestive behavior. Figure 25.1 shows daily food consumption and body weight of the lactating dam during the first 17 days of lactation.

Similar alterations in food and water intake are obtained in mice. Figure 25.2 illustrates the daily food, water, and lead intake of lactating mice drinking 0.5% lead acetate-containing water. Again maternal ingestive behavior is disrupted. Panel [A] shows the solid food consumption by control dams (hatched bars) and the somewhat smaller intake of food by those drinking leaded water (dotted bars). Panel [B] shows the fluid consumption. There is a significant difference in the volume of fluid intake. Panel [C] illustrates the daily lead consumption (mg) as shown by the height of the bars and the cumulative ingestion by the connected solid circles. By the 18th day of lactation the nursing mouse has consumed 800 mg of lead or about 24 g/kg body weight. As observed in our earlier experience with the rat, ingestion of considerable quantities of lead by the dam does not result in overt signs of lead poisoning in her. However, ingestive behavior is disrupted.

Figure 25.3 illustrates that under normal dietary conditions the fluid to food consumption ratio is about 1.8:1.0, but when drinking 5 mg/ml lead acetate in water, this ratio decreases to 1.1:1.0.

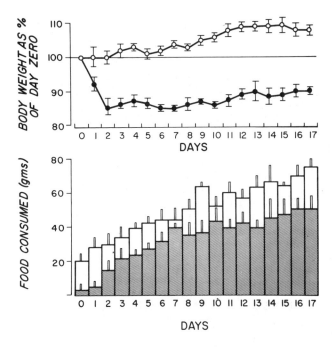

Figure 25.1 Daily food consumption and body weight of lactating rats eating normal diet (open bars or circles) or 5% lead acetate-containing diet (shaded bars or circles).

Lead intake at this level, in conjunction with the disruption in food and water intake, undoubtedly produces both quantitative and qualitative changes in the dam's milk supply. We have not undertaken a detailed study of milk composition in these highly lead-exposed rats and mice. However, we have initiated investigations into trace metal content of milk when dams ingest much lower quantities of lead, *i.e.*, 0.02 to 0.20% lead acetate in drinking water.

Table 25.2 illustrates the effect of lead ingestion on zinc and copper concentration in dam's milk. This exposure level produces no disruption in food and water intake by the dam. However, lead appears to depress zinc concentrations (33%) and copper concentrations (28%) during the early stages of lactation. Since trace metals are ordinarily present in their highest concentrations during the first three days of lactation, greater lead-related zinc depression might be seen on day 2 or 3 of lactation. The essential role of such trace metals in brain development and function is well-documented.[38]

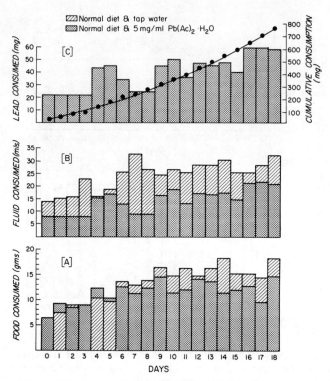

Figure 25.2   Daily food [A], fluid [B] and lead [C] intake of control and lead-exposed lactating mice.

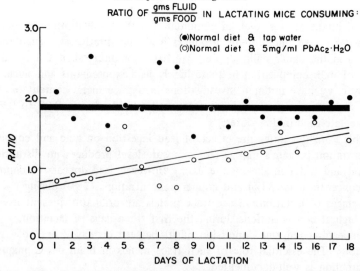

Figure 25.3   Ratio of water intake to food intake in control and lead-exposed lactating mice.

Table 25.2   Zinc[a] and Copper[b] Content of Dam's Milk (ppm)

Days of Lactation	% Pb(Ac)$_2$ in Drinking Water		
	Tap Water	0.02%	0.20%
Zinc			
5	17 ± 1	13 ± 0.0	13 ± 0.9
10	13 ± 2	14 ± 0.2	12 ± 0.3
15	11 ± 1	12 ± 0.1	11 ± 0.8
20	10 ± 2	11 ± 3.0	8
Copper			
5	2.50	2.11	1.81
10	2.36	2.22	2.01
15	2.45	2.25	2.34
20	1.81	1.75	1.80

[a]Each value represents the average obtained from 3 dams.
[b]Each value is a pooled milk sample from 3 dams.

The pre- and postweaning lead exposure level obtained in these models also requires evaluation. None of these studies took into account the *total* daily exposure of the neonate. By monitoring the amount of leaded diet or leaded water consumed we can readily establish the level of postweaning lead exposure. In studies where neonatal rats are weaned to maternal diet containing 5.0% lead acetate (27,300 ppm Pb) the young weanlings are in fact exposed to 5000 μg Pb/g body weight/day. When mice wean onto the dam's drinking water, which contains 0.5% lead acetate, the daily lead intake is approximately 600 μg Pb/g body weight/day. These are extremely high exposure levels, especially when one considers that the exposure often is maintained for life.[9,18,21,22,25,26,34]

These exposure levels in adult rodents are known to produce serious disruptions in the renal function and erythropoiesis. Until recently a methodology was not available for estimating the degree of exposure during the preweaning period when the pups consume lead via milk. Nor was it known how these exposure levels related to postweaning exposure levels. We have developed a way by which one can make a fairly good approximation of the volume of milk, and consequently the amount of lead, consumed each day.[39] Our theoretical estimates of daily milk consumption are in good agreement with our expectations based on limited reports of milk production in rodents.[40] Experimental validation of our theoretical estimates employing a 24-hr cross-fostering technique has confirmed the general validity of our theoretical estimates.[41]

Employing this methodology we have established the daily exposure of the Pentschew model wherein neonatal rats suckle dams producing 40 ppm Pb in their milk, while consuming a diet containing 31,000 ppm lead. Prior to weaning, the exposure to the neonate is about 1.0 mg/kg/day (Figure 25.4 upper solid curve). Following weaning to the dam's

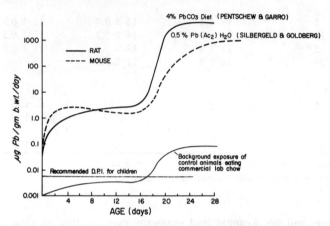

Figure 25.4 Daily lead exposure levels in rats and mice during pre- and postweaning periods.

lead-containing diet the exposure is equivalent to 5 g lead/kg/day. The transition begins about day 16 when pups begin to gain access to maternal food and water supplies, and ends when the dam is removed from the neonate's environment. It should be pointed out that the ability of the adult rat to tolerate such high exposure levels is in part due to the low (<1%) intestinal absorption of lead by the adult rat. However, the young neonate absorbs more than 50% of the ingested dose.[42]

The "hyperactive" mouse model described by Silbergeld and Goldberg[9,21] is illustrated by the upper broken line of Figure 25.4 and demonstrates the similarity in exposure levels to that found in rats when employing Pentschew and Garro's[1] procedure. These mice produce milk containing about 15 ppm Pb, which is less than that seen in the Pentschew model. However, the high metabolic rate of neonatal mice is reflected in a higher intake of milk per gram body weight. This results in a daily lead exposure rate in mice approximating that seen in the Pentschew rat model.

These estimates indicate that neonatal rats suckling a nonlead-exposed dam have a daily lead exposure of < 3 μg Pb/kg/day (Figure 25.4, lowest solid line). Note that exposure increases upon weaning onto normal laboratory chow, which often contains considerable quantities of lead.[43]

As a frame of reference, the recommended daily permissible intake (DPI) for children less than 1 year of age—4 μg Pb/kg/day[44]—is also shown in Figure 25.4.

The exposure level or external dose is of course only one of several important descriptive indices. Of greater importance is the internal dose as reflected by blood- and brain-lead concentrations. During the 21-day suckling period, the neonatal rodent absorbs in excess of 50% of the ingested lead. Furthermore, immature renal function results in low excretion rates. These two factors combine to produce a very high body burden of lead during the lactation period. During a short period of time immediately following weaning, the absorptive capacity of the gas-trointestinal tract decreases markedly and renal function approaches that seen in a mature adult. This greatly reduces the body burden, which results from a given level exposure.

These factors become apparent when one compares the daily exposure level pre- and postweaning with resultant blood-lead levels. Twenty-one-day-old mice, suckling dam's drinking 0.5% lead acetate, are exposed to about 1 μg of lead/g body weight/day with a resultant blood-lead concentration of 190 μg%. Forty-day-old mice now being exposed to about 600 μg of lead/g body weight/day via drinking water have blood-lead concentrations of about 120 μg%. Thus blood-lead concentrations fall in spite of a 600-fold increase in exposure levels. The practice of reporting blood-lead concentrations in the adult at the time of behavioral or neurochemical testing is somewhat misleading since it does not reflect the higher blood-lead concentrations attained during critical periods of brain development. These extreme daily exposure levels in conjunction with the disruption in maternal ingestive behavior and alterations in milk quality interact in some manner to produce profound retardation in normal growth rates. The magnitude of growth retardation in neonatal rats and mice can be seen in Figure 25.5.

At day 21, a time at which artificial weaning is usually imposed, the difference in body weight between control animals and lead-exposed animals is considerable. Figure 25.5 shows a 46% depression in the Pentschew rat model. Silbergeld and Goldberg[9] report a 40% depression in body weight of 21-day-old offspring of mice drinking 0.5% lead acetate in water. We consistently find a 35-45% depression at day 21, using this model. However, a difference in body weight is no longer detectable in mice surviving to 100 days of age. This apparent "catch-up" by the lead-treated mice may be a reflection of decreasing lead absorption with increasing age. However, it may also be a reflection of a biased sample.

At these exposure levels, the mice appear to be more susceptible to infection and a considerable percentage of the mice die as a direct or

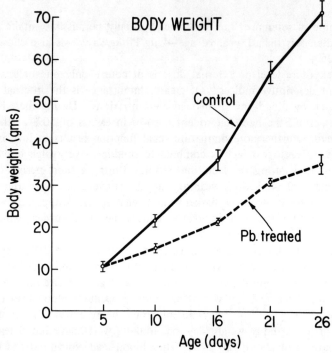

Figure 25.5 Body weight in grams of lead exposed (5% lead acetate) and control neonatal rats during the suckling period.

indirect result of lead exposure. Presumably, those that die are those that are most adversely affected by lead exposure. Survivors may reflect less weight depression and lower blood-lead concentrations than those that died earlier.

UNDERNUTRITION, BEHAVIOR AND NEUROCHEMISTRY

It has been well-documented that these levels of growth retardation during critical periods of brain development have demonstrable effects on neurochemistry and potentially irreversible effects on the behavior of the adult. A review[38] of the effects of experimental undernutrition on the nervous system reports numerous cases wherein enzymes involved in myelin formation, neurotransmitter metabolism, glycolysis and Krebs cycle enzymes can be affected. More specifically, Sereni et al.[45] report decreases in the ontogenetic appearance of normal levels of norepinephrine and 5-hydroxytryptamine as well as acetylcholinesterase in undernourished rats. These effects were only demonstrable during the first 14 days after parturition. Likewise, Adlard and Dobbing[46] report reduced AChE activity in whole brain of 21-day-old rats undernourished during fetal life and lactation. In contrast, these same investigators[47] report elevated AChE activity in adult rats after undernutrition in early life. The picture is even more complex if one considers effects of undernutrition on regional or subcellular neurochemistry.

Obviously, no firm conclusions can be drawn pertaining to the relationship between malnutrition and neurotransmitter metabolism. This is largely due to the diversity of experimental designs used to produce malnutrition. However, it is quite apparent that nutritional status, especially during early development, is an important variable influencing the outcome and interpretation of neurochemical studies.

Undernutrition also affects immediate as well as long-term behavioral functioning. The type, duration and timing of undernutrition as well as the age of the animal at testing can influence the observed effect on behavior. Randt and Derby[48] report behavioral changes in mice undernourished during gestation and lactation and subjected to nutritional rehabilitation. They found alterations in specific types of learning, and in alteration in arousal level reflected by an increase in locomotor activity. Likewise, Castellano and Oliverio[49] reported that undernutrition produced by rearing mice in small, intermediate or large litters results in ontogenetic retardation as well as impaired avoidance learning and a 2-fold increase in exploratory activity after 45 days of rehabilitation.

LEAD EXPOSURE AND LOCOMOTOR ACTIVITY

Undoubtedly, much of the current interest in the effects of lead on the neurochemistry and behavior of neonatally lead-exposed rodents stems from the initial reports of hyperactivity, altered neurochemistry and altered pharmacological drug responses from the laboratories of Michaelson[18,33,34] and Silbergeld and Goldberg.[21] The report of hyperactivity in the rat[18,33] at 25 to 28 days of age has been confirmed by another laboratory.[35] However, it appears that this particular behavioral effect is transient in nature and is not demonstrable in adult rats. This transient hyperactivity may well reflect a maturational lag in the occurrence of the normal activity spurt that is seen in normal weanling rats at about 20 to 22 days of age.[50] Whether this maturational lag is a direct lead effect or an indirect effect brought about by undernutrition remains to be determined.

Of greater interest and clinical importance are the reports of sustained hyperactivity in lead-exposed mice.[9] In Silbergeld and Goldberg's[9] study, mice were exposed to lead from birth by suckling dams drinking a solution of lead acetate (0.2, 0.5 and 1%). Upon weaning, the young were continued on the same solution that had been supplied to their mothers. Growth and development of the offspring were monitored from birth to 60 days of age. Growth rates were retarded in the lead-treated offspring.

Spontaneous motor activity of offspring was measured between 40 and 60 days of age and treated mice were reported to be more than three times as active as age-matched controls. It should be noted that control mice were not matched for early growth retardation.

The authors provided no information as to food and water consumption by the nursing dam, daily and cumulative lead exposure, or blood- and brain-lead content.[9] In a subsequent report,[36] lead-exposed mice and control animals were given drugs used in the treatment and diagnosis of minimal brain dysfunction (MBD) hyperactivity in children: d-amphetamine, methylphenidate and phenobarbital. Lead-treated hyperactive mice were found to respond paradoxically to the drugs. That is, stimulants suppressed activity while depressants increased their levels of motor activity.

Because of the significant implications of these reports, we attempted to replicate their findings. At the same time we attempted to document the nutritional status, lead exposure level and resultant blood- and brain-lead concentrations both prior to and following weaning. Some of these data appear in Figures 25.2, 25.3 and 25.4 and Table 25.3. We have

Table 25.3   Lead Concentration[a] in Mice as a Function of Age and Treatment

| | Content of Lead in Dam's Water | | | |
| | ≤0.05 ppm Pb | | 2780 ppm Pb | |
Age (days)	Blood	Brain	Blood	Brain
20	15	5	190	200
40	17	5	120	306
100	4	4	143	584

[a]Pooled samples: 4-5 mice per sample, reported as μg%.

Continuous exposure: during first 3 weeks via maternal milk and postweaning via dam's water supply.

attempted to replicate the reported lead-induced hyperactivity on four separate occasions and we have failed on each attempt to find any statistically significant alteration in activity level (see Table 25.4). These replication attempts have been carried out using the same strain of mouse, the same age mouse, the same exposure levels, the same type activity-monitoring devices and the same testing protocol. While we were

Table 25.4 Locomotor Activity in 35-Day-Old Mice

Time (Min)	Content of Lead in Dam's Water	
	<0.05 ppm (N = 23)	2780 ppm (N = 13)
0-30	770 ± 34	658 ± 53
30-60	462 ± 39	370 ± 58
60-90	350 ± 48	192 ± 46
90-120	203 ± 49	191 ± 44
120-150	289 ± 57	202 ± 66
150-180	323 ± 48	225 ± 62

unsuccessful in finding hyperactivity, we did find an attenuated response to amphetamine. This attenuation of the stimulant action of amphetamine has been observed in a number of laboratories[32,35] although confirmation of the paradoxical drug effects has not been forthcoming.

Since Silbergeld and Goldberg's[36] study was not controlled for weight and, as indicated previously, undernutrition can alter brain chemistry and locomotor activity levels, the question arose as to whether or not undernutrition might interact in some manner to produce the results reported. We therefore examined the effects of *undernutrition alone* on locomotor activity and response to stimulants and depressant drugs. A large spectrum of growth rates was achieved by raising neonatal mice in both normal size (8 pups) and large size (16 pups) litters.

Between 35 and 45 days of age all mice were tested in locomotor activity cages similar in size and design to those used by Silbergeld and Goldberg.[9] Likewise the testing protocol was similar[36] —2 hr of predrug recording to establish habituation rates and baseline levels of activity and 2 hr of recording following the i.p. administration of either 10 mg/kg of amphetamine or 20 mg/kg of phenobarbital. An examination of baseline activity levels revealed a strong negative correlation between activity level and body weight, *i.e.*, the more undernourished the animal the higher its predrug activity level. Highest activity levels were obtained in those mice whose body weights were about 45% of control body weights.

The magnitude of the increase in activity was the same as that obtained by Silbergeld and Goldberg in their lead-exposed mice, *i.e.*, a 2- to 3-fold increase. The response of these mice to drugs was entirely unexpected. The mice exhibited a strong positive correlation between body weight and response to amphetamine. The postdrug activity level of highly undernourished mice was actually below predrug baseline levels, an apparently paradoxical response. A similar paradoxical effect was obtained when these same mice were challenged with phenobarbital. The more severely undernourished the animal, the greater was the increase in activity obtained during the first hour following the administration of the sedative.

Visual observation of these animals following drug administration has lead us to formulate the following explanation of these data: early neonatal undernutrition results in either an increase in the amount of drug reaching CNS or a change in the sensitivity of the CNS to these drugs. This results in a shift of the normal-dose-response curve to the left. Following the administration of a high dose of amphetamine (10 mg/kg), the normal-body-weight mice are seen to increase their amount of coordinated locomotor activity while undernourished mice exhibit a greater drug response by entering into stereotyped motor activities that prevent the occurrence *and recording* of coordinated locomotor activity, thereby giving the impression of a paradoxical response to amphetamine. A similar case can be made for the phenobarbital data. Sedatives and anesthetics are characterized by an initial period of excitation. Phenobarbital is a long-acting sedative with a proportionately long excitation period. More than one-half of the 2 hr postdrug recording period is taken up by this excitatory phase of normal drug action. The undernourished mice exhibit a greater drug response than controls, including a greater initial period of excitation.

Figure 25.6 provides a comparison between the response to methylphenidate obtained in lead-exposed mice by Silbergeld and Goldberg[36] and the amphetamine response obtained by us in mice undernourished to the same extent as the lead-exposed mice of Silbergeld and Goldberg.[9]

There are no published data available that would permit a direct comparison between the effects of either amphetamine or phenobarbital in lead-exposed and undernourished mice. It is not our intent to suggest that all of the data reported by Silbergeld and Goldberg can be accounted for by undernutrition. However, the data do suggest that a very important variable, nutritional status, has not been controlled. Age-matched controls are not sufficient.

CONCLUSION

The more dramatic harmful effects of pediatric lead encephalopathy are well recognized. Ample supporting evidence of a dangerous body burden can always be found when the blood lead exceeds 80 to 100 μg lead/100 ml. The central nervous system is a prime target following acute high-level exposures. Inhibition of heme synthesis and proximal tubular injury can also be detected in these children.

EFFECT OF METHYLPHENIDATE (40 MG/KG): EKS-C☐, EKS-Pb▨
AND d-AMPHETAMINE (10 MG/KG) NORMAL▥
UNDERNOURISHED▤ ON MOTOR ACTIVITY IN MICE

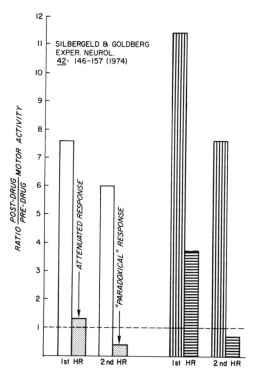

Figure 25.6 Ratio of postdrug activity to predrug baseline activity in lead-exposed (left panel) and undernourished mice (right panel).

Until recently lead poisoning has been defined as a public health problem only for those children living in inner-city metropolitan slum areas. However, the definition of the population at risk needs reevaluation. The concentration of inorganic lead in our immediate environment is on the increase. Young children are being chronically exposed to low levels of lead in their diet, in the air they breathe, and in the dirt and dust that are found in their play areas. This chronic low-level exposure is being reflected in elevated blood-lead levels in the range of 30 to 60 μg%. Furthermore, recent studies indicate that such elevated blood-lead levels are not uncommon in children growing up in rural areas. Therefore the population at risk as a result of undue lead exposure is not restricted to just those children living in the inner city.

A major question from the public health point of view is, what effect does excessive lead absorption have on mental development among those who never develop encephalopathy or any other overt symptoms of poisoning? At present there is good reason to believe that adverse effects might be particularly marked when exposure occurs during the period of central nervous system development in early childhood. However, we have very little reliable information concerning the potential neurotoxic effects of chronic low-level lead exposures, even though there have been indications from clinical studies that such exposures during early childhood may produce behavioral and intellectual impairment.

Investigators have attempted to use experimental animals to investigate the neurological, biochemical and behavioral aspects of neonatal lead exposure. However, previous animal models have employed unrealistic exposure levels and resultant body burdens. Furthermore, the interpretation of results has been seriously compromised by the profound growth retardation produced by these exposure levels.

Animal models used to examine the biochemical and behavioral consequences of a chronic low-level lead exposure in neonatal rats and mice should be well-defined with respect to lead exposure level, duration of exposure, lead body burden, and nutritional status. Because of the documented alterations in maternal ingestive behavior and resultant undernutrition in these highly lead-exposed neonates, as well as the documented and complex effects of undernutrition on neurochemistry and behavior, it is recommended that data derived from these models be viewed with healthy skepticism.

Since behavioral effects such as learning deficits, decreased general activity levels and altered habituation rates have been reported at much lower exposure levels[31,35] for relatively short exposure periods (10-20 days) and at blood-lead concentrations that more closely approximate the human pediatric population, it would be of value to conduct neurochemical studies in these animals and not in the severely poisoned rat or mouse that has been used for the majority of previous studies.

ACKNOWLEDGMENTS

The work for this study was supported in part by USPHS NIH Research Grant NIEHS-ES-01077, communicated by I. A. Michaelson; by Post-Doctoral Fellowship Grant NIEHS-ES-02614 and International Lead and Zinc Research Organization LH-245, for R. L. Bornschein; and by Training Grant NIEHS-ES-00127, for D. A. Fox.

REFERENCES

1. Pentschew, A. and F. Garro. "Lead-Encephalo-Myelopathy of the Suckling Rat and Its Implications on the Porphyrinopathic Nervous Diseases," *Acta Neuropathologica* 6:266 (1966).
2. Pentschew, A., F. Garro and P. Schweda. "Systemized Dysoric Encephalopathy in the Suckling Rat Produced by Lead," *Proc. V Int. Congress Neuropathology*, Zurich, Amsterdam (1965), Int. Kongr. Nr. 100, *Excerpta Medica* (1966).
3. Lampert, P., F. Garro and A. Pentschew. "Lead Encephalopathy in Suckling Rats," *Proc. Symp. Brain Edema,* Vienna (1965).
4. Thomas, J., D. Dallenbach and M. Thomas. "Considerations on the Development of Experimental Lead Encephalopathy," *Virchows Arch. Abt. A. Path. Anat.* 352:61 (1971).
5. Michaelson, I. A. "Effects of Inorganic Lead on RNA, DNA and Protein Content in the Developing Neonatal Rat Brain," *Toxicol. Appl. Pharmacol.* 26:539 (1973).
6. Krigman, M., M. Druṣe, T. Traylor, M. Wilson, L. Newell and E. Hogan. "Lead Encephalopathy in the Developing Rat: Effect Upon Myelination," *J. Neuropath. Exper. Neurol.* 33:55 (1974).
7. Clasen, R., J. Hartmann, A. Starr, P. Coogan, S. Pandolfi, I. Laing, R. Becker and G. Hass. "Electron Microscopic and Chemical Studies of the Vascular Changes and Edema of Lead Encephalopathy," *Amer. J. Pathol.* 74:215 (1974).
8. Rosenblum, W. and M. Johnson. "Neuropathologic Changes Produced in Suckling Mice by Adding Lead to the Maternal Diet," *Arch. Pathol.* 85:640 (1968).
9. Silbergeld, E. and A. Goldberg. "A Lead-Induced Behavioral Disorder," *Life Sci.* 13:1275 (1973).
10. Bull, R., P. Stanaszek, J. O'Neill and S. Lutkenhoff. "Specificity of the Effects of Lead on Brain Energy Metabolism for Substrates Donating a Cytoplasmic Reducing Equivalent," *Environ. Health Persp.* 12:89 (1975).
11. Brown, D., A. Klein and R. Louis-Ferdinand. "Effect of Lead on Behavioral, Morphological and Biochemical Indices of Development in the Neonatal Rat Brain," *Soc. Toxicol. Abstr.* 1976(237):197 (1976).
12. Grant, L., G. Breese, J. Howard, M. Krigman and P. Mushak. "Neurobiology of Lead-Intoxication in the Developing Rat," *Fed. Proc.* 35:503 (1976).
13. Goldstein, G., A. Asbury and I. Diamond. "Pathogenesis of Lead Encephalopathy. Uptake of Lead and Reaction of Brain Capillaries," *Arch. Neurol.* 31:382 (1974).
14. Holtzman, D. and J. Hsu. "Early Effects of Inorganic Lead on Immature Rat Brain Mitochondrial Respiration," *Pediat. Res.* 10: 70 (1976).
15. Krall, A., C. Pesavento, S. Harmon and R. Packer. "Elevation of Norepinephrine Levels and Inhibition of Mitochondrial Oxidative Phosphorylation in Cerebellum of Lead Intoxicated Suckling Rats," *Fed. Proc.* 31:655 (1972).

16. Millar, J., V. Battistini, R. Cumming, F. Carswell and A. Goldberg. "Lead and δ-Aminolaevulinic Acid Dehydratase Levels in Mentally Retarded Children and in Lead-Poisoned Suckling Rats," *Lancet.* II:695 (1970).

17. Modak, A., S. Weintraub and W. Stavinoha. "Effect of Chronic Ingestion of Lead on the Central Cholinergic System in Rat Brain Regions," *Toxicol. Appl. Pharmacol.* 34:340 (1975).

18. Sauerhoff, M. and I. A. Michaelson. "Hyperactivity and Brain Catecholamines in Lead-Exposed Developing Rats," *Science* 182: 1022 (1973).

19. Sobotka, T., R. Brodie and M. Cook. "Psychophysiologic Effects of Early Lead Exposure," *Toxicol.* 5:175 (1975).

20. Modak, A., S. Weintraub, W. Stavihoha and R. Purdy. "Effects of Chronic Lead Ingestion on Total Acetylcholine Content of Mouse Brain," *Soc. Toxicol. Abstr.* 1976(161):133 (1976).

21. Silbergeld, E. and A. Goldberg. "Pharmacological and Neurochemical Investigations of Lead-Induced Hyperactivity," *Neuropharmacol.* 14:431 (1975).

22. Silbergeld, E. and J. Chisolm. "Lead Poisoning: Altered Urinary Catecholamine Metabolites as Indicators of Intoxication in Mice and Children," *Science* 192:153 (1976).

23. Gerber, G., A. Leonard, A. Mazanowska, J. Deroo, and J. Decock. "Biochemical Parameters in Mice Given Different Doses of Lead in the Drinking Water," *Proc. Intl. Symp. Environmental Health Aspects of Lead,* Amsterdam (1972).

24. Michaelson, I. A. and M. Sauerhoff. "The Effect of Chronically Ingested Inorganic Lead on Brain Levels of Fe, Zn, Cu, and Mn of 25-Day-Old Rat," *Life Sci.* 13:417 (1973).

25. Silbergeld, E., P. Carroll and A. Goldberg. "Monoamines in Lead-Induced Hyperactivity," *Pharmacologist* 17:212 (1975).

26. Golter, M. and I. A. Michaelson. "Growth, Behavior and Brain Catecholamines in Lead-Exposed Neonatal Rats: A Reappraisal," *Science* 187:359 (1975).

27. Michaelson, I. A., R. Greenland and W. Roth. "Effect of Inorganic Lead on Norepinephrine and Dopamine Turnover in Brain of Developing Rat," *Fed. Proc.* 33:578 (1976).

28. Brown, S., N. Dragann and W. Vogel. "Effects of Lead Acetate on Learning and Memory in Rats," *Arch. Environ. Health* 22:370 (1971).

29. Shapiro, M., M. Tritschler and A. Ulm. "Lead Contamination: Chronic and Acute Behavioral Effects in the Albino Rat," *Bull. Psychon. Soc.* 2:94 (1973).

30. Snowden, C. "Learning Deficits in Lead-Injected Rats," *Pharmacol. Biochem. Behavior* 1:599 (1973).

31. Brown, D. "Neonatal Lead Exposure in the Rat: Decreased Learning as a Function of Age and Blood Lead Concentrations," *Toxicol. Appl. Pharmacol.* 32:628 (1975).

32. Sobotka, T. and M. Cook. "Postnatal Lead Acetate Exposure in Rats: Possible Relationship to Minimal Brain Dysfunction," *Amer. J. Mental Deficiency* 79:5 (1974).

33. Michaelson, I. A. and W. Sauerhoff. "An Improved Model of Lead-Induced Brain Dysfunction in the Suckling Rat," *Toxicol. Appl. Pharmacol.* 28:88 (1974).

34. Michaelson, I. A. and M. Sauerhoff. "Animal Models of Human Disease: Severe and Milk Lead Encephalopathy in the Neonatal Rat," *Environ. Health Persp.* 7:201 (1974).

35. Reiter, L., G. Anderson, J. Laskey and D. Cahill. "Developmental and Behavioral Changes in the Rat During Chronic Exposure to Lead," *Environ. Health Persp.* 12:119 (1975).

36. Silbergeld, E. and A. Goldberg. "Lead-Induced Behavioral Dysfunction: An Animal Model of Hyperactivity," *Exper. Neurol.* 42:146 (1974).

37. Maker, H., G. Lehrer and D. Silides. "The Effect of Lead on Mouse Brain Development," *Environ. Res.* 10:76 (1975).

38. Dodge, P., A. Prensdy, R. Feigin and S. Holmes. *Nutrition and the Developing Nervous System* (St. Louis: The C. V. Mosby Co., 1975).

39. Fox, D., I. A. Michaelson and R. L. Bornschein. "A Method for Estimating Degree of Exposure to Toxic Agents Transmitted to Neonates via Maternal Milk: Lead," *Pharmacologist* 17:121 (1975).

40. Yagil, R., Z. Etzion and G. Berlyne. "Changes in Rat Milk Quantity and Quality Due to Variations in Litter Size and High Ambient Temperature," *Lab. Animal Sci.* 26:33 (1976).

41. Michaelson, I. A., R. Bornschein and D. Fox. "Verification of Theoretical Estimation of Daily Lead Exposure in Suckling Neonatal Rodents," *Pharmacologist* 18:125 (1976).

42. Kostial, K., I. Simonivic and M. Pisonic. "Lead Absorption from the Intestine in Newborn Rats," *Nature* 233:564 (1971).

43. Fox, J., F. Aldrich and G. Boylen. "Lead in Animal Foods," *J. Toxicol. Environ. Health* 1:461 (1976).

44. Barltrop, D. "Sources and Significance of Environmental Lead for Children," *Proc. Intl. Symp. Environmental Health Aspects of Lead* Amsterdam (1972).

45. Serini, F., N. Principi, L. Perletti and L. P. Sereni. "Undernutrition and the Developing Rat Brain. I. Influence on Acetylcholinesterase and Succinic Acid Dehydrogenase Activities and on Norepinephrine and 5-OH-Tryptamine Tissue Concentration," *Biol. Neonate* 10:254 (1966).

46. Adlard, B. P. F. and J. Dobbing. "Vulnerability of Developing Brain. III. Development of Four Enzymes in the Brains of Normal and Undernourished Rats," *Brain Res.* 28:97 (1971).

47. Adlard, B. P. F. and J. Dobbing. "Elevated Acetylcholinesterase Activity in Adult Rat Brain After Undernutrition in Early Life," *Brain Res.* 30:198 (1971).

48. Randt, C. T. and B. Derby. "Behavioral and Brain Correlations in Early Life Nutritional Deprivation," *Arch. Neurol.* 28:167 (1973).

49. Castellano, C. and A. Oliverio. "Early Malnutrition and Postnatal Changes in Brain and Behavior in the Mouse," *Brain Res.* 101:317 (1976).

50. Campbell, B. A., L. D. Lytle and H. C. Fibiger. "Ontogeny of Adrenergic Arousal and Cholinergic Inhibitory Mechanisms in the Rat," *Science* 166:635 (1969).

EPILOG

Wellington Moore

Health Effects Research Laboratory
U.S. Environmental Protection Agency
Cincinnati, Ohio 45268

I would like to thank all of the participants for this stimulating conference. It has been a very good conference and we owe special thanks to the different chairmen for running the program and to the program committees for arranging the details of this symposium. As indicated by several speakers, there is a need for a correlation between the morphological and biochemical findings. In the selection of the presentations, a special effort was made to bring together people interested in the morphological effects as well as those people interested in the biochemical effects of pollutant exposure. The program committee selected people with particular expertise in these areas.

Dr. Barth, the keynote speaker, briefly touched on the environmental concerns of EPA and the efforts of EPA to solve the problems. EPA has been given certain regulatory functions in the establishment of criteria and standards. He pointed out to us the complexity of this job and the complexity of the effects of environmental pollutants on biological systems. In addition, he stressed the need for continuing research. We have discussed at this meeting NO_2, ozone, and trace metals which occur naturally and we have no clear-cut evidence and very few studies on the long-term effects of exposure to these pollutants at relevant environmental levels. The chronic effects associated with interactions among these pollutants is also an area of major concern. In addition, there is considerable geographical variability as indicated by several speakers, and it was pointed out that people traveling from an area of low exposure to areas of high exposure may experience some discomfort.

It is clear that the assessment of the biological effects of long-term and even lifetime exposure to ambient levels of environmental pollutants

461

is an exceedingly difficult one. Papers presented at this meeting have certainly indicated some of the effects even when we talk about acute studies. Speakers have also pointed out the development of tolerance following exposure and have stressed the variation of response among individuals and between species. One individual in the meeting posed the question, "Is there an adaptive phenomenon in which no further injury occurs? If so, what are the conditions that mediate and what are the threshold levels?" Another interesting topic which requires considerable research involves the interactions of different pollutants and the influence of these interactions on biological response. A question discussed in our session concerning the influence of certain pollutants upon the individual response to different drugs needs further investigation. I should also point out the need for information on the reaction between pollutants and infectious agents and how they impact upon the human population. We can cite many more examples of interactions and the need for research in all these areas. Today we have discussed some of the interactions of the essential trace elements and their influence upon heavy metal toxicity. These discussions have pointed out the importance of nutrition in altering the vulnerability of the human population to pollutant exposure. As pointed out by Dr. Petering, it is impossible to eliminate heavy metal exposure; however, it may be practical to make minor changes in our dietary intake that would greatly lessen the deleterious effects of exposure. The value of the kinetic approach to the study of potential environmental problems has been stressed. I think this is an area EPA has to seriously consider because we must not only show that biological effects occur, but we must assess how likely they are to occur in real-life situations. Finally, I think we can say there were many other good ideas that should be mentioned, but time does not permit. In closing, on behalf of Dr. Garner, I would like to again thank all of you attending and I would like to say it has been a very informative symposium.

SYMPOSIUM COMMITTEE

Dr. R. John Garner,
General Chairman
Director of Health Effects Research
  Laboratory
U.S. Environmental Protection
  Agency
Health Effects Research Laboratory
Cincinnati, Ohio 45268

Dr. S.D. Lee, Chairman
Organizing Committee
U.S. Environmental Protection
  Agency
Health Effects Research Laboratory
Cincinnati, Ohio 45268

Dr. R. Bull, Organizing Committee
U.S. Environmental Protection
  Agency
Health Effects Research Laboratory
Cincinnati, Ohio 45268

Dr. H. Petering,
Organizing Committee
Department of Environmental Health
College of Medicine
University of Cincinnati
Cincinnati, Ohio 45267

Dr. J.F. Stara, Chairman
Program Committee
U.S. Environmental Protection
  Agency
Health Effects Research Laboratory
Cincinnati, Ohio 45268

Dr. V. N. Finelli, Program Committee
Department of Environmental
  Health
College of Medicine
University of Cincinnati
Cincinnati, Ohio 45267

Dr. D. Tierney, Program Committee
U.C.L.A. School of Medicine
Center for Health Sciences
Los Angeles, California 90024

Dr. R. Bhatnagar
Program Committee
Laboratory of Connective Tissue
  Biochemistry
School of Dentistry 630 S
University of California
San Francisco, California 94143

476

CONTRIBUTORS

R.C. Aloia
Departments of Anesthesiology and Bio-
chemistry
Loma Linda University
Loma Linda, California 92354

D.S. Barth
Deputy Assistant Administrator for
Health and Ecological Effects
U.S. Environmental Protection Agency
Washington, D.C. 20460

R.S. Bhatnagar
Laboratory of Connective Tissue Bio-
chemistry
School of Dentistry 630 S
University of California
San Francisco, California 94143

R.L. Bornschein
Department of Environmental Health
College of Medicine
University of Cincinnati
Cincinnati, Ohio 45267

G.P. Brierley
Department of Physiological Chemistry
College of Medicine
Ohio State University
Columbus, Ohio 43210

R.D. Buckley
USC–Rancho Los Amigos Hospital
7601 East Imperial Highway
Downey, California 90242

D.R. Buhler
Department of Agricultural Chemistry
and Environmental Health Science
Center
Oregon State University
Corvallis, Oregon 97331

R.J. Bull
U.S. Environmental Protection Agency
Health Effects Research Laboratory
Cincinnati, Ohio 45268

F.L. Cerklewski
Department of Environmental Health
College of Medicine
University of Cincinnati
Cincinnati, Ohio 45267

D.P. Chang
California Primate Research Center and
Department of Veterinary Pathology
University of California
Davis, California 95616

465

M. Chvapil
Department of Surgery
University of Arizona
Tucson, Arizona 85724

K. Clark
USC–Rancho Los Amigos Hospital
7601 East Imperial Highway
Downey, California 90242

R.G. Crystal
Pulmonary Branch
National Heart, Lung, and Blood
 Institute
Building 10, Room 6N260
Bethesda, Maryland 20014

D.L. Dungworth
California Primate Research Center and
 Department of Veterinary Pathology
University of California
Davis, California 95616

N.A. Elson
Pulmonary Branch
National Heart, Lung, and Blood
 Institute
Building 10, Room 6N260
Bethesda, Maryland 20014

M.J. Evans
Stanford Research Institute
333 Ravenswood Avenue
Menlo Park, California 94025

V.N. Finelli
Department of Environmental Health
College of Medicine
University of Cincinnati
Cincinnati, Ohio 45267

J.A. Foster
Boston University
School of Medicine
80 East Concord Street
Boston, Massachusetts 02118

D.A. Fox
Department of Environmental Health
College of Medicine
University of Cincinnati
Cincinnati, Ohio 45267

C. Franzblau
Boston University
School of Medicine
80 East Concord Street
Boston, Massachusetts 02118

B.A. Freeman
Department of Biochemistry
University of California
Riverside, California 92502

G. Freeman
Stanford Research Institute
333 Ravenswood Avenue
Menlo Park, California 94025

E.M. Gause
Southwest Foundation for Research
 and Education
P.O. Box 28147
8848 West Commerce Street
San Antonio, Texas 78284

A.M. Goldberg
The Johns Hopkins University
Department of Environmental Medicine
School of Hygiene and Public Health
615 N. Wolfe Street
Baltimore, Maryland 21205

N.D. Greene
Southwest Foundation for Research
  and Education
P.O. Box 28147
8848 West Commerce Street
San Antonio, Texas 78284

A.D. Hacker
The Center for the Health Sciences
University of California
Los Angeles, California 90024

J.D. Hackney
USC–Rancho Los Amigos Hospital
7601 East Imperial Highway
Downey, California 90242

M.Z. Hussain
Laboratory of Connective Tissue
  Biochemistry
School of Dentistry 630 Sciences
University of California
San Francisco, California 94143

J.L. Johnson
Department of Biochemistry
Duke University Medical Center
Durham, North Carolina 27710

L. -Y. Lee
Cardiovascular Research Institute and
  Department of Medicine and Physiology
University of California
San Francisco Medical Center
San Francisco, California 94143

S.D. Lee
U.S. Environmental Protection Agency
Health Effects Research Laboratory
Cincinnati, Ohio 45268

R. Loch
Department of Environmental Health
College of Medicine
University of Cincinnati
Cincinnati, Ohio 45267

M.L. Meltz
Southwest Foundation for Research
  and Education
P.O. Box 28147
8848 West Commerce Street
San Antonio, Texas 78284

I.A. Michaelson
Department of Environmental Health
College of Medicine
University of Cincinnati
Cincinnati, Ohio 45267

P.F. Moore
California Primate Research Center and
  Department of Veterinary Pathology
University of California
Davis, California 95616

W. Moore
U.S. Environmental Protection Agency
Health Effects Research Laboratory
Cincinnati, Ohio 45268

J.B. Mudd
Department of Biochemistry
University of California
Riverside, California 92502

L. Murthy
Department of Environmental Health
College of Medicine
University of Cincinnati
Cincinnati, Ohio 45267

M.G. Mustafa
The Center for the Health Sciences
University of California
Los Angeles, California 90024

J.A. Nadel
Cardiovascular Research Institute and
   Departments of Medicine and Physiology
University of California
San Francisco Medical Center
San Francisco, California 94143

J.J. Ospital
The Center for the Health Sciences
University of California
Los Angeles, California 90024

D.H. Petering
Department of Chemistry
University of Wisconsin–Milwaukee
Milwaukee, Wisconsin 53201

H.G. Petering
Department of Environmental Health
College of Medicine
University of Cincinnati
Cincinnati, Ohio 45267

C. Posin
USC–Rancho Los Amigos Hospital
7601 East Imperial Highway
Downey, California 90242

K.V. Rajagopalan
Department of Biochemistry
Duke University Medical Center
Durham, North Carolina 27710

R.A. Rimerman
Department of Agricultural Chemistry and
   Environmental Health Sciences Center
Oregon State University
Corvallis, Oregon 97331

G. Rouser
Division of Neurosciences
City of Hope National Medical Center
Duarte, California 91010

C.J. Allen-Rowlands
Southwest Foundation for Research
   and Education
P.O. Box 28147
8848 West Commerce Street
San Antonio, Texas 78284

J.R. Rowlands
Southwest Foundation for Research
   and Education
P.O. Box 28147
8848 West Commerce Street
San Antonio, Texas 78284

L.W. Schwartz
California Primate Research Center and
   Department of Veterinary Pathology
University of California
Davis, California 95616

B.K. Tarkington
California Primate Research Center and
   Department of Veterinary Pathology
University of California
Davis, California 95616

W.S. Tyler
California Primate Research Center and
   Department of Veterinary Pathology
University of California
Davis, California 95616

P.D. Whanger
Department of Agricultural Chemistry
   and Environmental Health Sciences
   Center
Oregon State University
Corvallis, Oregon 97331

H.P. Witschi
Départment de Pharmacologie
Faculté de Médecine
Université de Montréal
Montréal, P.Q., Canada

INDEX

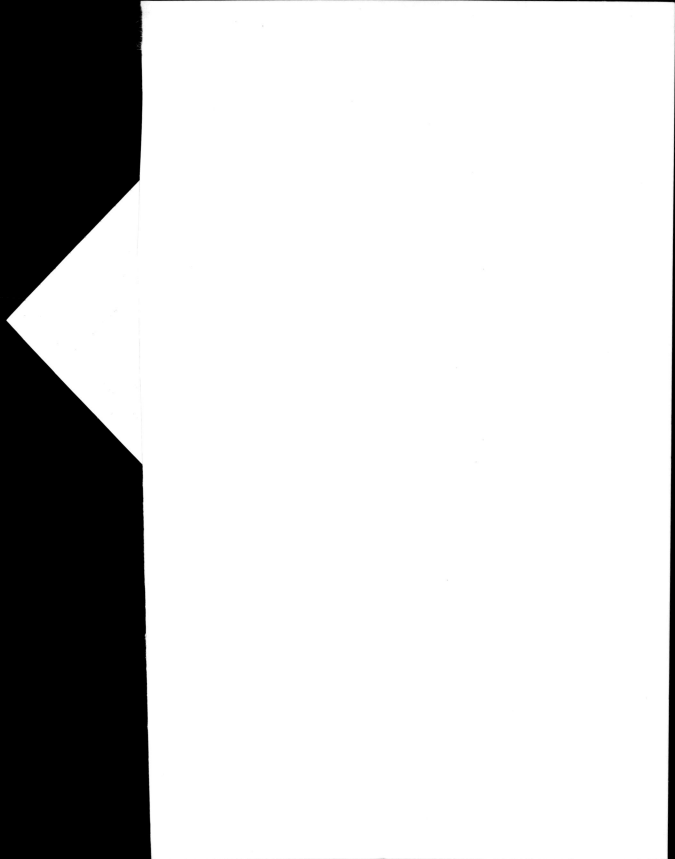

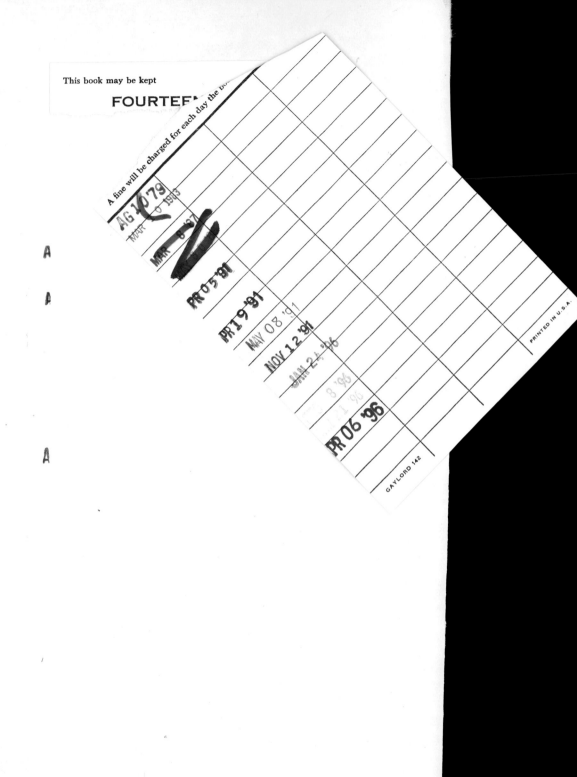

This book may be kept

FOURTEF

A fine will be charged for each day the bo

AG 10 79

MAR 8 1983

PR 05 '91

PR 19 91

MAY 08 '91

NOV 12 91

JAN 24 96

8 '96

PR 06 '96

A

A

A

PRINTED IN U.S.A.

GAYLORD 142